Novel Drug Delivery System

Novel Drug Delivery System

Victor Cardenas
Afsan Bhadelia

Kruger Brentt
Publishers
2025

Kruger Brentt Publishers UK. LTD.
Company Number 9728962

Regd. Office: 68 St Margarets Road, Edgware, Middlesex HA8 9UU

ISBN: 978-1-78715-415-5

For information on all our publications visit our website at http://krugerbrentt.com/

PREFACE

"Novel Drug Delivery Systems" represents a comprehensive exploration into the design, development, and applications of innovative drug delivery technologies, offering insights into the latest advancements, challenges, and opportunities in this rapidly evolving field. This book serves as an essential resource for researchers, scientists, clinicians, and pharmaceutical industry professionals seeking to enhance drug efficacy, improve patient compliance, and overcome limitations associated with conventional drug delivery approaches.

Effective drug delivery plays a pivotal role in optimizing therapeutic outcomes while minimizing adverse effects and maximizing patient comfort and convenience. Novel drug delivery systems offer a range of sophisticated approaches to target specific tissues or cells, control drug release kinetics, and enhance drug stability and bioavailability.

As editors of this volume, we have endeavored to compile a diverse array of perspectives, methodologies, and case studies from leading experts and practitioners in the field of drug delivery. Through a blend of theoretical foundations, practical insights, and real-world applications, this book covers a wide range of topics, including nanotechnology-based drug delivery, controlled-release formulations, transdermal delivery systems, targeted drug delivery strategies, and personalized medicine approaches.

Our overarching goal in presenting this book is to provide readers with a comprehensive understanding of the principles and applications of novel drug delivery systems. By offering insights into the latest advancements, best practices, and emerging trends in drug delivery research and development, we aim to inspire innovation, collaboration, and excellence in the design and implementation of next-generation drug delivery technologies.

We extend our sincere gratitude to all the contributors who have generously shared their expertise, experiences, and insights in the field of novel drug delivery systems. It is our hope that this book will serve as a valuable reference and guide for researchers, scientists, clinicians, and industry professionals as they strive to translate cutting-edge drug delivery concepts into clinical practice and improve the lives of patients worldwide.

Victor Cardenas

Afsan Bhadelia

CONTENTS

1 Chapter

INTELLIGENT DELIVERY MECHANISMS UTILIZING SHAPE MEMORY AND SELF-FOLDING POLYMERS

1. INTRODUCTION: AN OVERVIEW

Polymers are a category of materials characterized by their versatility, encompassing both industrial substances like synthetic plastics and biopolymers. The qualities of polymers, whether synthetic or naturally occurring, are determined by the nature of the constituent monomers, their sequence, the overall polymer length, and the types of bonds present in their structure. Over the past two decades, a novel class of polymers has been identified that demonstrates intriguing features, specifically shape memory and self-folding. Polymers with these characteristics are currently the focus of rigorous investigation for their prospective applications in the biomedical field and medication delivery systems. This chapter will initially present the basics of shape memory, followed by a synopsis of the research conducted in this domain. This section introduces the notion of self-folding and polymer origami, a subset of self-folding. Recent research in this dynamic field is given, together with a specific future outlook on shape memory and self-folding polymers.

2. SHAPE MEMORY ALLOYS

Shape memory materials (SMMs) exhibit plastic deformation (temporary shape) upon the application of an external stimulus and can revert to their original shape from this temporary configuration. This phenomenon is often referred to as the "shape memory effect" (SME) [1]. form memory polymers (SMPs) are a category of form memory materials that react to external stimuli by providing mechanical action. The network elasticity of the shape memory polymer dictates whether the SMP retains one or several shapes [2]. Dual-shape memory polymers, which will be detailed subsequently, are the initial shape memory polymers (SMPs). The temporary shape of the shape memory polymer (SMP) remains constant until an external stimulus is supplied to initiate shape recovery. Temperature, light, electric fields, magnetic fields, pH, particular ions, or enzymes can serve as stimuli to alter the configurations of shape memory polymers. The transformation in shape can occur swiftly from a transitory form to a permanent one [3–6]. Figure 1 delineates the correlation among polymer composition, structure, stimuli, and shape memory functionality. In the late 1970s, CdF Chimie Company (France) pioneered the development of the first shape memory polymer, known as polynorbornene. One year later, it was designated as Norsorex by Nippon Zeon Company (Japan) and subsequently marketed [7]. Kurare TP-301 and Asmer, other commercial shape memory polymers, were manufactured by Kurare Corporation (Japan) and Asahi Company (Japan), respectively [8]. Mitsubishi Heavy Industries developed a widely utilized polyurethane (PU)-based shape memory polymer (SMP) [4]. A significant category of shape memory materials is shape memory alloys (SMAs). Nevertheless, form memory alloys possess drawbacks compared to other shape memory materials, including elevated manufacturing costs, toxicity, restricted recovery, and complex surgical challenges. Recently, form memory polymers, ceramics, and hydrogels have gained preference due to their benefits over shape memory metals [9].

3. SHAPE MEMORY POLYMERS

The shape memory effect can be achieved by integrating polymer structure and morphology through processing and programming techniques. The material qualities are unrelated to SME [10]. The distinctive characteristics and primary benefits of SMP materials are outlined below:

SMPs are lightweight and allow substantially higher elongations, which have properties for various technical applications [11].

- SMPs have wide range of glass transition temperatures from -70°C to +100°C.
- Since they have a wide range of glass transition temperatures, their stiffness can be tailored. Also, SMPs can be processed easily [12].
- SMPs have shape recovery property up to 400% of plastic strain. (Shape memory alloys have 7–8%).
- Between the glassy and rubbery states of SMPs, large reversible changes of elastic modulus can be observed (as high as 500 times) [13].
- Shape memory polymers have high elastic deformation (strain up to more than 200% for most of the materials). They have low density and biodegradable materials.
- Most of the SMPs are biocompatible materials which allow them to be used in potential medical applications.
- SMPs are easy to process. They are applicable to molding or extrusion. They have low cost [13].
- Shape memory polymers have low thermal conductivity compared to shape memory alloys. This feature can be useful if shape memory foams are used a as insulation materials [14,15].
- They can use many external stimuli and triggers. There are many alternative ways to actuate shape recovery such as light, magnetic field, electricity, and water [16].

As mentioned previously, shape memory polymers and their composites can recover their original shapes after large deformation when subjected to an external stimulus [17]. This external stimulus can be temperature [18,19], magnetism [20–22], moisture [23], or light [18,24].

Thermally Induced Shape Memory Polymers

Among these shape memory polymers, the thermoresponsive SMPs are the most common type [25,26]. Thermally induced shape memory polymers have a wide range of applications in biomedical fields, [27] such as drug delivery, implanting, suture, and wound healing [28].

The general thermomechanical cycle of thermoresponsive shape memory polymers consists of the following steps at a macroscopic level:

1. Programming
2. Storage
3. Recovery [29].

This cycle is depicted in Figure 1. The first step is the fabrication of the shape memory polymers into an original shape. Second, the polymer is heated above the thermal transition temperature (T_{trans}) (this temperature can be either melting temperature T_m or glass transition temperature T_g). When the polymer is at its T_{trans}, an applied external force deforms it, and it is cooled below thermal transition temperature. When it is cooled, the applied force is removed in order to preserve the temporarily pre-deformed shape. In the last step, the pre-deformed shape memory polymer is heated above T_{trans}, and shape recovery is observed, and SMP attains its original shape.

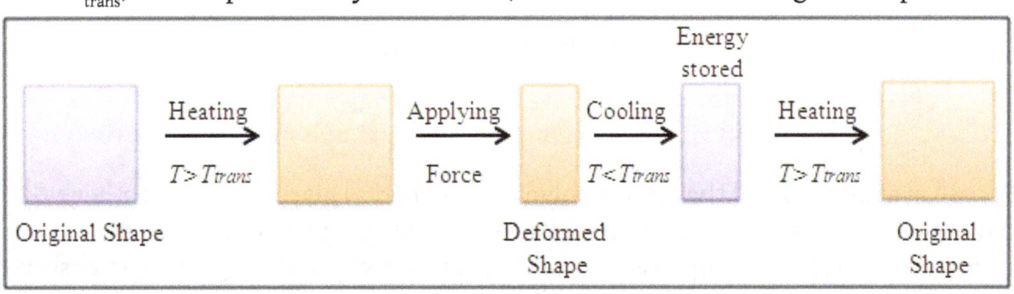

Figure 1. Thermomechanical cycle of thermoresponsive shape memory polymers.

At the molecular level, shape memory polymers exhibit the shape memory effect through their two components: cross-links and switching segments. These SMPs may comprise chemically cross-linked networks or physically cross-linked copolymers. Physically cross-linked copolymers typically consist of linear block copolymers with rigid and switchable segments. Their permanent configuration is maintained by hard segments, while the temporary configuration is determined by switching segments [30]. Cross-links are established through covalent bonding and physical interactions, such as molecular entanglements [5,31]. Reshaping covalently cross-linked shape memory polymers is challenging due to the fixation of their shape by covalent bonds. These polymers are referred to as thermosets [32]. Polymer comprises two distinct domains in the context of physical cross-linking. The domain comprises two components: hard and reversible switching segments. The hard section, functioning as the net point, is associated with the highest thermal transition temperature. Reversible switching segments or molecular switches are associated with the second highest thermal transition temperature. These polymers are referred to as thermoplastics [33]. Figure 2 illustrates the rigid and flexible parts throughout the shape memory phenomenon. The lines represent net points, whereas the square dots indicate the switching segments.

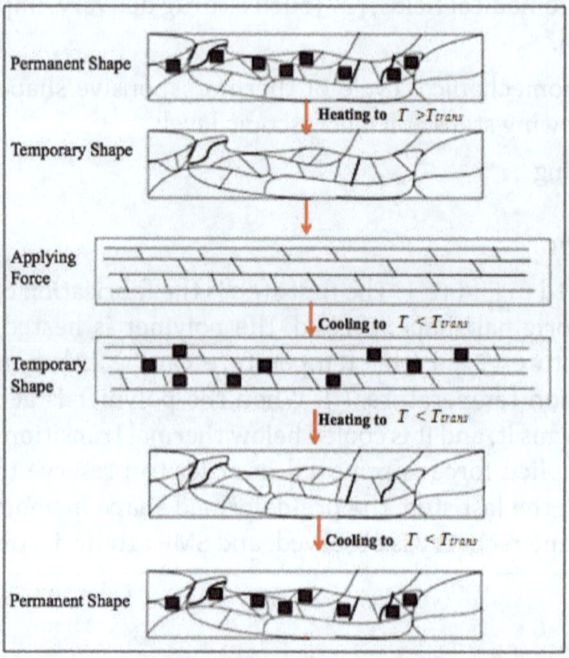

Figure 2. Hard and soft segments during shape memory effect.

Rousseau et al. reported that epoxy polymers (neopentyl glycol diglycidyl ether NGDE) have tunable glass transition temperatures by changing the cross-link density and chain flexibility. Ranging up to 89°C, excellent shape fixity and recovery were observed [34].

Zhou et al. reported that PDLLA/HA (poly D,L-lactide co-glycolide/hydroxyapatite) composites have desirable shape memory effects and the amount of HA particles in composites played an important role during the shape memory recovery. Since PDLLA has remarkable properties such as shape memory effect, biodegradability, biocompatibility, easier availability, and osteoconductivity of HA, these composites have potential in biomedical applications such as minimally invasive surgery (MIS) and bone and tissue repair [35].

Lendlein et al. developed a thermoresponsive shape memory polymer which consists of oligo(ε-caprolactone) diol (OGL) and crystallizable oligo(p-dioxanone) (ODX) as switching and hard segments, respectively. A fiber of this thermoplastic SMP was used to close the wound by loosely knotting the fiber and then when temperature increased to T_{trans}, the suture shrinks and the knot is tightened. So, they suggested that this type of material could be used in order to design new surgical devices [10].

In another study, Ashby et al. reported that poly(ε-caprolactone) (PCL) and poly(octylene adipate-co-meso-2,5-diazodipate) shape memory polymers were actuated by switching temperature. This new developed SMP would have potential applications in the biomedical field [36].

3.1. One-Way (Dual) Shape Memory Effect (1W-SME)

When an external stimulus is applied on SMP, the temporary shape becomes permanent shape. In order to obtain the temporary shape again, another external force or stress is required. This procedure shows that shape memory behavior is nonreversible or "one-way", and it has a wide range of applications [37].

The most basic procedure of polymer shape memory effect is described in Figure 1. First, the shape memory polymer is heated to a transition temperature or deformation temperature (T_d), which resulted in softening of the material. Second, a deformation force is applied on SMP (i.e., loading or stress). Third, the SMP is cooled down under the load. Then, load is removed and the deformed shape is fixed, which is the temporary shape. After shape fixing, shape recovery is obtained by reheating the temporary shaped SMP to a recovery temperature (T_r) when no stress is applied on it. Finally, the original (permanent) shape of SMP is recovered [38]. If a shape memory process follows this procedure, it is called as dual-shape memory effect.

The thermal transition temperature, which is associated with switching domains, has various types. The melting transition ($T_{trans} = T_m$), liquid crystalline transition ($T_{trans} = T_{LC}$), or a glass transition ($T_{trans} = T_g$) can be taken as thermal transition temperature. However, mostly, melting and liquid crystalline phase transitions are designated to relatively small temperatures [39].

If we take a look at the macroscopic shape of shape memory polymer, when it has a permanent shape, its molecular chains are thermodynamically stable because of the highest entropy of SMP conformation. When SMP is heated above T_{trans}, chain mobility is triggered. Due to the lower entropy state and macroscopic shape change after applied stress, chain conformations of SMP are changed. Finally, when the SMP is cooled below T_{trans}, molecular chain segments freeze by kinetically trapping of lower entropy state. As a result of this, macroscopic shape fixity is obtained. In the last step, when heating the deformed SMP above T_{trans}, when there is no stress applied, the chain mobility is activated again. So, molecular chains regain their highest entropy. The one-way shape memory effect is illustrated in Figure 3 briefly.

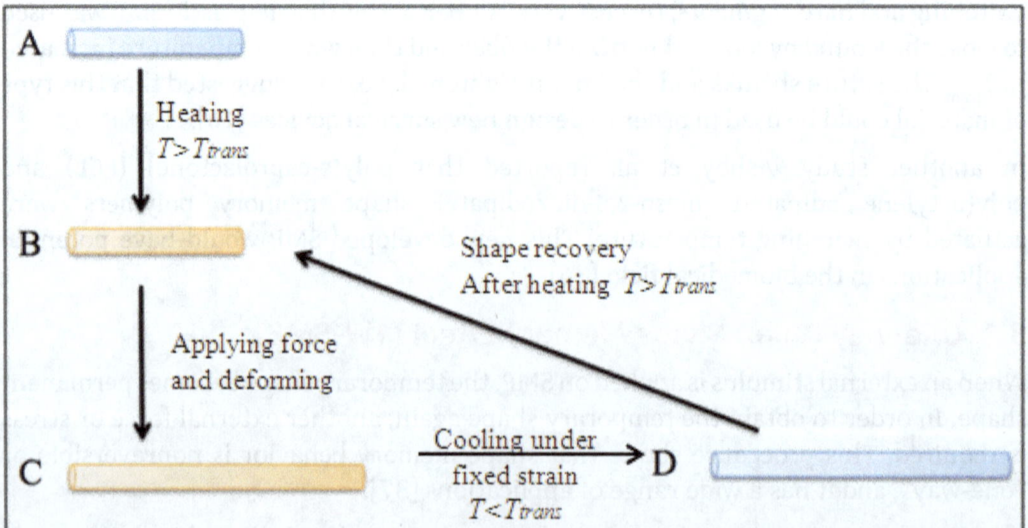

Figure 3. One-way shape memory effect.

Basically, shape memory polymers are able to change their shapes between original and temporary shape under applied stress which is a type of one-way shape memory effect. Another type of one-way shape memory effect is triple shape memory effect. The main difference of triple shape memory effect (TSME) is having one intermediate shape between its original and temporary shapes. If there is more than one intermediate shape, it is called multiple shape memory effect for a more complicated motion generation [40]. Polymers blends, grafting and blocking copolymers, SMP hybrids, and polymer laminates are some of the ways of managing the triple shape memory effects [41]. Figure 4 shows the basic procedure of triple shape memory effect. As mentioned in the figure, there are two different thermal transition temperatures which are $T_{low,1}$ and $T_{low,2}$. This is attributed to the two segregated crystalline domains in the original shape [42].

Kumar et al. reported that grafted polymer network contains crystallizable poly(ethylene glycol) (PEG) side chains, and poly (ε-caprolactone) (PCL) shows triple shape memory effect [43]. The triple shape memory behavior of crystalline polyurethane was observed by Hu et al. [44]. Also, polyalkenemer and polyolefin-based polymer blends were used by Cuevas et al. in order to develop triple shape memory polymers which were two semicrystalline polymers (poly(cyclooctene) (PCO) and polyethylene (PE)) [42]. Xie et al. developed polymeric bilayers that consisted of two dual-shape memory polymers, and this new shape memory polymer bilayer shows triple shape memory effect [45]. Furthermore, Xie reported that perfluorosulphonic acid ionomer (PFSA) is able to show tunable shape memory effect which includes dual, triple, and quadruple without any change in the material composition [46].

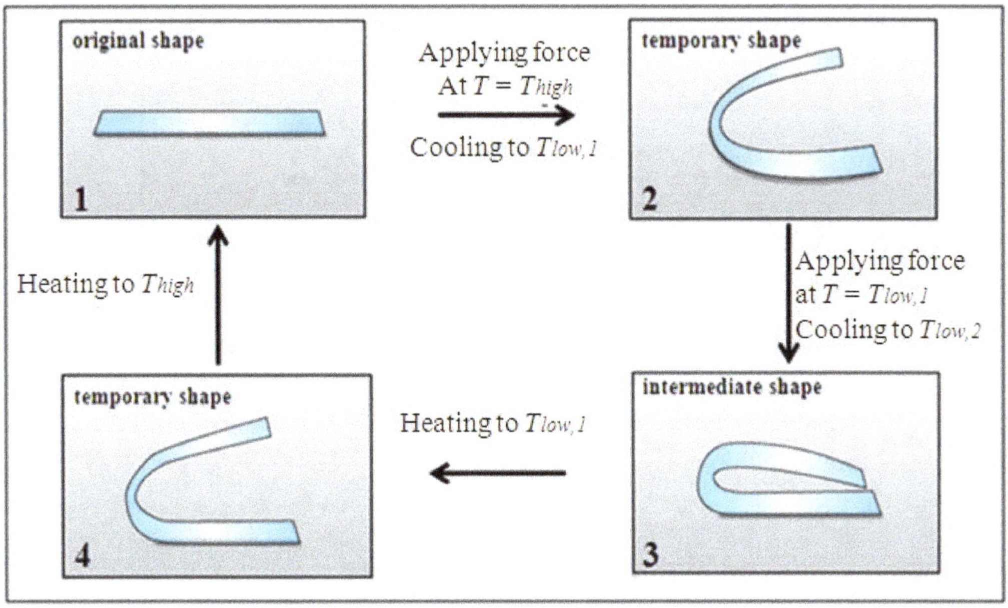

Figure 4. Triple shape memory effect.

3.2. Two-Way Shape Memory Effect (2W-SME)

Most of the typical SMPs show one-way shape memory effect. A different type of SME which is the two-way shape memory effect can be observed in liquid crystalline elastomers and photo-actuated deformation polymers [47].

2W-SME can be quite useful; however, its high cost represents an obstacle for its widespread use. In 2W-SME process, a crystallization-induced elongation and melting-induced contraction is observed during cooling and heating, respectively. This condition originated from the formation of liquid crystalline structure [48]. The comparison of 2W-SME and 1W-SME is shown in Figure 5 briefly.

Chen et al. reported that the two-way shape memory behavior of SMP laminate was observed by bending upon heating from 25°C to 60°C and reverse bending upon cooling from 60°C to 25°C. Laminated layers were prepared from shape memory exhibiting polyurethane [49].

Zhou et al. developed self-folding poly(octylene adipate) (POA). Besides showing conventional one-way irreversible shape memory, this SMP is able to form one-way reversible shape memory during heating and two-way reversible shape memory upon heating and cooling cycles. The chemical cross-links of this semicrystalline elastomer are responsible for the memorization of the original shape, whereas the physical network constructs the temporary shape [50].

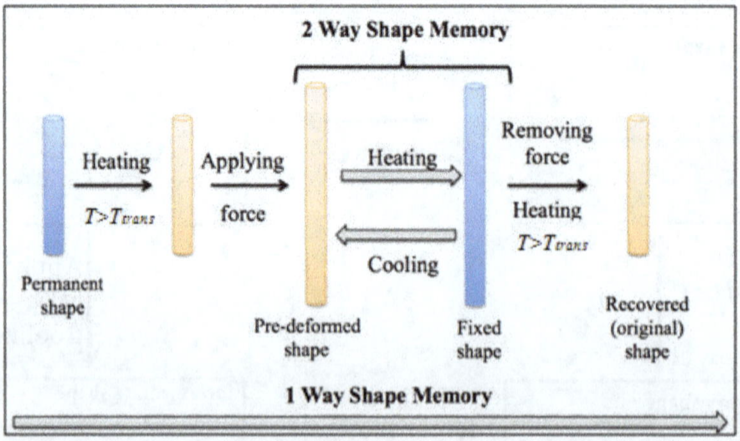

Figure 5. Comparison of two-way shape memory effect and one-way shape memory effect.

Magnetically Induced Shape Memory Polymers

Certain magnetic materials tend to respond to magnetic fields and are capable of maintaining their magnetic properties after the external magnetic field is removed. Such magnetic particles are called as ferrimagnetic of ferromagnetic materials which are iron, nickel, cobalt, and some of their alloys [51]. Some magnetic materials such as iron oxides (Fe_3O_4, Fe_2O_3, etc.), when below a certain nanometer size, do not have any remaining magnetization once the external magnetic field is removed. These are superparamagnetic materials and can be preferred over ferromagnetic ones depending on the application.

Shape memory can be induced by the application of an external magnetic field due to magnetic heating. So magnetic induction is a type of thermal induction, where temperature change is driven by magnetic field due to the presence of magnetic material in the nanocomposite.

The magnetic SMP has several advantages:

1. By using magnetic heating, possible danger of overheating can be eliminated.
2. Since heat is not given to the system externally, any complex-shaped device can be actuated virtually.
3. This method is convenient for medical devices which can be actuated inside the human body, since they can be controlled in a wireless manner [52].

Hilt et al. reported that magnetic field can be used in order to heat the SMPs by remote heating. This heating method relies on magnetic nanoparticles within the polymer matrix in order to create heat via power loss when exposed to an alternating magnetic field [53].

According to the study of Razzaq et al., by changing the magnetic field parameters and amount of the Fe_3O_4 in the polyurethane polymer matrix, shape recovery of the helical bended strip of polyurethane filled with 20% volume microsized magnetite was observed [54].

Magnetically inducing method is an indirect method. So this method can be useful if shape memory polymer cannot be actuated by direct heating methods. However, Zhou et al. reported that for cross-linked poly(ε-caprolactone) polymers, magnetite composite shows better reactivity to hot water than alternating magnetic field [55].

In the research study of Schmidt, polymer network composites were implemented with different contents of superparamagnetic nanoparticles (Fe_3O_4) and butyl acrylate cross-linked with oligo (ε-caprolactone) dimethacrylate. As it can be seen in Figure 3, the permanent shape is deformed by heating above T_{trans}. Then by cooling the temporary shape, the crystalline phase of oligo(ε-caprolactone) segments makes the polymer to become stable. Induction heating of magnetic nanoparticles in electromagnetic field leads to temperature increase inside the matrix. By magnetically heating above the T_{trans}, the original (permanent) shape is recovered [56].

Zhou et al. reported that poly (D,L-lactide) /magnetite (Fe_3O_4) nanocomposites show excellent shape memory effect when an alternating magnetic field was applied as a stimulus. Since PDLLA is biocompatible, these nanocomposites show potential for application as magnetically controlled smart implants in biomedical field [57].

According to the study of Puig et al., 8 wt% oleic acid-stabilized magnetic nanoparticles exhibited a temperature increase of 25°C at its surface when exposed to an alternating magnetic field in biomedical applications. Also, this temperature was enough to actuate the shape memory of the nanocomposite [58].

Electro-Active Shape Memory Polymers

As observed, shape memory effect is usually induced by thermal stimulation by heating above the transition temperature of the polymers, such as the glass transition temperature or melting temperature. However, some other stimulating sources, such as electric field, may also be used in order to trigger polymers with shape memory [59].

Electricity can be used as a stimulus which enables resistive actuation of shape memory polymer filled with conductive fillers. By passing an electrical current, shape memory effect can be actuated easily in these nanocomposites. To date, most of the studies regarding electroactive SMPs composite are focused on thermoplastic SMP resins [60]. As a result of these, in recent studies, most of the electroactive shape memory polymers are well-dispersed carbon nanotube (CNT)-reinforced thermoplastic polyurethane (TPU) resin nanocomposites [61–63].

According to the study of Leng et al., thermoset styrene-based shape memory polymer nanocomposite filled with different amounts of nanosized carbon powder shows that with increasing nanocarbon powder amount, electrical conductivity increases. Also, it was reported that 10 vol.% nanocarbon powder shows good electroactive shape recovery property [64].

Zhou and coworkers fabricate cross-linked poly(ε-caprolactone) (cPCL) and conductive multiwalled carbon nanotubes (MWNTs). These nanocomposites exhibit excellent shape memory properties under the direct thermal and electrical stimulations. Therefore it was reported that this composite might be a promising prospect in biomedical applications [65].

Jung et al. obtained electroactive shape memory polymer composites by using polyurethane and three kinds of fillers. When polyurethane-multiwalled carbon nanotube composite is lightly coated with polypyrrole (PPy), new nanocomposite shows good electroactive shape memory properties when an electric voltage is applied [66].

Water-Induced Shape Memory Polymers

As a trigger mechanism, water can be used for shape transition of shape memory polymers or shape memory polymer composites. Since solvent or water molecules can penetrate into the amorphous areas of shape memory polymers, this can result in a plasticizing effect on SMP molecules. Therefore the flexibility of the molecule increases and shape recovery is observed [67].

Chen et al. reported that water-induced poly(methacrylic acid)-grafted clay and thermoplastic polyurethane composite was developed with shape memory effect. Also, this new polymer–clay composite responds to pH changes and mechanically adaptive properties when water is exposed [68].

The polymer composite composed of carbon nanotubes and shape memory polyurethane (SMPU) was developed by Luo et al. The new and developed composite has shape memory-enhanced water-sensing property which can be used in smart polymer applications such as sensory materials [69].

Aqueous environments can be used as a trigger of shape memory effect. Nöchel et al. used different grafted copolymer networks (named CLEG) which consist of different ratios of the hydrophobic cross-linker poly(ε-caprolactone) diisocyanoethyl methacrylate (PCLDIMA) and hydrophilic poly(ethylene glycol) monomethyl ether monomethacrylate (PEGMA). The shape memory properties of this new hydrogel were studied by bending and uniaxial elongation experiments in the aqueous environments. As a result, CLEG has dual-shape capability and degradability and could be promising materials in biomedical applications [70].

Paakinaho et al. reported that the shape memory property of orientation-programmed PDLLA in an aqueous environment at 37°C was triggered by the combined effect of water molecules and thermal activation [71]. Mendez et al. developed new water-activated biomimetric nanocomposites by adding rigid cotton cellulose nanowhiskers (CNWs) into a rubbery polyurethane matrix. At a specific concentration of CNW, aqueous swelling and shape memory behavior were observed [72].

4. SELF-FOLDING POLYMERS

Self-folding is the ability of a material to fold and unfold without the external effects. Also without any external interference, such as human control, self-folding can be attributed to the self-assembly mechanism. These mechanisms can be patterned templates or thin films which can be folded, curved, or rolled-up to become spirals, tubes, and cylindrical tubes [73,74]. Self-folding can occur spontaneously or in response to stimuli such as light, pH [75], temperature, magnetic field, or solvent [76,77]. In Figure 6, self-folding mechanism which is provided by hinges is shown briefly.

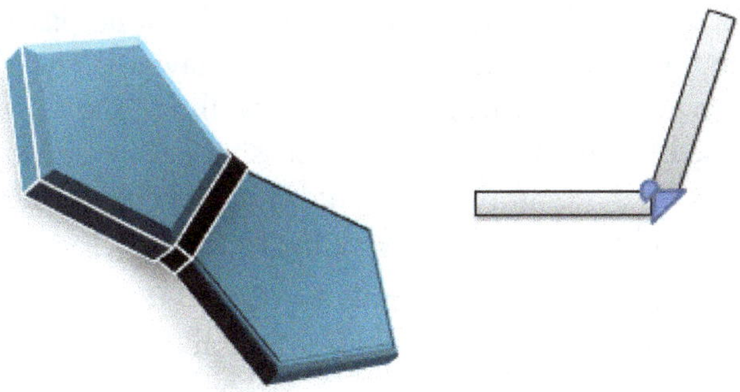

Figure 6. Illustration of 3D and 2D self-folding mechanism.

Self-folding films have become attractive recently since there is a variety of polymers which are sensitive to different stimuli, and they can fold by responding external signals. Many polymers are able to change their properties with pH and temperature. For biotechnological applications, biodegradable and biocompatible polymers are favorable choices and are frequently encountered. Polymers can also undergo considerable and reversible changes of volume that allow design of systems with reversible folding [78]. Thermoresponsive self-folding films can be designed using continuous thermal expansion, melting shape memory transition of polymers which demonstrate the low critical solution temperature (LCST) in solutions [79].

Luchnikov et al. reported that a polymer bilayer consisting of a polystyrene (PS) layer on top of a poly(4-vinyl pyridine) (P4VP) layer is formed on the polished surface on the silicon wafer or other substrates (e.g., a glass slide) by means of dip or spin coating. Rolling, in this system, is achieved due to the swelling of the P4VP in a water solution of an acid, due to protonation of the pyridine rings [80]. In another study of Ionov, self-rolling due to swelling was observed. Fully biodegradable polysuccinimide shows self-rolling response with its polymer bilayers, and this results in the formation of microtubes [81].

Ionov et al. demonstrated a self-folding polymeric bilayer consisting of poly(methyl methacrylate) copolymer and poly(N-isopropylacrylamide) copolymer which can encapsulate an oily liquid. This new developed bilayer can be expressed as an anisotropic capsule, and the folding behavior is observed due to the swelling difference of the layers of the polymer film. Self-healing materials and drug delivery design are featured possible application areas of this approach [82]. A representative illustration of self-folding polymeric bilayer is shown in Figure 7.

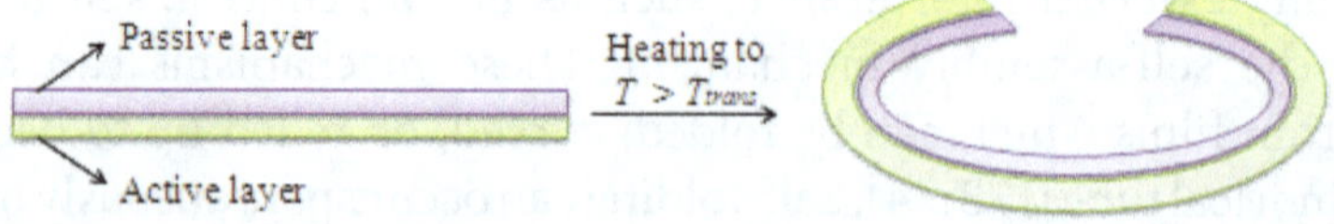

Figure 7. Self-folding procedure of thermoresponsive polymeric bilayer.

Ionov et al. studied two different sets of thermoresponsive polymeric bilayer behaviors to different stimuli. Polymeric bilayers were selected as one passive layer which is hydrophobic or random copolymer, and the active layer is the thermoresponsive hydrogel. Thermoresponsive hydrogels show swelling and shrink response to increased or decreased temperature, whereas passive layers prevent swelling of the active layer. In this manner, nonuniform expand/shrink behavior is achieved. In other words, folding and unfolding can be observed due to swelling [83].

Huang et al. developed a heat-responsive poly lactic acid (PLA) structure which would provide good uses for customized deployable/retractable and biodegradable implant devices for individual patients [84].

Lee et al. developed that self-folding oral delivery device which is capable of providing enhanced mucoadhesion, drug protection, and targeted multidirectional delivery. The device is composed of three layers which are backing layer, a foldable bilayer, and a mucoadhesive layer entrapped with drugs. The swelling bilayer was made of pH-sensitive hydrogel cross-linked poly(methyacrylic acid) (PMAA) which swells during contact with body fluid whereas non-swelling layer is poly(hydroxyethyl methacrylate) (PHEMA), and it acts as a diffusion barrier in order to minimize drug leakage in the intestine. When mucoadhesive drug layer is attached on the bilayer, self-folding device attaches to the mucus first and then curls into the mucus due to the different swelling of the bilayered structure, leading to enhanced mucoadhesion [85].

Temperature-stimulated liquid crystal elastomer–polystyrene bilayers which can show complex shape changing behavior such as helical twisting, reversible folding, and patterned wrinkles were developed by Agrawal et al. Tailoring was achieved by changing film thickness and overall aspect ratio [86].

Huck et al. reported that microscale, quasi-2D composite objects are fabricated which can respond to the addition of salt and pH changes [87].

Schenning et al. developed accordion-like striped actuators made of liquid crystal polymer films, which show response to the pH or temperature. These actuators would be used in medical systems and microrobotics [88]. Another liquid crystal shape memory actuator was developed by Park et al. which shows different swelling behavior between its UV exposed and non-UV exposed sides [89].

Visible light-induced graphene oxide/poly(vinylidenefluoride-hexafluoro propylene) (PVDF-HFP) nanocomposite films were produced by Yu et al. Tumbler movement was observed on the films due to the photothermal effect of graphene oxide and shape memory effect of PVDF-HFP. This behavior can be improved for full-plastic devices actuated by visible light [90].

Ionov et al. developed self-assembled porous scaffolds with uniaxial tubular pores. By producing rectangular polymer bilayers which include hydrophopic (poly methyl-methacrylate-co-benzophenoneacylate) and stimuli-responding hydrophilic polymer (poly N-isopropylacrylamide-co-acylic acid co-benzophenoeacylate), pH-dependent rolling of bilayers was observed. Also, these bilayers are capable of controlled self-assembly [91].

5. POLYMER ORIGAMI

The phrase origami originates from the Japanese words 'ori,' signifying 'to fold,' and 'kami,' denoting 'paper.' Origami is the internationally acknowledged Japanese art of paper folding. Currently, origami surpasses simple paper artistry and is employed in technological applications to create three-dimensional objects. To obtain these items, it is essential to provide fold pattern sequences to fabricate the desired object from a flat sheet. [93].

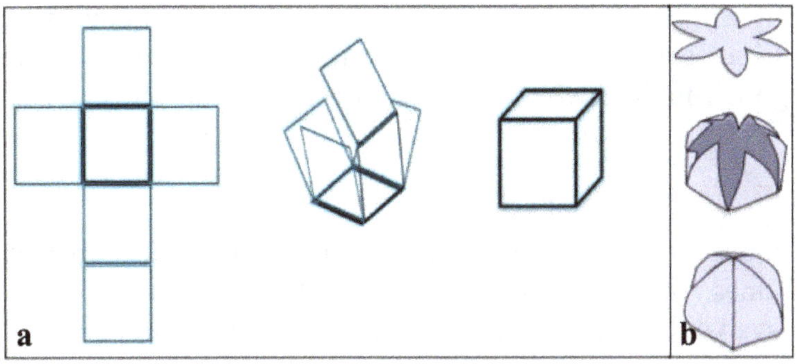

Figure 8. Origami folding sequence of a cubic structure (a), illustration of polymer origami self-folding (b).

Origami facilitates the construction of intricate structures, in contrast to bilayers, which can only flex in a single direction or undergo several folds. The configuration of self-folded structures is influenced by the initial geometry of the film, the radius of curvature (which is contingent upon the layer thickness), and the existence of a substrate [94]. Figure 8(a) illustrates a conventional origami folding structure. Polymer origami structures are utilized in space structure solar arrays, automobile airbags, shopping bags and cartons, photovoltaic cells, and biological applications [93].

Various stimuli can be employed to activate the material's self-folding properties and origami folding. Gracias et al. reported that self-folding functional microgrippers, which integrate a swellable, photo-cross-linked N-isopropylacrylamide-co-acrylic acid soft hydrogel with a non-swellable, hard-segmented polymer (polypropylene fumarate, PPF), exhibit a thermomechanical response to the hydrogel, enabling their application in surgical contexts [95].

In a study, Baroud et al. manually excised a geometric shape from a polymethylsiloxane membrane layer situated on a hydrophobic surface. Upon the addition of a water droplet to a membrane and subsequent evaporation, the diminishing water volume causes the thin membrane sheet to envelop the liquid, resulting in a three-dimensional pattern that illustrates the interplay between elasticity and capillarity [96]. This approach is illustrated in Figure 8(b).

Gracias et al. created three-dimensional (3D) microfabricated nanoliter containers by thermally actuating a two-dimensional (2D) structure to fold into a 3D configuration, resembling polymer origami. The 2D template incorporates intelligent hinges. Researchers proposed that this novel production technique will be employed for the advancement of microscale biomedical devices in the future [97].

Ryu exhibited photo-origami that activates both flat and curved surfaces of polymer films to produce three-dimensional shapes at a macroscopic scale by a technique of localized photo-induced stress relaxation. Photo-origami is propelled by an amorphous, covalently crosslinked polymer of pentaerythritol tetra(3-mercaptopropionate) (PETMP), 2-methylene-propane-1,3-di(thioethylvinylether) (MDTVE), and ethylene glycol di(3-mercaptopropionate) (EGDMP). [93]. Gracias et al. created photo-cross-linked polyethylene glycol (PEG)-based bio-origami hydrogel bilayers capable of self-folding in aqueous solutions. The newly created bilayers preserve various types of tissues through self-folding, which could be enhanced in the field of tissue engineering [98].

6. SMART POLYMERS AS DRUG CARRIERS

The primary application of shape memory polymers is in medication delivery systems. Certain medicines, owing to their limited solubility in the bloodstream, exhibit enhanced bioavailability when administered via a carrier system. This may facilitate the prolonged release of the medication, which is advantageous if the drug is intended to be eluted over an extended duration. Various drug delivery technologies have been developed, including liposomal systems and biodegradable polymeric systems. Polymers provide a diverse array of customizable features suitable for the intended drug elution system. Smart polymers are a distinct category of materials suitable for the construction of innovative drug delivery systems. Criteria such as drug loading capacity, aqueous environmental conditions, drug release patterns, and degradation behavior dictate the appropriateness of shape memory polymers as matrix materials for drug release or carrier applications. [99].

Based on the requirements defined by a specific application, such polymer systems will allow selecting one specific polymer out of a larger number of related materials without the need to change to a totally different material chemistry. In addition to adjustable thermal properties, polymer systems can also be helpful to realize demanded mechanical properties or desired degradation rates of SMP implants [100].

For biomedical applications of SMPs, the capability to change their shape should be established at relevant conditions, i.e., T_{sw} (switching temperature) of the SMP device should be close to or at reasonable levels above body temperature. To meet this goal, the thermal properties such as T_g or the melting temperature T_m that account for the shape memory effect need to be adjusted. Polymer systems as families of materials, in which different properties and functions can ideally be tailored over a wide range independent from each other, may allow the adjustment of T_{sw} by polymer chemistry, which make them good candidates as drug carriers [101].

About the controlled drug release ability of shape-memory polymers, Ohya et al. reported that chemically cross-linked networks of branched oligo(ε-caprolactone) polymer can perform sustained release of theophylline drug over a month without initial burst release in Phosphate Buffer Saline (PBS) at 37°C [102].

According to the study of Ameer et al., hydroxyl-dominant (HD) polydiolcitrates (HD polymers) can perform the subsequent release of hydrophobic dichlorofluororescein (DCF) drug. This means polydiolcitrate elastomers could benefit from smart biodegradable materials for tissue engineering applications [103].

Such systems are ideal for minimally invasive surgery where implants are inserted through a small incision, and after self-anchoring, they start to release a pharmacological agent. Dobrzyński et al. developed a shape memory polymer based on L-lactide, glycolide, and trimethylene carbonate in order to obtain double layer systems for paclitaxel drug delivery that paves the way for drug eluting stents [104].

Lendlein et al. reported that oligo (caprolactone-co-glycolide) dimethacrylate was combined with drug, and its activation was obtained between 28-42°C where shape memory effect was pronounced at body temperature. In this study, diffusion-controlled drug release was observed independent from polymer degradation [105].

Gong et al. reported that biodegradable polymeric cross-linked poly(ε-caprolactone) (cPCL) and poly(sebacic anhydride) (PSA) were developed, and release accumulation of drug can be enhanced by adding PSA into cPCL matrix. This shape memory polymer could be used as potential drug-eluting stents in biomedical field [106].

7. POTENTIAL BIOMEDICAL APPLICATIONS OF SMART POLYMERS

During the past decade, biomedical applications of shape memory materials became a very active area of research [107].

As mentioned in the previous section, the progress in surgical techniques, especially in minimally invasive surgery, allows these materials to be used widely in biomedical applications of polymers.

These smart materials are enabled to insert a bulky device in the body through a small keyhole incision in a temporarily fixed shape. After a precise position by the surgeon, such smart materials gain their application-relevant shape on demand [108].

Zhang et al. demonstrated a new nanofibrous, biomimetic, shape memory, and biodegradable poly(D,L-lactide-*co*-trimethylene carbonate) by electrospinning which would be applicable for MIS implantation [109].

Nelson et al. developed hydrogel bilayers composed of N-isopropylacrylamide with polyethyleneglycol diacrylate. By using the expansion difference of these layers due to swelling, self-folding behavior was observed. These new devices are switchable and show reversible shape transition against external stimuli. These layers were designed for different purposes in order to demonstrate microstructures which can preserve magnetic alginate microbeads when they have folded structures. After exposing to NIR laser source, microbeads are capable of being released from the microstructures. So, this method offers a solution for drug and cell delivery systems [110].

Tai et al. demonstrated an origami technique by constructing 3D spherical structure from 2D parylene-C (PA-C) film for intraocular implantation application [111]. Maitland et al. developed an SMP adapter in order to reduce the hemodynamic stress which arises from impingement of dialysis needle in an arteriovenous graft [112].

The most effective areas of biomedical applications of shape memory polymers are intravascular stents, treating aneurysm occlusion and clot removal.

7.1. Intravascular Stents

Intravascular stents are predominantly used in main arteries or peripheral arteries, in the treatment of cardiovascular diseases (CVDs) which is the number one cause of death globally: more people die annually from CVDs than from any other cause [113]. First-generation stents are metallic, whereas second-generation ones are polymer-coated drug-eluting metallic stents. New-generation stents are biodegradable polymers that are also drug eluting. The potential advantages of pure polymer stents compared to bare metal stents include increased biocompatibility, biodegradability, increased drug loading, enhanced compliance matching, reduced cost, ease of fabrication for patient-specific devices, molecular surface engineering, and the use of shape memory effect [114].

Metallic stents are effective in hindering acute occlusion and reducing late restenosis after coronary angioplasty; however, many concerns still remain. Compared with metallic stents, poly-L-lactic acid (PLLA) stents are biodegradable and can deliver drugs locally, and these were developed by Igaki and Tamai. It was reported that feasibility, safety, and effectiveness of PLLA-biodegradable stents were verified in humans [115].

Wagner et al. reported that shape memory thermoplastic polyurethane is developed as a self-expandable stent, and it can be used as a drug delivery system [116].

A polymer system consists of *tert*-butyl acrylate, and poly(ethylene glycol) dimethylacrylate is improved which meets specific needs of minimally invasive cardiovascular devices by Gall and his coworkers. In this study, it was found that 10 wt% cross-linked polymer network can be stored unconstrained at room temperature and can be activated at body temperature which can be fabricated as a stent [117].

Chen et al. developed shape memory chitosan-based films (chitosan/PEO/glycerol) which are used to produce biodegradable stents. Chitosan cross-linked with epoxy compound stent's most remarkable property shows rapid expansion from a crimped state by using the hydration in an aqueous environment as a stimulant. By using minimally invasive surgery techniques, this stent can be placed into an artery. In another study of Chen and coworkers, genipin cross-linked chitosan-based stents were developed. The possibility of using this newly developed genipin stent as a drug delivery vehicle was also examined by loading an anti-proliferation drug, sirolimus. Findings showed that the genipin stent with enhanced mechanical strength can be used as an attractive stent platform for local drug delivery [118,119].

Maitland et al. performed the design and fabrication of an SMP stent (MM5520 thermoplastic polyurethane) which was triggered by photothermal actuation at 40–45°C [120].

Wang and coworkers developed fully biodegradable polymeric stent that can self-expand at body temperatures (37°C), using the concept of elastic memory. This self-expansion is necessary in fully polymeric stents, to overcome the problem of elastic recoil following balloon expansion in a body vessel. Bilayered biodegradable stent prototypes were produced from poly-L-lactic acid and polyglycolic acid (PLGA) polymers [121].

7.2. Aneurysm Treatment

An aneurysm is a formation of balloon-like bulge in an artery. This bulge is formed when a part of artery wall becomes weak which results in unusual widening. Aneurysms can occur in any of the artery; however, the most common ones are aortic, cerebral (in the brain), popliteal (in the leg, behind knee), mesenteric (in the intestine), and splenic artery aneurysm (in the spleen). Almost 13,000 Americans die annually from aortic aneurysms. Surgery is the possible option for the treatment of large aortic aneurysms [122,123].

Shape memory polymer foams are the most attractive materials for aneurysm treatment by using them as a filling device in the artery [124]. Wilson and his coworkers showed that the shape memory polymer foam which includes hexamethylene diisocyanate (HDI), N,N,N',N'-tetrakis(2-hydroxypropyl)ethylenediamine (HPED), and triethanolamine (TEA) can be laser deployed in an *in vitro* aneurysm model. In this study, 10-mm aneurysm was treated with a new developed device [125].

In the study of Wong et al., shape memory polymer Calomer™ was investigated as a candidate for aneurysm coils. In this work, shape memory polymer coils spread inside a simulated aneurysm model proved that the typical hemodynamic forces do not prevent the shape recovery process [126].

Maitland et al. developed shape memory polyurethane foam with high porosity which makes it convenient for intracranial aneurysm treatments. Adding 4% tungsten into this foam improves radioopacity. Inherent radioopacity makes the material to be visualized by using conventional patient imaging modalities such as fluoroscopy in order to deliver it safely [127].

Another shape memory polymer foam based on hexamethylenediisocyanate, triethanolamine, and tetrakis(2-hydroxyl propyl)ethylenediamine was developed by Maitland et al. which is found to be suitable for aneurysm treatment [128].

Raymonda et al. developed a non-cytotoxic, non-mutagenic, and poorly thrombogenic polyurethane-based foam called cold hibernated elastic memory (CHEM) for endovascular procedures. The shape memory property and possibly modifying T_g or the size of the pores let this material for developing new tools including embolic agents that could completely replace the aneurysmal cavity, without intervening thrombus, to prevent recanalization and recurrences after the endovascular treatment of aneurysms [129].

7.3. Clot Removal

When blood does not flow smoothly in the blood vessels, it can begin to coagulate and/or blood clots. A blood clot, or thrombus, may continue to grow, blocking the blood supply to certain parts of the body and causing damage to tissues and organs. Some medical intervention is often required to remove the clots. It is estimated that each year thrombosis affects as many as 900,000 people in the USA and kills up to 100,000 [130,131].

Maitland et al. reported that a prototype endovascular electromechanical clot extraction device was fabricated using a combination of shape memory polymer and shape memory nickel–titanium alloy (nitinol). This preliminary study suggests that SMP–nitinol device may have an application in the treatment of acute stroke or other thromboembolic diseases [132].

Also, Maitland and coworkers aimed to evaluate the feasibility of utilizing a system of SMP acrylates for a thrombectomy device by determining an optimal cross-link density that provides both adequate recovery stress for blood clot removal and sufficient strain capacity to enable catheter delivery. They have reported an acrylic SMP system with glass transitions above body temperature in the range of 65–75°C with tailorable recovery stresses that were controlled by varying the cross-link density. From the four different material compositions evaluated, devices with 15 mole% bisphenol A(BPA) gave the most favorable outcome [133].

Wilson et al. reported that coil, umbrella, and microgripper-shaped polyurethane microactuators are used to treat stroke by activating this shape memory polymer with laser to remove clots. The actuation of the devices was obtained between 65 and85°C [134].

8. CONCISE SUMMARY

This chapter summarizes novel smart polymeric materials, including shape memory polymers, self-folding polymers, and polymer origami structures, along with their prospective uses. Shape memory polymers are a category of smart materials that can restore their original shape after deformation by being cooled below their transition temperature. Subsequently, upon reheating to the specified transition temperature, the restoration to the original shape is evident. They can be synthesized from polymeric materials or by blending with network-based polymers. Owing to their superior biocompatibility, shape memory polymers (SMPs) serve as promising components in biomedical applications, including polymer vascular stents utilizing SMPs for drug delivery systems, intelligent surgical sutures, laser-activated SMP microactuators for clot removal in blood vessels, and implants for minimally invasive surgery. Currently, SMP development is advancing swiftly, particularly in clinical applications. Advancing biomedical applications beyond medical devices will be accomplished by integrating shape memory polymers with suitable materials. In the context of minimally invasive surgery, implants must be capable of executing intricate movements. These movements must be executed by a material capable of undergoing programmed shifts repeatedly, such as shape memory polymers (SMPs). SMPs would be necessary for individual patients as they are tailored to specific ailments. Shape memory polymers are seen as a prospective technique to avert undesirable consequences in biomedical treatments, offering advantages over shape memory alloy materials due to their biodegradability. Due to their versatility, SMPs will continue to evolve owing to their intriguing prospective applications.

REFERENCES

1. Huang W.M, Ding Z, Wang C.C, Wei J, Zhao Y, Purnawali H. Shape Memory Materials. Materials Today; 2010, 13(7-8): 54–61.
2. Mather P.T, Luo X, Rousseau I.A. Shape Memory Polymer Research. Annual Review of Material Research; 2009, 39: 445–471.
3. Konstanze K. Julich-Gruner, Löwenberg C, Neffe A.T, Behl M, Lendlein A. Recent Trends in the Chemistry of Shape Memory Polymers. Macromolecular Chemistry and Physics; 2013, 214(5): 527–536.
4. Serrano M.C, Ameer G.A. Recent Insights into the Biomedical Applications of Shape Memory Polymers. Macromolecular Bioscience; 2012, 12(9): 1156–1171.
5. Meng Q, Hu J. A Review of Shape Memory Polymer Composites and Blends. Composites: Part A; 2009, 40: 1661–1672.
6. Lendlein A, Kelch S. Shape-Memory Polymers. Angewandte Chemie International Edition; 2002, 41: 2034–2057.
7. Hiltz J.A. Shape Memory Polymers Literature Review. Defence R&D Canada Technical Memorandum; 2002, 127.
8. Liang C, Rogers C.A, Malafeew E. Investigation of Shape Memory Polymers and Their Hybrid Composites. Journal of Intelligent Material Systems and Structures; 1997, 8(4): 380–386.
9. Ahmed N, Kausar A, Muhammad B. Advances in Shape Memory Polyurethanes and Composites: A Review. Polymer-Plastics Technology and Engineering; 2015, 54: 1410–1423.
10. Lendlein A, Langer R. Biodegradable, Elastic Shape-Memory Polymers for Potential Biomedical Applications. Science; 2002, 296 (5573): 1673-1676.
11. Behl M, Zotzmann J, Lendlein A. Shape-Memory Polymers and Shape-Changing Polymers. Advance in Polymer Science; 2009, 226: 1–40.

12. Liu C, Qin H, Mather P.T. Review of Progress in Shape – Memory Polymers. Journal of Materials Chemistry; 2007, 17: 1543–1558.
13. Sokolowski W, Metcalfe A, Hayashi S, Yahia L, Raymond J. Medical Applications of Shape Memory Polymers. Biomedical Materials; 2007, 2: 23–27.
14. Monkman G.J. Advances in Shape Memory Polymer Actuation. Mechatronics; 2000, 10: 489–498.
15. Witold M, Sokolowski A, Chmielewski B, Hayashi S, Yamada T. Cold Hibernated Elastic Memory (CHEM) Self-deployable Structures. SPIE Conference on Electroactive Polymer Actuators and Devices; 1999.
16. Hu J, Zhu Y, Huang H, Lu J. Recent Advances in Shape – Memory Polymers: Structure, Mechanism, Functionality, Modeling and Applications. Progress in Polymer Science; 2012, 37: 1720–1763.
17. Leng J, Lan X, Liu Y, Dua S. Shape-Memory Polymers and Their Composites: Stimulus Methods and Applications. Progress in Materials Science; 2011, 56: 1077–1135.
18. Kumpfer J.R, Rowan S.J. Thermo-, Photo- and Chemo-Responsive Shape-Memory Properties From Photo - Crosslinked Metallo - Supramolecular Polymers. Journal of the American Chemical Society; 2011, 133: 12866–12874.
19. Leng J.S, Lan X, Liu Y.J, Du S.Y, Huang W.M, Liu N, Phee S.J, Yuan Q. Electrical Conductivity of Thermoresponsive Shape - Memory Polymer with Embedded Micron Sized Ni Powder Chains. Applied Physics Letters; 2008, 92 (1).
20. Mohr R, Kratz K, Weigel T, Lucka-Gabor M, Moneke M, Lendlein A. Initiation of Shape - Memory Effect by Inductive Heating of Magnetic Nanoparticles in Thermoplastic Polymers. Proceedings of the National Academy of Sciences; 2006, 103 (10): 3540–3545.
21. Razzaq M.Y, Behl M, Nöchel U, Lendlein A. Magnetically Controlled Shape -Memory Effects of Hybrid Nanocomposites from Oligo(w-pentadelactone) and Covalently Integrated Magnetite Nanoparticles. Polymer; 2014, 55: 5953–5960.
22. Xia S, Li X, Wang Y, Pan Y, Zeng Z, Ding X, Peng Y. A Remote Activated Shape Memory Polymer Network Employing Vinyl Capped Fe_3O_4 Nanoparticles as Netpoints for Durable Performance. Smart Materials and Structures; 2014, 23(8).
23. Huang W.M,Yang B, Zhao Y, Ding Z. Thermo-Moisture Responsive Polyurethane Shape-Memory Polymer and Composites: A Review. Journal of Materials Chemistry; 2010, 20: 3367–3381.
24. Lendlein A, Jiang H, Jünger O, Langer R. Light Induced Shape Memory Polymers. Nature; 2005, 434: 879–882.
25. Huang W.M, Zhao Y, Wang C.C, Ding Z, Purnawali H, Tang C, Zhang J.L. Thermo/Chemo - Responsive Shape Memory Effect in Polymers: A Sketch of Working Mechanisms, Fundamentals and Optimization. Journal of Polymer Research; 2012, 19(9952).
26. Chatterjee T, Dey P, Nando, Naskar K. Thermo - Responsive Shape Memory Polymer Blends Based on Alpha Olefin and Ethylene Propylene Diene Rubber, Polymer; 2015, 78: 180–192.
27. Langer R, Tirrel D.A. Designing Materials for Biology and Medicine, Nature; 2004, 428: 487–492.
28. Xue L, Dai S, Li Z. Synthesis and Characterization of Elastic Star Shape-Memory Polymers as Self Expandable Drug-Eluting Stents. Journal of Materials Chemistry; 2012, 22: 7403–7411.

29. Yakachi C.M. Shape Memory and Shape Changing Polymers. Polymer Reviews; 2013, 53: 1–3.
30. Sokolowski W, Metcalfe A, Hayashi S, Yahia L, Raymond J. Biomedical Materials; 2007, 2: 23–27.
31. Razzaq M.R, Anhalt M, Frorman L, Weidenfeller B Mechanical Spectroscopy of Magnetite Filled Polyurethane Shape Memory Polymers. Materials Science and Engineering; 2007, 471: 57–62.
32. Ebara M. Shape-Memory Surfaces for Cell Mechanobiology. Science and Technology of Advance Materials; 2015, 16(1).
33. Behl M, Lendlein A. Shape Memory Polymers. Materials Today; 2007, 10(4): 20–28.
34. Xie T, Rousseau I.A. Facile Tailoring of Thermal Transition Temperatures of Epoxy Shape Memory Polymers. Polymer; 2009, 50, 1852–1856.
35. Zheng X, Zhou S, Li X, Weng J. Shape Memory Properties of Poly(D,L-lactide)/ Hydroxyapatite Composites. Biomaterials; 2006, 27: 4288–4295.
36. Brosnan S.M, Jackson A.S, Wang Y, Ashby V.S. Shape Memory Particles Capable of Controlled Geometric and Chemical Asymmetry Made from Aliphatic Polyesters. Macromolecular Rapid Communications; 2014, 35: 1653–1660.
37. Pandini S, Baldi F, Paderni K, Messori M, Toselli M, Pilati F, Gianoncelli A, Brisotto M, Bontempi E, Riccò T. One-way and Two-way Shape Memory Behavior of Semi-Crystalline Networks Based on Sol-gel Cross Linked Poly(ε-caprolactone). Polymer; 2013, 54: 4253–4265.
38. Xie T. Recent Advances in Polymer Shape Memory. Polymer; 2011, 52: 4985–5000.
39. Behl M, Razzaq M.R, Lendlein A. Multifunctional Shape-Memory Polymers. Advanced Materials; 2010, 22: 3388–3410.
40. Wu X, Huang W.M, Zhao Y, Ding Z, Tang C, Zhang J. Mechanisms of the Shape Memory Effect in Polymeric Materials. Polymers; 2013, 5: 1169–1202.
41. Li X, Zhu Y, Dong Y, Liu M, Ni Q, Fu Y. Epoxy Resin Composite Bilayers with Triple - Shape Memory Effect. Hindawi Publishing Corporation Journal of Nanomaterials; 2015.
42. Cuevas J.M, Rubio R, Germán L,Villas J.L, Rodriguez M, León L.M. Triple Shape Memory Effect of Covalently Crosslinked Polyalkenamer Based Semicrystalline Polymer Blends. Soft Matter; 2012, 8: 4928–4935.
43. Kumar U.N, Kratz K, Behl M, Lendlein A. Shape - Memory Properties of Magnetically Active Triple - Shape Nanocomposites Based on a Grafted Polymer Network with Two Crystallizable Switching Segments. Express Polymer Letters; 2012, 6(1): 26–40.
44. Chen S, Hu J, Yuen C, Chan L, Zhuo H. Triple Shape Memory Effect in Multiple Crystalline Polyurethanes. Polymers for Advanced Technologies; 2010, 21: 377–380.
45. Xie T, Xiao X, Cheng Y. Revealing Triple-Shape Memory Effect by Polymer Bilayers. Macromolecular Rapid Communications; 2009, 30: 1823–1827.
46. Xie T. Tunable Polymer Multi- Shape Memory Effect. Nature; 2010, 464: 267–270.
47. Basit A, L'Hostis G, Pae M.J, Durand B. Thermally Activated Composite with Two-Way and Multi-Shape Memory Effects. Materials; 2013, 6: 4031–4045.
48. Li J, Rodgers W.R, Xie T. Semicrystalline Two-Way Shape Memory Elastomer, Polymer; 2011, 52: 5320, 5325.
49. Chen S, Hu J, Zhuo H, Zhu Y. Two-way Shape Memory Effect in Polymer Laminates. Materials Letters; 2008, 62: 4088–4090.

50. Zhou J, Turner S.A, Brosnan S.M, Li Q, Cartillo J.Y, Nykypanchuk D, Gang O, Ashby V.S, Dobrynin A.V, Sheiko S.S. Shapeshifting: Reversible Shape Memory in Semicrystalline Elastomers. Macromolecules; 2014, 47: 1768–1776.

51. Madbouly S.A, Lendlein A. Shape – Memory Polymer Composites. Advanced Polymer Science; 2010, 226: 41–95.

52. Leng J, Lu H, Liu Y, Huang W.M, Du S. Shape-Memory Polymers- A Class of Novel Smart Materials. Mrs Bulletin; 2009, 34.

53. Yakachi C.M, Satarkar N.S, Gall K, Likos R, Hilt J.Z. Shape- Memory Polymer Networks with Fe_3O_4 Nanocomposites for Remote Activation, Journal of Applied Polymer Science; 2002,112: 3166–3176.

54. Razzaq M.Y, Anhalt M, Frormann L, Weidenfeller B. Thermal, electrical and magnetic studies of magnetite filled polyurethane shape memory polymers. Materials Science and Engineering A; 2007, 444: 227–235.

55. Yu X, Zhou S, Zheng X, Guo T, Xiao Y, Song B. A Biodegradable Shape-Memory Nanocomposite with Excellent Magnetism Sensitivity. Nanotechnology; 2009, 20(23).

56. Schmidt A.M. Electromagnetic Activation of Shape Memory Polymer Networks Containing Magnetic Nanoparticles. Macromolecules Rapid Communications; 2006, 27: 1168–1172.

57. Zheng X, Zhou S, Xiao Y, Yu X, Li X, Wu P. Shape Memory Effect of Poly(D,L-lactide)/Fe_3O_4 Nanocomposites by Inductive Heating of Magnetic Nanoparticles. Colloids and Surfaces B: Biointerfaces; 2009, 71: 67–72.

58. Puig J, Hoppe C.E, Fasce L.A, Pérez C.J, Piñeiro-Redondo Y, Bañobre-López M, López-Quintela M.A, Rivas J, Williams R.J.J. Superparamagnetic Nanocomposites Based on the Dispersion of Oleic Acid-Stabilized Magnetite Nanoparticles in a Diglycidylether of Bisphenol A-Based Epoxy Matrix: Magnetic Hyperthermia and Shape Memory. The Journal of Physical Chemistry C; 2012, 116: 13421–13428.

59. Cho J.W, Kim J.W, Jung Y.C, Goo N.S. Electroactive Shape-Memory Polyurethane Composites Incorporating Carbon Nanotubes. Macromolecular Rapid Communications; 2005, 26: 412–416.

60. Liu Y, Lv H, Lan X, Leng J, Du S. Review of Electro-Active Shape-Memory Polymer Composite, Composites Science and Technology; 2009, 69: 2064–2068.

61. Yoo H.J, Jung Y.C, Sahoo N.G, Cho J.W. Polyurethane-Carbon Nanotube Nanocomposites Prepared by In-Situ Polymerization with Electroactive Shape Memory. Journal of Macromolecular Science, Part B: Physics; 2006, 45: 441–451.

62. Jung Y.C, Yoo H.J, Kim Y.A, Cho J.W, Endo M. Electroactive Shape Memory Performance of Polyurethane Composite Having Homogenously Dispersed and Covalently Crosslinked Carbon Nanotubes, Carbon; 2010, 48: 1598–1603.

63. Sahoo N.G, Jung Y.C, Cho J.W. Electroactive Shape Memory Effect of Polyurethane Composites Filled with Carbon Nanotubes and Conducting Polymer. Materials and Manufacturing Processes; 2007, 22: 419–423.

64. Leng J, Lan X, Liu Y, Du S. Electroactive Thermoset Shape Memory Polymer Nanocomposite Filled with Nanocarbon Powders. Smart Materials; 2009, 18.

65. Xiao Y, Zhou S, Wang L, Gong T. Electro-Active Shape Memory Properties of Poly(ε-caprolatone)/Functionalized Multiwalled Nanotune Nanocomposite. Applied Materials and Interfaces; 2010, 2(12): 3506–3514.

66. Sahoo N.G, Yung Y.C, Yoo H.J, Cho J.W. Influence of Carbon Nanotubes and Polypyrrole on the Thermal, Mechanical and Electroactive Shape-Memory Properties of Polyurethane Nanocomposites, Composites Science and Technology; 2007, 67: 1920–1929.
67. Meng H, Li G. A review of stimuli-responsive shape memory polymer composites. Polymer; 2013, 54: 2199–2221.
68. Wu T, O'Kelly K, Chen B. Poly(methacrylic acid)-Grafted Clay–Thermoplastic Elastomer Composites with Water-Induced Shape-Memory Effects. Journal of Polymer Science, Part B: Polymer Physics; 2013, 51: 1513–1522
69. Luo H, Ma Y, Li W, Yi G, Cheng X, Ji W, Zu X, Yuan S, Li J. Shape Memory-Enhanced Water Sensing of Conductive Polymer Composites, Materials Letters; 2015, 161: 189–192.
70. Nöchel U, Reddy C.S, Uttamchand N.K, Kratz K, Behl M, Lendlein A. Shape-Memory Properties of Hydrogels Having a Poly(ε-caprolactone) Crosslinker and Switching Segment in an Aqueous Environment, European Polymer Journal; 2013, 49: 2457–2466.
71. Paakinaho K, Hukka T.I, Kastinen T, Kellomäki M. Demonstrating the Mechanism and Efficacy of Water-Induced Shape Memory and the Influence of Water on the Thermal Properties of Oriented Poly (d,l-lactide). Journal of Applied Polymer Science; 2013: 4209–4213.
72. Mendez J, Annamalai P.K, Eichhorn S.J, Rusli R, Rowan S.J, Foster E.J, Weder C. Bioinspired Mechanically Adaptive Polymer Nanocomposites with Water-Activated Shape-Memory Effect. Macromolecules; 2011, 44: 6827–6835.
73. Hernandez E.A, Hartl D.J, Malak Jr R.J, Lagoudas D.C. Origami- Inspired Active Structures: A Synthesis and Review. Smart Material Structures; 2014, 23(9).
74. Gracias D.H. Stimuli Responsive Self-Folding Using Thin Polymer Films, Current Opinion in Chemical Engineering; 2013: 112–119.
75. Azam A, Laflin K.E, Jamal M, Fernandes R, Gracias D.H. Self - Folding Micropatterned Polymeric Containers. Biomedical Microdevices; 2011: 51–58.
76. Guan J, He H, Hansford D.J, Lee L.J. Self-Folding of Three-Dimensional Hydrogel Microstructures. Journal of Physical Chemistry B; 2005, 109(49): 23134–23137.
77. Fernandes R, Gracias D.H. Self-Folding Polymeric Containers for Encapsulation and Delivery of Drugs, Advanced Drug Delivery Reviews; 2012, 64: 1579–1589.
78. Ionov L. 3D Microfabrication Using Stimuli-Responsive Self-Folding Polymer Films. Polymer Reviews; 2013, 53: 92–107.
79. Zakharchenko S, Sperling E, Ionov L. Fully Biodegradable Self-Rolled Polymer Tubes: A Candidate for Tissue Engineering Scaffolds. Biomacromolecules; 2011, 12: 2211–2215.
80. Luchnikov V, Ionov L, Stamm M. Self-Rolled Polymer Tubes: Novel Tools for Microfluidics, Microbiology, and Drug-Delivery Systems. Macromolecular Rapid Communications; 2011, 32: 1943–1952.
81. Ionov L. Soft Microorigami: Self-Folding Polymer Films. Soft Matter; 2011, 7: 6786–6791.
82. Zakharchenko S, Ionov L. Anisotropic Liquid Microcapsules from Biomimetic Self-Folding Polymer Films. ACS Applied Materials and Interfaces; 2015, 7(23): 12367–12372.
83. Stoychev G, Zakharchenko S, Turcaud S, Dunlop J.W, Ionov L, Shape-Programmed Folding of Stimuli-Responsive Polymer Bilayers. ACS Nano; 2012, 6(5): 3925–3934.
84. Huang W.M, Lu H.B, Zhao Y, Ding Z, Wang C.C, Zhang J.L, Sun L, Fu J, Gao X.Y. Instability/ Collapse of Polymeric Materials and Their Structures in Stimulus - Induced Shape/ Surface Morphology Switching. Materials and Design; 2014, 59, 176–192.

85. He H, Guan J, Lee J.L. An Oral Delivery Device Based on Self-Folding Hydrogels. Journal of Controlled Release; 2006, 110: 339–346.

86. Agrawal A, Yun T, Pesek S.L, Chapman W.G, Verduzco R. Shape-Responsive Liquid Crystal Elastomer Bilayers. Soft Matter; 2014, 10: 1411–1415.

87. Kelby T.S, Wang M, Huck W.T.S. Controlled Folding of 2D Au–Polymer Brush Composites into 3D Microstructures. Advanced Functional Materials; 2011, 21: 652–657.

88. De Haan L.T, Gimenez-Pinto V, Konya A, Nguyen T, Verjans J.M.N, Sánchez-Somolinos C, Selinger J.V, Selinger R.L.B, Broer D.J, Schenning A.P.H.J. Accordion-like Actuators of Multiple 3D Patterned Liquid Crystal Polymer Films. Advanced Functional Materials; 2014, 24: 1251–1258.

89. Kamal T, Park S. Shape-Responsive Actuator from a Single Layer of a Liquid-Crystal Polymer. Applied Material Interfaces; 2014, 6: 18048–18054.

90. Yu L, Yu H. Light-Powered Tumbler Movement of Graphene Oxide/Polymer Nanocomposites. Applied Material Interfaces; 2015, 7(6): 3834–3839.

91. Zacharchenko S, Puretskiy N, Stoychev G, Waurisch C, Hickey S.G, Eychmüller A, Sommer J, Ionov L. Stimuli-Responsive Hierarchically Self-Assembled 3D Porous Polymer-Based Structures with Aligned Pores. Journal of Material Chemistry B; 2013, 1: 1786–1793.

92. Fei L.J, Sujan D. Origami Theory and Its Applications: A Literature Review. International Scholarly and Scientific Research & Innovation; 2013, 7(1).

93. Ryu J, D'Amato M, Cui X, Long K.N, Qi H.J. Photo-origami- Bending and Folding Polymers with Light. Applied Physics Letter; 2012, 100.

94. Ionov L. Polymer Origami: Programming the Folding with Shape, e-Polymers; 2014,14(2): 109–114.

95. Breger J.C, Yoon C, Xiao R, Kwan H.R, Wang M.O, Fisher J.P, Nguyen T.D, Gracias D.H. Self-Folding Thermo-Magnetically Responsive Soft Microgrippers. Applied Material Interfaces; 2015, 7: 3398–3405.

96. Py C, Reverdy P, Doppler L, Bico J, Roman B, Baroud C.N. Capillary Origami: Spontaneous Wrapping of a Droplet with an Elastic Sheet. Physical Review Letters; 2007, 98.

97. Randall C.L, Leong T.G, Bassik N, Gracias D.H. 3D Lithographically Fabricated Nanoliter Containers for Drug Delivery. Advanced Drug Delivery Reviews; 2007, 59: 1547–156.

98. Jamal M, Kadam S.S, Xiao R, Jivan F, Onn T, Fernandes R, Nguyen T.D, Gracias D.H. Bio-Origami Hydrogel Scaffolds Composed of Photocrosslinked PEG Bilayers. Advanced Healthcare Materials; 2013, 2: 1142–1150.

99. Wischke C, Neffe A.T, Steuer S, Lendlein A. Evaluation of a Degradable Shape-Memory Polymer Network as Matrix for Controlled Drug Release. Journal of Controlled Release; 2009, 138: 243–250.

100. Wischke C, Behl M, Lendlein A. Drug-Releasing Shape-Memory Polymers- The Role of Morphology, Processing Effects, and Matrix Degradation. Expert Opinion on Drug Delivery; 2013, 10(9).

101. Lendlein A, Wischke C. How to Accelerate Biomaterial Development? Strategies to Support the Application of Novel Polymer-Based Biomaterials in Implantable Devices. Expert Review of Medical Devices; 2011, 8(5): 533–537.

102. Nagahama K, Ueda Y, Ouchi T, Ohya Y. Biodegradable Shape-Memory Polymers Exhibiting Sharp Thermal Transitions and Controlled Drug Release. Biomacromolecules; 2009, 10: 1789–1794.

103. Serrano M.C, Carbajal L, Ameer A.G. Novel Biodegradable Shape-Memory Elastomers with Drug-Releasing Capabilities. Advanced Materials; 2011, 23: 2211–2215.
104. Musial-Kulik M, Kasperczyk J, Smola A, Dobrzyński P. Double Layer Paclitaxel Delivery Systems Based on Bioresorbable Terpolymer with Shape Memory Properties. International Journal of Pharmaceutics; 2014, 465: 291–298.
105. Wischke C, Neffe A.T, Steuer S, Lendlein A. Comparing Techniques for Drug Loading of Shape-Memory Polymer Networks – Effect on Their Functionalities. European Journal of Pharmaceutical Sciences; 2010, 41: 136–147.
106. Xiao Y, Zhou S, Wang L, Zheng X, Gong T. Crosslinked Poly(ε-caprolactone)/Poly(Sebacic Anhydride) Composites Combining Biodegradation. Controlled Drug Release and Shape Memory Effect. Composites: Part B; 2010, 41: 537–542.
107. Lendlein A, Behl M, Hiebl B, Wischke C. Shape-Memory Polymers as a Technology Platform for Biomedical Applications. Expert Review of Medical Devices; 2010, 7 (3): 357–379.
108. Wischke C, Lendlein A. Shape-Memory Polymers as Drug Carriers-A Multifunctional System. Pharmaceutical Research; 2010, 27(4).
109. Bao M, Lou X, Zhou Q, Dong W, Yuan H, Zhang Y. Electrospun Biomimetic Fibrous Scaffold from Shape Memory Polymer of PDLLA-co-TMC for Bone Tissue Engineering. Applied Material Interfaces; 2014, 6: 2611–2621.
110. Fusco S, Sakar M.S, Kennedy S, Peters C, Pene S, Mooney D, Nelson B.J. Self-Folding Mobile Microrobots for Biomedical Applications, Robotics and Automation (ICRA). IEEE International Conference; 2014: 3777–3782.
111. Liu Y, Park J, Lang R.J, Emami-Neyestanak A, Pellegrino S, Humayun M.S, Tai Y. Parylene Origami Structure for Intraocular Implantation. Solid-State Sensors, Actuators and Microsystems; 2013: 1549–1552
112. Ortega J.M, Small IV W, Wilson T.S, Bennett W.J, Loge J.M, Maitland D.J. A Shape Memory Polymer Dialysis Needle Adapter for the Reduction of Hemodynamic Stress within Arteriovenous Grafts. IEEE Transactions on Biomedical Engineering; 2007, 54(9): 1722–17244.
113. World Health Organization. Global Status Report on Noncommunicable Diseases; 2014.
114. Yakacki C.M, Gall K. Shape – Memory Polymers for Biomedical Applications. Advanced Polymer Science; 2010, 147–175.
115. Tamai H, Igaki K, Kyo E, Kosuga K, Kawashima A, Matsui S, Komori H, Tsuji T, Motohara S, Uehata H. Initial and 6-Month Results of Biodegradable Poly l-Lactic Acid Coronary Stents in Humans. Circulation; 2000, 102: 399–404.
116. Wache H.M, Tartakorwska D.J, Hentrich A, Wagner M.H. Development of a Polymer Stent with Shape Memory Effect as a Drug Delivery System. Journal of Materials Science: Materials in Medicine; 2003, 14: 109–112.
117. Yakacki C.M, Shandas R, Lanning C, Rech B, Eckstein A, Gall K. Unconstrained Recovery Characterization of Shape-Memory Polymer Networks for Cardiovascular Applications. Biomaterials; 2007, 28: 2255–2263.
118. Chen M, Tsai H, Chang Y, Lai W, Mi F, Liu C, Wong H, Sung H. Rapidly Self-Expandable Polymeric Stents with a Shape-Memory Property. Biomacromolecules; 2007, 8: 2274–2280.
119. Chen M, Liu C, Tsai H, Lai W, Chang Y, Sung H. Mechanical Properties, Drug Eluting Characteristics and in Vivo Performance of a Genipin-Crosslinked Chitosan Polymeric Stent. Biomaterials; 2009, 30: 5560–5571.

120. Baer G.M, Small IV W, Wilson T.S, Benett W.J, Matthews D.L, Hartman J, Maitland D.J. Fabrication and in Vitro Deployment of a Laser-Activated Shape Memory Polymer Vascular Stent. BioMedical Engineering OnLine; 2007, 6(43).

121. Venkatraman S.S, Tan L.P, Joso J.F.D, Boey Y.C.F, Wang X. Biodegradable Stents with Elastic Memory. Biomaterials; 2006, 27: 1573–1578.

122. American Heart Association, What Is an Aneurysm?; 2015.

123. National Heart, Lung and Blood Institute (NIS), What is an Aneurysm?; 2011.

124. Small IV W, Buckley P.R, Wilson T.S, Benett W.J, Hartman J, Saloner D, Maitland D.J. Shape Memory Polymer Stent with Expandable Foam: A New Concept for Endovascular Embolization of Fusiform Aneurysms. IEEE Transactions on Biomedical Engineering; 2007, 54(6).

125. Maitland D.J, Small IV W, Ortega J.M, Buckley P.R, Rodriguez J, Hartmana J, Wilson T.S. Prototype Laser-Activated Shape Memory Polymer Foam Device for Embolic Treatment of Aneurysms. Journal of Biomedical Optics; 2007, 12(3).

126. Hampikian J.M, Heaton B.C, Tong F.C, Zhang Z, Wong C.P. Mechanical and Radiographic Properties of a Shape Memory Polymer Composite for Intracranial Aneurysm Coils. Materials Science and Engineering C; 2006, 26: 1373–1379.

127. Rodriguez J.N, Yu Y, Miller M.W, Wilson T.S, Hartman J, Clubb F.J, Gentry B, Maitland D.J. Opacification of Shape Memory Polymer Foam Designed for Treatment of Intracranial Aneurysms. Annual Biomedical Engineering; 2012, 40(4): 883–897.

128. Singhal P, Wilson T.S, Maitland D.J. Controlling the Physical Properties of Random Network Based Shape Memory Polymer Foams. Materials Research Society Symposium Proceddings; 2010, 1274.

129. Metcalfe A, Desfaitsa A, Salazkina I, Yahiab L, Sokolowskic W.M, Raymonda J. Cold Hibernated Elastic Memory Foams for Endovascular Interventions. Biomaterials; 2003, 24: 491–497.

130. Beckman M.G, Hooper W.C, Critchley S.E, Ortel T.L. Venous Thromboembolism: A Public Health Concern. American Journal of Preventing Medicine; 2010, 38(4): 494–501.

131. Raskob G.E, Silverstein R, Bratzler D.W, Heit J.A, White R.H. Surveillance for Deep Vein Thrombosis and Pulmonary Embolism: Recommendations from a National Workshop. American Journal of Preventing Medicine; 2010, 38(4): 502–109.

132. Hartman J, Small IV W, Wilson T.S, Brock J, Buckley P.R, Benett W.J, Loge J.M, Maitland D.J. Embolectomy in a Rabbit Acute Arterial Occlusion Model Using a Novel Electromechanical Extraction Device. American Journal of Neuroradiol; 2007, 28: 872–874.

133. Muschenborn A.D, Hearon K, Volk B.L, Conway J.W, Maitland D.J. Feasibility of Crosslinked Acrylic Shape Memory Polymer for a Thrombectomy Device. Smart Materials Research; 2014.

134. Maitland D.J, Metzger M.F, Schumann D, Lee A, Wilson T.S. Photothermal Properties of Shape Memory Polymer Micro-Actuators for Treating Stroke. Lasers in Surgery and Medicine; 2002, 30: 1–11.

2

Chapter

UNDERSTANDING SMART DRUG DELIVERY SYSTEMS: AN IN-DEPTH EXAMINATION OF THERAPEUTIC TARGETING APPROACHES

1. INTRODUCTION: AN OVERVIEW

The Smart Drug distribution System (SDDS) is a sophisticated approach to Drug Targeted (DT) distribution. The cognitive enhancer administered by this system must meet the following criteria: 1) augment the dosages of the administered pharmacological agent to the specific tissue/cells/organs of interest, 2) resist degradation by bodily fluids, 3) mitigate adverse effects by enhancing the therapeutic efficacy, 4) ensure the absorption of the delivered drug traverses a biological membrane, and 5) facilitate the release of the drug in suitable dosages to the targeted area. The primary objective of a drug delivery system is to localize and preserve drug characteristics, ensure a designated delivery route, specifically target the intended site, minimize drug adverse effects, and extend drug contact with affected tissue. The targeted delivery system sustains the necessary drug concentration in plasma and tissues at specific areas, hence preventing harm to normal tissues or cells caused by the drug. The DT delivery system is intricate and necessitates the integration of multiple fields, including biology, chemistry, and engineering [1–3].

Nanoparticle-based drug delivery systems are designed based on the specific characteristics of target cells, transport carriers, the type of indicators related to drug binding to specific ligands, and receptors influenced by physical components. Ideally, DT delivery systems must be non-immunogenic, non-toxic, chemically and physically stable under both *in vitro* and *in vivo* conditions, exhibit targeted drug distribution to specific tissues, cells, or organs, ensure uniform capillary distribution, maintain a predictable and controllable drug release rate, and minimize drug leakage during transit [3–5]. Carriers employed for targeted medication delivery must be readily biodegradable or easily excreted from the body without causing any adverse effects. The development of the targeted delivery system should be uncomplicated, reproducible, and economically viable. The drawbacks of traditional medications render customized distribution an appealing focus for our work. Conventional pharmaceuticals exhibit diminished solubility of administered doses, inadequate absorption, reduced half-life, necessitate extensive distribution volumes, possess lower specificity, and have a narrower therapeutic index; these limitations are substantially addressed by tailored drug delivery systems [1–3].

This chapter encompasses: 1) the classifications of nanoparticles utilized for internal targeted drug delivery systems based on size, shape, and composition (metallic, biological, polymeric, and lipidic); 2) a detailed illustration of the mechanisms and strategies employed in targeted drug delivery systems; 3) an introduction to organ-specific targeted drug delivery mechanisms; 4) an explanation of therapeutic strategies for drug delivery and targeting actions; 5) an elucidation of the significance and desirable attributes of targeted delivery; 6) and ultimately, a validation of a concise overview of future challenges and trends in drug targeted delivery systems aimed at enhancing therapeutic efficiency and drug functionality in the treatment of cancer and genetic disorders.

2. STRATEGIES FOR TARGETED DRUG DELIVERY SYSTEMS

Targeted drug distribution enhances therapeutic efficacy by mitigating the adverse effects associated with the medication. The delivery of pharmaceuticals to malignant tissue is enhanced, while the normal tissue remains unaffected. Various methodologies of targeted drug delivery systems, including passive, active, dual, combination, inverse, double, and physical targeting, are being extensively employed in therapeutic applications.

2.1. Passive Targeting System

Passive targeting denotes the aggregation of a drug-carrier system or drug delivery to a specific location, which can be ascribed to the chemical, physical, pharmacological, and biological characteristics of the disease. The dimensions and surface characteristics of the drug-targeted nanoparticles must be meticulously regulated to avoid absorption by the reticuloendothelial system, hence enhancing targeting efficacy and prolonging circulation time. Accelerated vascularization facilitates the growth of tumor tissue, resulting in a compromised or permeable structure that increases the absorption of harmful chemotherapeutic agents. Few medications can be administered as inactive compounds or prodrugs, so allowing their conversion into highly active forms upon exposure to malignant tissue. Passive targeting additionally incorporates tailored medicine delivery to the tumor site via multiple invasive techniques.

2.1.1. Leaky Vasculature

Polymer nanoparticles demonstrate improved retention and permeability for targeted administration in tumor cells [6]. The capillary endothelium in tumor tissue is disordered and increases permeability to macromolecules compared to normal tissues.

This process facilitates extravasation of polymeric nanoparticles into the tumor interstitium for targeted medication administration. The tumor bed has insufficient lymphatic outflow, leading to medication buildup and improving targeted therapies. A chemotherapeutic agent is associated with a particular nanoparticle or nanocarrier via a linker that might enhance the concentration of therapeutic medications within malignant cells. These unique properties of polymer-drug conjugates alter drug concentration in malignant tissues at levels 10 to 100 times greater than that of free drugs.

2.1.2. Tumor Micro-environment

The medication is conjugated to a cancer-specific molecule and delivered in an active form. Upon reaching its ultimate target, the cancerous milieu transforms the prodrug into a reactive and dynamic agent, known as malignant cell-activated prodrug therapy. Malignant tissue is marked by vascular disarray and sporadic alterations in the basement membrane, which promote the spread of atypical cells to normal cells. The inadequate delivery of nutrients and the alteration of lymphatic networks fail to effectively eliminate cellular waste products. A tumor cell accumulates protons, resulting in a reduction of the physiological pH within the cells [7]. The constituents of the extracellular matrix, including macrophages, fibroblasts, and collagen fibers, are also heightened in malignant tissues. Matrix metalloproteinase-2 exacerbates the breakdown of tumor bed membranes and the extracellular matrix. A recent study by Mansour et al. [8] on a water-soluble maleimide derivative of doxorubicin, which includes a matrix metalloproteinase-2-specific peptide sequence, demonstrated that this drug conjugate-polymer complex exhibited a high affinity for cysteine-34 of the circulating bound form of albumin. Doxorubicin was effectively cleaved by matrix metalloproteinase-2 from the bound form of albumin. The redox potential and altered pH have been identified as triggers for medication release at the tumor site [9] for targeted therapy.

2.1.3. Direct (Local) Drug Application

Direct application of the drug to the cancer cells permits the drug to react directly with the malignant cells without systematic blood circulation. Various methodologies have been used to improve the anticancer drug for targeted delivery for tumors such as intraperitoneal, intravesical injection, and administration of various chemotherapeutic agents. These methodologies require introducing higher concentrations of anticancer agents that is not always possible. Localized targeted drug delivery by intratumoral direction is a modified and attractive methodology, which has been used and tested [10]. Localized administration of anticancer drug mitomycin surface of the malignant tissue leads to an increased concentration of the drug and decreased toxicity at the targeted tumor site [11]. Onyx-0115 is a type 2/5 chimeric adenovirus improved by attenuation of the E1B-55 kDa gene [12]. Its complex with some other proteins binds and inactivates the p53 gene. This drug has been administered by various methods, most of which permit the drug to be applied directly into the malignant cells. Onyx-0115 is used in clinical trials through intratumoral administration to treat head and neck cancer [13], intratumoral via endoscopic ultrasound for pancreatic cancer [14], via hepatic artery for metastatic colorectal cancer [15], intraperitoneal (IP) administration in ovarian cancer [16], and intratumoral under radiographic guidance for advanced sarcomas [17]. Recently, a polymer, poly (lactic-co-glycolic acid), linked with Tacrolimus (FK506) entrapped in pH-sensitive microspheres [18] was administered rectally or orally to colitis animals. The experimental animals showed the released nanoparticles and drug concentration into the tumor environment was different from its surrounding tissues. The drug permeability level in malignant tissues was 3-fold higher than normal tissue when nanoparticles were used as drug carriers. Direct targeted delivery of antitumor drugs into the malignant tissue inhibited the drug from circulating in the blood. The drawback of direct targeted delivery of drugs into the tumor is highly invasive and localization in some type of tumors is not feasible and can be problematic.

2.2. Active Targeting System

"Active targeting" means specific interactions between drug/drug carrier and the target cells, commonly through specific ligand-receptor interactions [19–23]. The ligand and receptor interactions are possible only when these components are in adjacent proximity (<0.5 nm). Specific ligand-receptor interaction for intracellular localization occurs after extravasations and blood circulation. Active targeting is favored as it controls a drug carrier/drug toward a target site (e.g., cruise missile). PEGylation increased the blood circulation time by altering the surface of the drug carrier with poly (ethylene glycol) and/or improving the enhanced permeability and retention (EPR) effect to augment the drug delivery to the targeted tumor site. Earlier reports show that targeting tumor ligands does not result in augmented accumulation of the nanoparticles in targeted tumor sites. The specific molecules in tumor cells or intracellular organelles enhance the active targeting pathways needs to active delivery of the drug into the entire tumor site [24–26]. Targeting a drug to a tumor site/specific area not only enhances the efficacy of therapeutic drugs, it also reduces the toxic effects associated with the drug and allows lower dosage of the drug for therapy. Active targeting is categorized into three approaches, these are: 1) targeting and restricting the circulation of nanoparticles to the capillary bed of a determined tumor targeted cell, site, tissue, or organ (cerebral ventricles, peritoneal cavity, compartmental targeting in lymphatics, plural cavity, joints, and eyes); 2) targeted delivery of the drug to a specific type of malignant cells/tissues and not to the normal healthy cells (specifically delivery of the nanoparticles to kupffer cells in the liver); and 3) targeting of nanoparticle delivery exactly to the intracellular site of targeted tumor cells (receptor-based ligand enters into a cell by endocytosis). The third approach is highly favored and used in guiding nanoparticles for targeted delivery through carbohydrates, receptors, and antigens.

2.2.1. Carbohydrate Targeted

The carbohydrate composition on the cell surface disrupts the communication between tumor cells and normal healthy cells, as well as with the extracellular matrix, facilitating metastatic growth and dissemination. The interaction between cells can be facilitated by tumor cell adhesion proteins and their carbohydrate counterparts known as lectins. Endogenous lectins are crucial in immune recognition of the "foreign patterns" present on the cell surface carbohydrates of cancer cells. It clearly illustrates that lectins disrupt the viability of malignant cells, endothelial adhesion/extracellular matrix interactions, and tumor tissue vascularization processes, which are crucial for metastatic growth and dissemination [27, 28]. This transmission of carbohydrate-ligand interaction can be enhanced by optimizing nanoparticles that encapsulate carbohydrate moieties aimed at targeting specific lectins (direct lectin targeting). As a result, targeted medication delivery methods have been developed utilizing the specific interaction between lectins and carbohydrates aimed at entire organs, which may pose risks to normal healthy cells. This constitutes a significant limitation of lectins that must be addressed for the advancement of "smart carrier" molecules in targeted medication delivery. Lectin exhibits a distinct affinity for the sugar moieties located on the surface of cancerous cells. Consequently, distinctive distinguishing traits appear to be an appealing mechanism for the enhanced delivery of targeted nano-drugs.

2.2.2. Receptor- and Antigen-directed Targeted

Human cancer cells have heightened expression of surface receptors or antigens, facilitating the effective uptake of nanoparticles via receptor-mediated endocytosis, hence allowing extracellular particles to penetrate the intracellular milieu. Drug-coated nanoparticles often infiltrate targeted tumor cells via ligand-receptor interactions. Upon reaching the specific region of the tumor cell surface, the targeted drug-coated nanoparticles may initiate cytosolic activity either following internalization or at the plasma membrane. The drug may detach from its carrier at the cell surface, in the extracellular space, or predominantly within lysosomes due to lysosomal enzymes, resulting in the release of the drug alone (without the carrier molecule) into the cytosol [30]. Upon the conclusion of drug delivery, the antigens or receptors must be reintroduced to the cell surface. This targeted drug delivery system incorporates key components, including a nano-carrier for drug conjugation and ligands-antibodies, thereby enhancing affinity for tumor cell surface antigens or receptors.

2.3. Dual Targeting System

The targeted drug delivery system is activated by stimuli, including temperature, pH, and redox conditions; certain malignancies exhibit two stimuli concurrently in the tumor-targeted environment. Modifications through a decrease in extracellular pH [31] and a minor increase in local temperature [32] would enhance the efficacy of drug delivery systems that utilize multiple external stimuli simultaneously. Nonetheless, the development of dual or multi-stimuli responsive nanocarriers for targeted tumor therapy continues to pose significant challenges. Currently, smart drug targeted delivery systems are attracting interest in thermo- and pH-sensitive triggered drug delivery mechanisms. Numerous hyper-branched polymers capable of integrating dual stimuli have been developed and may have viable applications in various cancers. Moreover, drug-targeted delivery methods that maintain sensitivity to dual stimuli have been developed. A prior investigation by Wu et al. [35] analyzed the release of 10-hydroxycamptothecin from dual stimuli-responsive nanoparticles. A hydrogel covered with vitamin B2, designed for intestine targeting and responsive to both thermal and pH stimuli, produced by Liu [36], shown significant thermo and pH sensitivity, making it appropriate for medication delivery to particular sites inside the gut. Additionally, thermo-sensitive hydrogels, pH-sensitive polymers, enzyme-degradable materials, redox dual-responsive micelles, and high-intensity focused ultrasound (HIFU) have been developed to facilitate sustained drug release in targeted delivery systems. Consequently, the detailed information regarding the dual sensitive system remains inadequately defined; yet, it offers a viable alternative for efficient targeted drug administration in biological applications.

2.4. Inverse Targeting System

Efforts to circumvent the passive absorption of colloidal carriers by reticuloendothelial systems are termed inverse targeting. The standard operation of reticuloendothelial systems is inhibited by the pre-injection of macromolecules like dextran sulfate or inert colloidal carriers. This focused methodology results in the saturation of reticuloendothelial systems and the impairment of the immune response, serving as an excellent strategy for administering targeted tumor therapeutics to organs beyond the reticuloendothelial system. Colloidal carrier systems, including vesicles, micellar solutions, liquid crystals, and nanoparticle dispersions composed of diminutive particles, exhibit significant potential for tailored drug delivery methods. The objective is to enhance the drug's coating and release characteristics, as well as its shelf life, while minimizing harmful effects. The combined drug with the colloidal system engaged in this microstructural manipulation may influence the molecular interactions of the drug, which possesses mesogenic and/or amphiphilic characteristics [39].

2.5. Stimuli-Responsive Drug Release Targeting System

Targeted tumor drug delivery systems must be biodegradable and harmless to healthy tissue while being deadly and highly effective against malignant cells. Rapid drug release from nanoparticles may result in premature discharge, causing systemic side effects; conversely, slow release may reduce the drug's potency at the target location and exacerbate multiple-drug resistance (MDR). Therefore, the release of the medicine for specific systems must be conducted in a systematic manner at the tumor location. The invention of stimuli-responsive drug carriers for targeted drug delivery is favored to enhance the efficacy and bioavailability of the medicine. Typical stimulus characteristics encompass temperature (thermal), pH, light intensity, magnetic field, redox potential (e.g., enzyme activity), glucose (ionic strength specific stimuli such as sugar concentration), and electrolyte concentrations, which are utilized to localize the drug-nanocarrier to the designated target site. The responses of nanocarriers encompass precipitation/dissolution, collapse/swelling, hydrophobic/hydrophilic transition, degradation, bond cleavage, and similar phenomena. Consequently, we assert that exterior stimuli-responsive systems (magnetic fields, light, and ultrasound) are less impactful, impractical, and economically unviable (i.e., costs, scalability) compared to internal stimuli-responsive systems (temperature, pH, redox potential, etc.).

3. ORGAN-BASED TARGETED DRUG DELIVERY

The concentration of the drug in a specific location or tissue pertains to targeted drug delivery, irrespective of the technique employed for site targeting and drug administration guidance. Successful drug target delivery encompasses several steps: the circulation of appropriately formulated drug-coated nanoparticles in the bloodstream at sufficient concentrations to reach the target site, retention of the nanoparticles at the site, release of the drug into the cells, and provision of adequate time for the drug's effective mechanism to operate. Targeted medicine distribution to certain locations inside the human body necessitates distinct delivery systems based on the chosen route.

4. NANOPARTICLES UTILIZED FOR TARGETED PHARMACEUTICAL DELIVERY

Nanoparticles, known as drug delivery vehicles or vectors, are the essential entities required for the effective delivery of the encapsulated medicine. A drug vehicle administers and preserves the therapeutic agent for transit to the specific spot or vicinity of the targeted tissue or region. These cars can perform certain roles due to minimal structural alterations. An optimal vehicle must be precisely and selectively identified by the target site while maintaining the functional specificity of the surface ligand without alteration. It must possess the ability to traverse barriers, be stable in interstitial fluid and plasma, and utilize non-toxic, non-immunogenic, and biodegradable components. Upon recognition of the carrier system by the target cells, the therapeutic drug moiety must be released at the designated spot. We additionally examine the characteristics and utilization of delivery trucks in Table 1. The targeting principles of metal, polymer, lipid, and biological nanoparticles utilized in treatments, along with prospective avenues in therapeutic research, are examined.

Table 1. Types of nanoparticles, properties and applications in medicine.

<table>
<tr><th colspan="3">Types and Description</th><th>Properties</th><th>Application</th><th>Examples</th></tr>
<tr><td colspan="3">Polymeric nanoparticles: Solid colloidal system with drug in various forms either encapsulated, adsorbed, etc. to form nanocapsules or nanospheres</td><td>Highly biocompatible and modifiable to make nanoparticle conjugates, e.g., polymeric magnetic nanoparticles, polymersomes, polyplexes, polymer hybrid system, modifiable surface properties High encapsulation of the drug and drug protection, prolonged drug delivery, and long shelf life</td><td>Wide range of targeted organs and cells, N-2(hydroxypropyl) methacrylamide (HPMA) polymer most widely used in theranoustics Polymeric micelles and water soluble polymers for improved drug delivery</td><td>Synthetic polymers such as PLGA, LPLA, PCL, and natural polymers such as Chitosan, Gelatin, Albumin, Sodium Alginate</td></tr>
<tr><td colspan="3">Dendrimers: Hyperbranched marcomolecules, densely packed to the periphery till they reach a “starburst effect”</td><td>Reduce viscosity of a solution, densely packed improved rheological properties, outermost dendrimeric surface can be both polar or hydrophobic capable or dissolving in different solvents</td><td>Used as contrast agents for MRI Vectors in gene therapy, soluble dendrimers able to solubilize acidic hydrophobic molecules and of fungus and bacteria</td><td>PAMAM dendrimer, PPI dendrimer, Techto dendrimer, Micellar dendrimer</td></tr>
<tr><td>Inorganic nanoparticles</td><td>Metallic</td><td>Gold nanoparticles (GNPs): Three shapes of GNPs are rods, shells, and spheres</td><td>These have a unique interaction with light, free electrons undergo oscillations in the presence of oscillating electromagnetic field of light</td><td>Biosensors, especially colorimetric biosensors, for detection of oligonucleotides immunosensors and redox enzyme biosensing</td><td>GNPs are conjugated with Silica, PEG, Chitosan, platinum tethered, gold-SPION hybrid</td></tr>
</table>

Types and Description			Properties	Application	Examples
		Carbon-based nanotubes: Well-ordered hollow graphitic nanomaterial either single- or multi-walled	Possibility of both covalent and non-covalent bonding Site specific delivery of proteins, peptides, nucleic acids, and other drugs	Used as an imaging agent Applications in malignancies of the brain, blood, colon, breast, liver, lymph nodes, cervical, and prostrate cancer	Multi-walled carbon nanotube (MWCNT) Single-walled carbon nanotube (SWCNT)
		Quantum Dots (QD): Uses the bandgap between valency and conduction electron bands, exciton is generated due to the difference in absorption energy and the spectral bandgap of the core semi- conductor	Exceptional physical features applied in optical imaging, strong absorbance, bright fluorescence	Unique optical features for in vitro and in vivo imaging especially biomedical fluorescent imaging, specifically used in the study of neuron and ganglia, used in photodynamic therapy especially to treat lung and gastrointestinal cancer, accurate recognition of molecular targets	Multi-spectral fluorescent Imaging – Quantum Dots (MSFI-QDs), Carbon dots, carbongenic-QDs, Silica-QD's, Zinc oxide-QDs,
	Metalloid	Silica based nanoparticles: Silica particles are good materials for nanoparticles because of its porosity and surface adaptability	Modifiable in size, porosity and structure Photophysical stability: does not absorb visible or uv light, biocompatibility, favorable colloidal properties, high porosity and extended surface area, relatively chemically inert, low cost of production, easily prepared and water dispersible	Application in combined therapy as they can transfer both genetic material and molecules of various sizes. Used as an optical contrast agent, can conjugate with antibodies, aptamers and polymers	Solid silica-based nanoparticles (SiNPs), Mesoporous silica nanoparticles (MSNs)

Types and Description			Properties	Application	Examples
	Magnetic	Iron oxide magnetic cores with changing shells are used	Some forms of iron oxide naturally occur in the body (maghemite, magnetite), thus reducing toxicity, various bindings, and interactions between the MNP and the drug are possible such as covalent, electrostatic, encapsulation, and adsorption	Used both in diagnosis and therapy concomitantly, Liver and spleen readily imbibe the MNP and can also be used in barin malignancies and it is able to cross the blood brain barrier	Iron oxide cores with shells of gold, polymer, dendrimers, and silane
Biological	Lipids	Homolipids, Heterolipids, complex- lipids	Increase in drug solubility, pharmokokinetics properties, reduced toxic effects	Applications in oral drug delivery, parenteral dug delivery, peptide and protein drug delivery, nasal vaccination, etc.	Solid lipid nanoparticles (SLN), Nanostructured lipid carriers (NLC), Lipid drug conjugates (LDC), Liposome, transferosomes, niosomes

4.1. Lipids-based Nanoparticles

Liposomes are diminutive, chemically engineered vesicles completely encased by phospholipid bilayer membranes, varying in size from 20 to 10,000 nm. Pharmaceutical compounds are encapsulated or intercalated within phospholipid bilayers, hence influencing the drug's localization through the physicochemical properties of lipids. A recent study reveals that lipid DOX-loaded nanoparticles possess potential as an effective targeted therapy for adriamycin-resistant breast cancer. Encapsulated therapeutic molecules within modified liposomes (utilizing transferrin [41] or antibodies [42, 43]) induce apoptosis in tumor cells [41–43]. Solid lipid nanocarriers are frequently employed for the treatment of chemotherapy-resistant tumors to deliver targeted medication.Self-assembled, hydrophobic interactions of amphiphilic block copolymers (5–50 nm) form supramolecular core-shell structures in aqueous solutions called micelles are gaining great attention in targeted drug delivery applications. Pluronic, phospholipid, polyester, and poly (L-amino acid) are the most often used micelles. Drug entrapped with block copolymer micelles and transported at high concentrations can exceed their intrinsic water-solubility. Furthermore, hydrophilic blocks form hydrogen bonds within the aqueous solution and form a compact shell that covers the micellar core protecting it against hydrolysis and enzymatic degradation with the help of hydrophobic core. Moreover, the reticuloendothelial system may prevent the recognition of the corona and eliminate the polymeric micelles from the blood circulation. The molecular weight, chemical composition, and block length ratios can be easily changed that control the size and morphology of the micelles. The cross linkable group with block copolymer can enhance the stability of the micelles and increase their temporal control. Polymeric micelles can be linked with various ligands, such as epidermal growth factors, antibody fragments, α-2-glycoprotein, folic acid, and transferrin, delivering the targeted anticancer drug to the tumor tissues/cells by passive and active mechanisms. Most of the anticancer drugs are poorly water soluble in nature, polymeric micelles deliver these anticancer drugs to the targeted tumor sites that selectively act only on targeted cells and do not affect the normal healthy cells. However, most of the polymeric micelles have been successfully established in targeted therapeutics and some are still at preclinical trials. Future studies need to pave the way for these therapies into clinical practice to increase the survival rate of cancer patients and enhance anticipation of cancer chemotherapy [45].

Niosomes are defined as nonionic surfactant vesicles that entrap both lipophilic and hydrophilic drugs in the vesicular membrane/aqueous phase. These are made up of lipid material possessing better stability than liposomes. Niosomes may be established as useful carriers for targeting the drugs to treat tumor, viral, parasitic, and other microbial diseases more effectively. Pharmacosomes are self-assembling components consisting of a pharmocon (active component) and a carrier molecule composed of amphipathic drugs. Drugs covalently linked to lipid molecules may be in colloidal dispersion as micelles or as ultrafine hexagonal aggregates used in targeted therapy. Ufasomes are single-chain fatty acid surfactant vesicles formed from double-chain amphiphiles and micelles. They are composed of lipid bilayer liposomes made of single-chain unsaturated fatty acids used in targeted drug delivery. Ufasome vesicles are colloidal suspensions of closed lipid bilayers consisting of ionized species (soap) and fatty acid molecules composed of more amphiphiles than micelles. These readily available fatty acids give ufasomes an advantage over liposomes. Cubosomes refer to liquid crystalline liposomes formed into cubic nanoparticles that are suitable for injection at the targeted site. Lipid droplets that allow easy penetration through the pores are called transferosomes, which are smaller than a droplet. Transferosomes is a supramolecular entity that can pass via permeability barriers and transport drug from one side to the other and is more elastic than a liposome.

4.2. Biological-based Nanoparticles

In addition to micelles, some groups of nanoparticles forming self-assembling structure are known as cell-penetrating peptides (CPPs). These molecules are applied in recognizing hydrophobic drugs and delivering biomolecules such as nucleic acids (siRNA, pDNA) intracellularly to the targeted cells. Furthermore, CPP drug delivery system is more constructive owing to its low toxicity, biocompatibility, structural stability, and easy preparation [46–49]. Addition to hydrophobic interaction, CPPs improve the nucleic acid delivery system. Both hydrophobic interactions and the electrostatic nature of CPPs contribute to its stable structure that can easily enter into the cells and deliver the siRNA.

Proteins are also important and promising agents for drug delivery that bioconjugate with drugs and deliver to the targeted sites (albumin-conjugated with paclitaxel named as abraxane). Albumin and paclitaxel linkage (abraxane) are prepared by homogenization under high pressure [50]. However abraxane is a more effective and less cytotoxic drug compared to conventional drugs. The drug is released from abraxane through the albumin receptor in blood vessels of the tumor cells [50, 51]. Bioconjugation of albumin-paclitaxel combination has been effectively used against lung cancer [50], breast cancer, [51] and gastric cancer [52].

4.3. Polymeric-based Nanoparticles

Polymers have good biocompatibility, are easily prepared, and morphologically manipulated into a variety of designs and structures. They possess bio-mimetic properties making it a widely used biomaterial. Polymers play an important role in smart drug delivery systems as they can effectively deliver chemotherapeutic drugs directly into the targeted site. The surface of polymeric nanoparticles has been functionalized by the alteration of nanoparticles through emulsification, adsorption, polymerization, functional surfactants, modulation of various forms of bio-conjugation, and covalently-bound functional molecules. Polymers are widely used in numerous therapeutic applications for targeting cancer, disorders of the central nervous system (CNS), and other bacterial and viral infections. Zhang et al. [53] reported that more than 26 nanoparticles based on their therapeutic action have been approved for clinical trials and a few more are in the pipeline. Polymeric nanoparticles possess characteristic properties that affect its bio-distribution, efficiently enhancing the delivery of targeted drug across the blood brain barrier compared to conventional drug treatments as well as other well-known drug carriers [54].

Microspheres are biocompatible polymers either particle or soluble in nature. Polymeric backbone carriers are *N*-(2-Hydroxypropyl) methacrylamide (HPMA) prepared by ficoll, dextrans, sepharose, or poly-L-lysine as core carrier system for chemotherapeutic drugs. Microspheres (30–200 μm) are larger than nanoparticles (0.2–0.5 μm) but have a smaller area for drug loading than soluble polymers. The drug incorporation of microsphere considerably affects its release rate. Once the drug is administered or systematically transported, it rapidly dispenses into the target site and is subsequently internalized by macrophages of the phagocytic system. Moreover, microspheres and nanoparticles are mostly used for cell-selective applications of drug delivery (oral delivery peptides and peptidomimetics) [55–58].

Dendrimers play a significant role in the delivery of different compounds such as tamsulosin, primaquine phosphate, 5-fluorouracil, doxorubicin, tropicamide, indomethacin, artemether, and pilocarpine as targeted drugs [59]. Bioconjugated dendrimers can deliver the targeted drug transdermally, intravenously, orally, and through the ophthalmic route, which proves the versatility and functionality of dendrimers [60].

4.4. Carbon-based Nanoparticles

The properties [61], application [62–68], and solubility nature [69] of carbon nanotubes are well-established nanocarriers for drug delivery. Jain et al. [70] reported that chemical modification of carbon nanotubes by carbohydrate D-galactose can generate a novel cascade of chemical functionalization of multi-walled carbon nanotubes (MWCNTs). Therefore, galactosylated MWCNTs are used to deliver the active ligands (such as galactose) as a bioactive(s) targeted drug to the tumor site (hepatic tissues) [70].

Carbon nanohorns related to carbon nanotubes belong to a new class of carbon materials. Single-walled carbon nanohorn (SWNH) aggregates consist of thousands of graphitic tubules (2–5 nm in diameter, similar structure to single-walled CNTs) having a spherical structure (50–100 nm in diameter). Based on the morphological features, nanohorns are divided into bud, dahlia, and seed types. SWNHs are non-metallic catalysts produced by laser ablation of a pure graphite target; however, its toxicity must be proactively investigated. Molecules completely composed of carbon are fullerene, spherical fullerenes are known as buckyballs. Fullerenes are similar to graphite structure consisting of stacked graphene sheets of connected hexagonal rings and pentagonal rings. Fullerene C60 is highly biocompatible with reduced toxicity and is used for targeted drug delivery for several diseases such as Parkinson's and HIV.

Nanoshells have a dielectric core covered with a thin metallic shell of gold-coated silica that is spherical in shape. These are used for early stages of cancer detection and treatment. Injected embedded drugs consist of cancer-targeted hydrogel polymers that are released at the tumor targeted site when exposed to laser (infrared).

4.5. Metal-based Nanoparticles

Metal-based nanoparticles are fascinating because the metal exhibits an important electronic and optical property and acts as an insulator or semiconductor [71–73]. Transition (Al, Co, Cu, Fe, Ni, Ti) and noble (Au and Ag) metal nanoparticles reveal a luminescence emission in the visible wavelength of light. Recent studies show metal linked with carbon nanotubets (Ag/CNT composites) are gaining increased attention due to their potential applications as optical limiters [74], catalyst [75], and advanced materials [76] capable of being used in bio-imaging of the cancer cells for targeted therapy [74].

Targeted drug delivery with gold nanoparticles possess a unique chemical and physical characteristic feature as they have strong binding interaction with proteins, thiols [77], aptamers [78], carboxylic acid [79], and disulfides linkages. These are widely used in tumor targeted delivery system for therapeutics. Gold particles can enter into targeted sites by phagocytosis, fluidphase endocytosis, and receptor-mediated endocytosis [80], depending upon the shape, size, surface charge, synthesis process, functionalized molecules, and surface coating toxicity of gold. Moreover, gold nanoparticles are considered to be non-toxic agents for drug delivery [81]. Gold nanoparticles possess a functional flexibility with prodrug molecules by covalent or non-covalent linkage enhancing the efficient transport of the drug into the targeted tumor sites. Gold nanoparticles can hold high drug concentration and deliver it to the specific targeted site via various routes of drug administration. Conventional drug side effects can be reduced by conjugated gold nanoparticles reducing the tumor survival rate.

5. THERAPEUTIC STRATEGIES FOR DRUG DELIVERY

5.1. Folate Targeting

Folate receptors (FRs) are overexpressed in various tumors (including leukemia, endometrial, ovarian, and kidney cancer), which binds vitamin folate and folate-drug conjugates with a high affinity [82]. Folate receptors are targets of various therapeutic strategies aimed at efficient delivery of chemotherapeutic drugs. Folate receptors also play a role in the uptake of antifolate drugs that are used for therapeutic intervention in malignant disorders. The salient features of folic acid for therapeutic strategies are: i) reasonable binding affinity to both diagnostic and targeted therapeutic agents; ii) its unique and high affinity for the folate receptor, even after binding to diagnostic and therapeutic cargo; and iii) the folate receptor in normal healthy tissues have limited scattering, despite its overexpression on both type of tumors cells (FR-α and FR-β isoforms) [83]. Earlier investigations [84] show that folate enter the cells through receptor-mediated endocytic process. Hence, folic acid is repeatedly used as a drug targeting ligand coated with delivery vehicles (polymeric nanoparticles, liposomes, dendrimers, and protein toxins) to selectively deliver targeted drugs into malignant cells.

We were the first to report that curcumin enhances the up-regulation of folate receptor β mRNA and protein levels in KG-1 cells by modulating the uptake and cytotoxicity of methotrexate. Notably, curcumin also augmented folate receptor β function as a transporter for radiolabeled folic acid and methotrexate in KG-1 cells. These reports optimized curcumin dosage and reduced the concentration of methotrexate resulting in the effective destruction of tumor cells. Therefore, amalgamation of non-toxic concentrations of methotrexate and curcumin may be a viable strategy for therapeutic intervention for leukemia using a folate receptor-targeted drug delivery system [85]. Shen et al. [86] reported that folate receptor-targeted drug conjugate had less communication with the cells and easily entered through overexpressed folate receptor of malignant cells by receptor-mediated endocytosis. Later the drug was transferred into lysosomes, wherein the active form of drug poly (amido amine)] dendrimers (PAMAM) was regenerated. The PAMAM left the lysosome and released anticancer drug camptothecin (CPT) in the nucleus. This modulation creates PAMAM dendrimers as valuable drug carriers for *in vivo* tumor cell nuclear drug targeted delivery. Folate receptor-targeted (nanoparticles) delivery systems, despite showing significant promising effects in human pathologies, enhance the tumor selectivity for tumor targeting. This modulatory strategy avoids possible obstacles, and we anticipate that folic acid will act as an essential candidate for receptor-targeted therapeutics in the near future.

5.2. Antibodies Targeting

Specific antigens are exclusively expressed on the surface of the cancer cells. Antibodies, especially monoclonal antibodies (mAb), can be produced to identify and specially bind to the antigens associated with tumor cells. In 1981, Milstein [87] developed an mAb that binds to malignant cells, a few functional classes of antibodies that possessed more binding and destroying activity in the tumor cells. Currently, numerous mAb-based tumor tissues targeting therapeutics has been effectively translated into clinical treatment such as trastuzumab, rituximab, cetuximab, and bevacizumab [88-91]. These mAb could be used as fragments or in their native state, generally having higher affinity toward tumor-associated antigens depicting its targeting efficacy. Moreover, the whole mAb are more beneficial than fragments to develop a higher binding affinity, owing to a synergic effect of having more than one binding site. Furthermore, the full or entire antibody sequences express more EPR effects that are maintained in cancer tissues, while in small fragments express less EPR effects that can easily be eliminated from blood circulation [92].

Recent investigations have attention on multi-functionalization of the nanoparticle surface with specific mAbs and encapsulation of therapeutic drugs into nanoparticles to sustain its targeting efficacy. Recent studies by Nobs et al. [93] shows poly-(lactic acid) (PLA) nanoparticles conjugated rituximab and trastuzumab exhibit six-fold enhances affinity and uptake compared with similar particles without mAb targeting molecules. The investigation of Miyano et al. [94] shows conjugated KG6Etrastuzumab (KG6E-amino acid dendrimer with surface modified by sixth-generation lysine dendrimer with glutamate –KG6Etrastuzumab) was expressively internalized and then transferred to lysosome for human epidermal growth factor receptor -2 (HER-2) positive cells (SKBR3), compared to HER2 – negative cells (MCF-7) indicates that KG6E-trastuzumab conjugates act as HER-2 targeting carriers in drug targeted delivery for cancer therapy. However, nanoparticles conjugated with mAbs still encounter numerous tasks and boundaries, owing to a "binding-site barrier" (decreased rate of penetration of nanocarriers due to high binding affinity) in solid tumors [95].

5.3. Glycoprotein Targeting

Serum glycoprotein transferrin (Tf) acts as a transporter to deliver the iron molecule into the cells via blood by binding to the transferrin receptor successfully that is being internalized through receptor-mediated endocytosis [96]. TfR is overexpressed on most of the tumor cells such as colon, pancreatic, lung, and bladder cancer cells due to increased metabolic rates. The TfR expression is 100 times greater in cancerous cells than normal healthy cells, this increase in expression is a result of a higher demand for iron in tumor cells, essential for their survival [97]. Tf has been often used as a drug targeting ligand in TfR-targeted drug delivery system for tumor cells. Direct conjugations of nanocarriers to Tf have enhanced intracellular drug delivery and efficient therapeutic outcome. Ishida et al. [98] demonstrated Tf conjugated with polyethyleneglycol (PEG)-liposomes exposed over prolonged periods in blood circulation but had reduced uptake via reticuloendothelial system (RES) in colon cancer. This proposes that Tf-conjugated nanoparticles were internalized by receptor-mediated endocytosis owing to specific ligand-receptor binding for cytoplasmic targeting to cancer cells. Tf-conjugated paclitaxel coated with poly (lactic-*co*-glycolic acid) (PLGA) nanoparticles showed enhanced suppression in cell growth than free paclitaxel in MCF-7 and MCF-7/Adr cells [99]. Doxorubicin (Dox)-coated, HAIYPRH (T7)-conjugated, PEG-modified polyamidoamine dendrimer (PAMAM-PEG-T7/Dox) nanoparticles was fabricated by Jiang et al. [100]. This modified targeted drug effectively accumulates in malignant cells via intravenous administration and can be internalized into cancer cells with Tf. These studies proved that Tf acts as a ligand for targeted drug delivery system in TfR overexpressed malignancies. However, TfR is also expressed in normal fast growing healthy cells (epithelial, fibroblast, and endothelial cells) that could lead to non-specific targeting and increase the cytotoxic effects reducing the efficacy of the targeted drug [101]. Furthermore, Tf with nanoparticles targeting ligands may improve drug delivery in tumor tissues and distribution in blood circulation similar to normal healthy cells expressing TfR (non-targeted systems) [102].

5.4. Oligonucleotide Targeting

Short, single-stranded RNA or DNA oligonucleotides designed *in vitro* from a huge number of random sequences around 1014–1015 that can identify the specific target sites are known as aptamers [103]. Aptamers possess high affinity and specificity features enhanced to bind a wide range of intracellular molecules, such as receptors, small molecule drugs, and proteins [104] specified for aptamer-based targeted cancer therapy. Although, aptamers and mAbs have similar and specific affinity against selected molecules, aptamers possess their own unique features: they can be synthesized in vitro without laboratory animals [105] and nanoparticle-conjugated aptamers very efficiently target the tumor tissue via active targeting pathway. Lupold et al. [106] established nanoparticle-conjugated aptamer (A10 aptamer) that target overexpressed transmembrane protein of prostate specific membrane antigen (PSMA) in various tumor tissues. Aptamers-doxorubicin (Apt-Dox) are conjugates that are also implemented (designed) for targeted delivery to malignant cells [107]. Furthermore, Huang et al. [107] demonstrated that Dox conjugated to DNA apatamer-sgc8c (sgc8c-Dox conjugate) retains its high binding affinity features increasing efficiency of internalization by tumor targeted cells. These characteristic features make targeted delivery of chemotherapeutic drugs more feasible with abundant targeting potencies. Furthermore, these therapeutic strategies give rise to a novel targeted drug delivery and provide promising approaches for future treatment.

5.5. Membrane Protein Targeting/Cell Surface Receptors Targeting

Integrin membrane glycoproteins are heterodimeric in nature composed of non-covalent bonding of α and β subunits; they play a major role in tumor malignancy and angiogenesis [107]. In tumor endothelium $\alpha_v\beta_3$ and $\alpha_v\beta_5$, integrins are overexpressed at the highest levels. Asparagine/glycine/arginine (NGR) and arginine/glycine/aspartic acid (RGD) are the largest number of tumor-homing peptides used to detect the corresponding receptors of integrins $\alpha_v\beta_3$ on tumor endothelial cells. Brooks et al. [109] reported that RGD vascular homing peptides enhanced intracellular targeted drug delivery accomplished via integrin-binding RGD and suppress the tumor growth. Recent studies described Dox-coated nanoparticles with cyclic RGD peptide ligand delivered the drug to targeted integrin $\alpha_v\beta_3$ and caused a decrease in survival rate of the tumor cells [110]. Moreover, investigations on paclitaxel entrapped liposomes with peptide consisting of specific ligand to alpha $_v$ integrins and specific motif to neuropilin-1 showed significant increase in paclitaxel uptake in targeted tumor cells (A549 and HUVEC) depicting the enhanced suppression of cell growth by dual targeted mechanism compared with single-targeted paclitaxel entrapped liposomes and paclitaxel injections (Taxol) alone [111]. Furthermore, investigations show that cyclic RGD peptide (cRGDyK) conjugated in PEG-b-PLGA micelles deliver the targeted hydrophobic drug into intracellular cancer cells and its neovasculature, enhancing the antiproliferative and cytotoxicity efficacy compared with cRGDyK-free non-targeted micelles [112]. However, targeted delivery to integrin glycoprotein meets many challenging tasks for therapeutic strategies. The most common are integrins receptors, which are extracellular and expressed in normal fast growing healthy epithelial cells other than tumor cells. Treatment with RGD also targets the normal functional integrin ($\alpha_5\beta_1$ and $\alpha_4\beta_1$) molecules, thus resulting in targets of nonspecific tumor cells [113].

6. SIGNIFICANT ROLE AND FUNCTIONAL PROPERTIES OF TARGETED DRUG DELIVERY

The application of nanoparticles in nanomedicine is for tailored medication delivery systems [114]. Over the past twenty years, researchers have elucidated the mechanisms of drug distribution and engineered pharmaceuticals for targeted administration. The majority of newly developed and already accessible therapeutic medicines (95%) exhibit suboptimal biopharmaceutical and pharmacokinetic properties [40]. The therapeutic index of biologically focused medications must be enhanced with appropriate nanotechnological applications for targeted distribution to malignant cells and tissues. Nanotechnological methods [114] facilitate the reevaluation of unsuccessful clinical trials of chemotherapeutic agents.

The targeted medication must be both safe and efficacious, ensuring adequate drug concentration in the body to provide an effective dosage at the designated tumor location. Chemotherapeutic targeted agents must exhibit significant toxicity and potent suppression of the proliferation of the targeted tumor tissue or cells. Numerous researchers have shown that biological poisons, protein macromolecules, and both hydrophobic and hydrophilic medicines are transported by nanocarriers. Nanostructured designs are potential elements that facilitate innovative chemotherapeutic agents for targeted delivery and elucidate the principles of component-specific drug delivery systems (Figure 1). Nanomedicine has consistently developed medication delivery systems that penetrate cells through intracellular pathways, thereby minimizing side effects. Nanoparticles possess a superior advantage over microparticles. They are suitable for intravenous targeted delivery, extensively utilized for precise drug release at specific sites, have extended blood circulation time to enhance drug extravasation, and yield positive results in targeted drug delivery for cancer treatment, central nervous system disorders, and immunodeficiency infections [115]. Additionally, 300 pharmaceutical businesses in the United States mostly concentrate on targeted medication delivery systems. Furthermore, medications can be administered via oral, pulmonary, ophthalmic, transmucosal, and implantation methods.

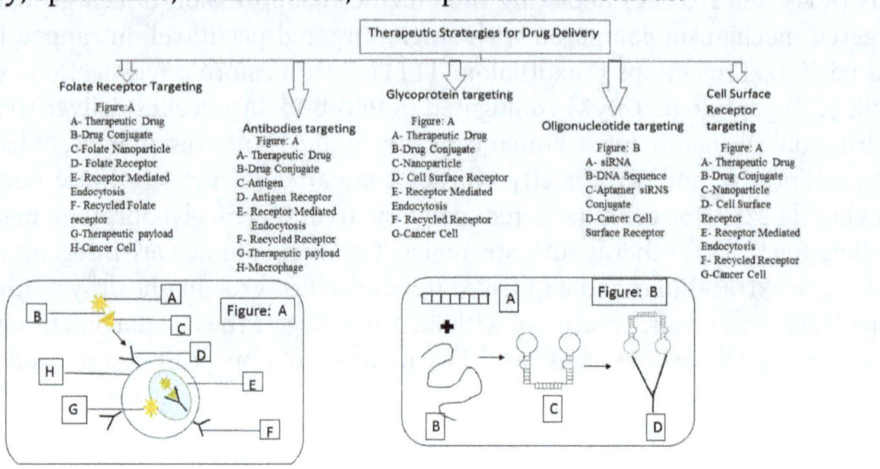

Figure 1. Schematic representation of components of targeted drug delivery

Nanomaterials are used in targeted drug delivery including metal-, biological-, lipid-, silicon-, carbon-, and polymer-based materials [114]. These technology-based medicines (nanomedicine platforms) can be multifunctional, also known as intelligent/smart drug system. We raise awareness of the physiological and functional challenges of therapeutic application and enlighten recent advances in our understanding and mechanism of tumor biology [116]. Nanoscale drug targeted delivery system is capable of enhancing pharmacokinetics and increasing the bio-distribution of therapeutic agents to targeted organs/tissues/cells with improved efficacy of the drug. The volume of drug distribution and toxicity is reduced, owing to drug accumulation at specific targeted sites and reduced concentration in normal healthy cells while using nanoscale carriers. It is designed to target cancer and inflammation sites through permeable vasculature. It is also biocompatible and made of biodegradable materials reported as safe replacement drug carriers than existing vehicles that may cause allergic reaction and peripheral neuropathy [40]. Few drugs have a very short half-life in blood circulation. The efficacy and stability of the drug can be increased by enclosing a drug with a nanocarrier to extend its short-half life. For example, a drug can be enclosed with a nanosized carrier (liposome).

Most of the drugs face difficulties in targeting tumor sites while crossing the blood brain barrier (BBB). Nanoparticle-coated drugs potentially penetrate BBB and are shown to potentially enhance the therapeutic concentration and index of anticancer drugs that have been delivered to the brain tumor. Its most noteworthy advantage is reduced toxicity and enhanced efficacy of the drug by guiding the drug to its target and retaining the drug concentration at the targeted site for a longer duration to increase its therapeutic action. [114]. Figure 2 explains the desirable therapeutic strategies of smart drug targeted delivery systems. Solid tumors possess vascular pores (vascular pore cut-off 380–780 nm) depending on various sizes, type of cancer, microenvironments, and proliferation rate. Thus, drug with the carrier molecules should be smaller than vascular pore cut-off size (diameter) to reach its targeted tumor sites. Normal healthy blood vessels do not permit drug-associated carrier molecules larger than 2–4nm size compared with unassociated drug molecules. Thus, nanomedicine has paved the way to enhance drug accumulation and its concentration in targeted cells/tissues/sites by extravasation and considerably diminishing its toxicity and distribution to normal healthy cells [40]. Ideal nanocarrier materials should be without any chemical modification and must fulfill the demands of biocompatibility, biodegradability, and release dynamics of targeted drugs [117, 118].

Nanocarriers essentially need to prolong exposure time in blood circulation and allow the nanocarriers to reach the targeted site through multiple pathways. Generally, nanoparticles possess a very short half-life, owing to natural immune/defense mechanisms of the human system that eradicate them after opsonisation by phagocytic mechanisms. Thus, the nanocarrier surface must be altered to be invisible to the opsonisation process.

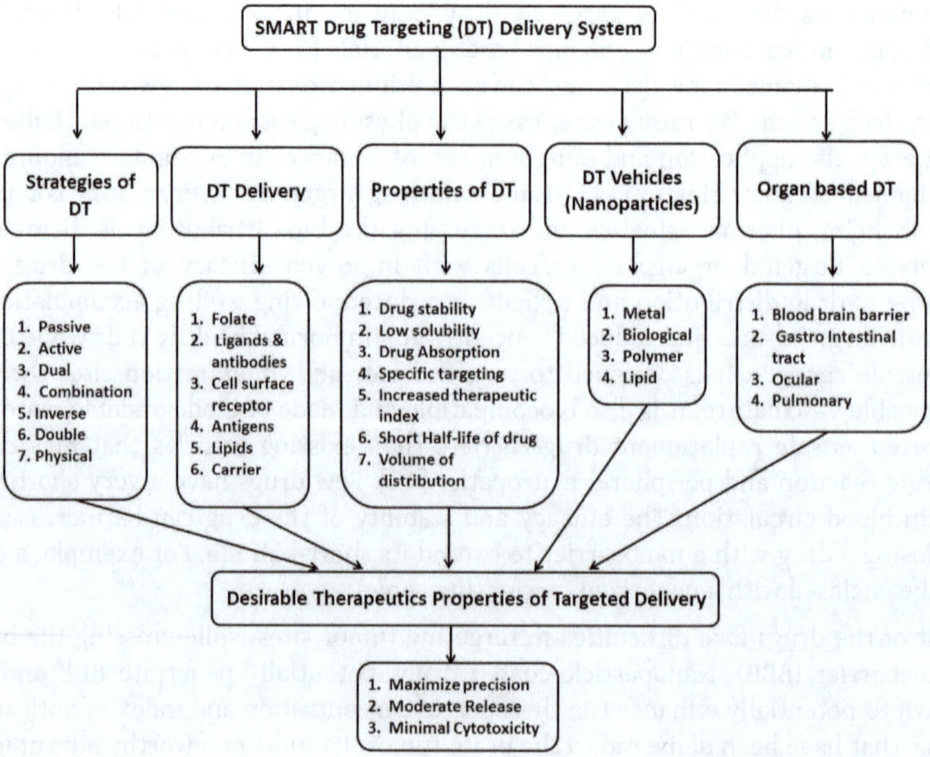

Figure 2. Schematic representation of SMART drug targeted strategies

Nanocarriers are naturally made up of macromolecular materials or entrapped lipids, adsorbed onto the surface of the nanoparticles or dissolved within the polymeric matrix. They are categorized into two types: nanospheres (matrix systems used to dispersing drug molecules) and nanocapsules (vesicular systems drugs that are surrounded by a membrane). Nanotechnology-based polymers are designed as top-down and bottom-up processes. The top-down method is initiated by breaking down larger objects into nanostructured molecules by over grinding, etching, or ball milling enhanced by laser or the addition of chemicals. However, this technique is time-consuming and repeatedly produces considerably wider particle size of distribution. This production method relies on systematic atom-by-atom or molecule-by-molecule arrangements, facilitating organized chemical reactions in either liquid or gas phases, hence ensuring the nucleation and development of nanoparticles. The bottom-up mechanism produces densely clustered aggregates of particles that remain intact during reconstitution [119]. Particles synthesized using sophisticated coacervation, salting-out, solvent emulsification diffusion, high-pressure homogenization, nanoprecipitation, supercritical fluid techniques, co-precipitation, fast expansion of supercritical solutions, supercritical antisolvent precipitation, and self-assembly processes [119]. The carriers utilized are polymeric nanoparticles, magnetic nanoparticles, metal and inorganic nanoparticles, quantum dots, polymeric micelles (PMs), solid lipid nanoparticles, and colloidal nanoliposomes.

7. TARGETED PHARMACOLOGICAL DELIVERY IN ONCOLOGICAL TREATMENT

A clear understanding of molecular mechanism of tumor proliferation, formation metastasis, invasion, and angiogenesis ensures a new mechanistic basis for targeted tumor drug discovery (targeted anticancer therapy). Exact blocking or altering of the molecular mechanism associated in the pathogenesis of tumor cell proliferation by targeted chemotherapeutic agents modify the natural process of the disease as well as improve therapeutic index with cytotoxic agents. Anticancer drug for targeted delivery system must meet a few requirements: a) the targeted drug must have minimal activity loss, b) it should destroy the targeted tumor cells, c) must be well-regulated and predicate the active form of drug release [120], and d) leakage of drug during transit must be minimal. Concurrently, therapeutic drugs with less dosage should be used during targeted therapy (minimal dose than the normal chemotherapy) with minimal side effects [120, 121]. Drugs are conjugated with nanocarriers and delivered to the receptor (outside) or inside the targeted tumor cells by a selective targeting mechanism [121]. The previous traditional process of administration of chemotherapy is an aggregation of drugs inside the tumor cells/tissues through EPR [122, 123, 117] as a result of the abnormal structure of blood vessels closer to the tumor tissues. Thus, the drug discharges easily to the tissues near the cancer cells [40, 123]. Furthermore, few drugs are used in conventional treatment such as methotrexate [124], paclitaxel [125], doxorubicin [126], gemcitabine [127] hexamethylmelamine [128], and cisplatin (DDP) or carboplatin (drugs based on platinum) [129]. The drug may be delivered to: a) the capillary bed of the active site, b) specific type of cells, c) intracellular region of tumour cells absent in normal healthy cells, and d) specific organ/tissues by complexion with the nanocarrier that recognizes the target. Conventional anticancer targeted therapy is composed of ligands (receptor, antibodies, and chemotherapeutic drugs) conjugated with nanocarriers, thus, the fabricated drug enables binding affinity with particular receptors of the targeted cancer cells. Overexpression of receptors in cancer cells enhances the binding affinity of the nanocarrier conjugated ligands to the receptor [121, 123, 117]. The targeted delivery system discharges the chemotherapeutic drugs directly to tumor cells and maintains prolonged circulation of the drugs with high concentration inside the tumor cells. However, targeted drugs cannot be released back to the blood stream because of the ligand and receptor binding affinity, the same principle that is used in immunogenicity [122].

8. OBSTACLES AND PROSPECTIVE PATHWAYS

The tailored delivery method for smart drugs is nearing optimal therapeutic options for cancer and other chronic diseases. Targeted drug delivery is a difficult method with numerous intricate elements; however, it has been effectively employed in the treatment of cancer and other chronic diseases. The optimal delivery strategy for targeted medication molecules to specific tissues, cells, or organs remains elusive and presents a formidable challenge inside the intricate cellular network of organisms. An optimal drug-targeted delivery system precisely administers the medication to the specific tumor location in the requisite amount. The reality, however, diverges significantly from the idealized scenario of bench-to-bedside care. The dose levels of medications administered to target areas are typically below 5%. Our endeavors should focus on enhancing modest medicine dosages administered to the target locations. Since chronic diseases and cancers cannot be eliminated by focusing solely on a single site, it may be essential to simultaneously treat numerous sites. Therefore, it may be beneficial to create a novel technology or a "magic shotgun" approach that delivers various medications to multiple targets for optimal therapeutic outcomes [130]. Modifying our existing targeted drug delivery systems will be a formidable job, as it will affect both the chosen tactics and the methods for identifying, altering, and evaluating the efficacy of these technologies. Moreover, unequivocal validation for recognizing novel methodologies and alterations does not inherently result in enhanced outcomes without substantial modifications to our existing protocols in targeted drug delivery research to achieve significant advancements in the future. The efficacy of drug delivery utilizing advanced nanomedicine technology will be constrained by extravasation and blood circulation dynamics. Selective ligands target tumor cell markers or receptors by receptor-ligand interaction, which happens subsequent to administration through extravasation and blood circulation. The receptor-ligand interaction will pose challenges for malignancies due to the cells' "over-expression" of specific surface indicators. The selectively targeted surface marker will also be present on the surface of non-cancerous cells due to the significant excess of cancer cell load. Excessive reliance on nanoparticles alone will be insufficient for substantial clinical advantages. Enhancement of targeted drug delivery systems necessitates a comprehensive understanding of the parameters governing blood distribution, temporal heterogeneity, tumor markers, energy characteristics of tumor spatiality, and the complexities of diffusional barriers in solid tumors. Furthermore, reliance on a single over-expressed tumor marker for targeted treatment management may be inadequate. Contemporary drug-targeted delivery and its approaches are based on a scientifically valid logic, although they have achieved limited success mostly due to the design of nanomaterials and pharmaceuticals based solely on biochemical and engineering principles. Currently available nanoparticles can enhance blood circulation duration and facilitate entry into malignant cells by potentially altering their interaction with tumor cell receptors. These intriguing nanoparticles address issues such as the aggressive manipulation of malignant cells and cancer heterogeneity. The optimal targeted delivery system for malignant and other therapies administers the medicine directly to the tumor site. Future efforts should concentrate on enhancing the delivery of a higher concentration of the medicine to the targeted spot. Eliminating malignant cells may require targeting numerous sites rather than focusing on a single location. Moreover, the integration of expertise in targeted medication delivery with advancements in molecular medicine would facilitate the understanding of the molecular and cellular mechanisms underlying diseases. Investigated new techniques should prioritize "bench-to-bedside" practices to minimize delays in therapeutic phases.

REFERENCES

1. Muller RH, Keck CM. Challenges and solutions for the delivery of biotech drugs—a review of drug nanocrystal technology and lipid nanoparticles. Journal of Biotechnology. 2004; 113(1–3):151–170.
2. Mark SW, Torchilin, Vladimir P. Drug delivery systems. Access Science, McGraw-Hill Companies, 2011.
3. Vyas SP, Khar RK. Basis of targeted drug delivery. In Targeted and controlled Drug Delivery, CBS Publishers and Distributors Reprint, 2008: 42–46, 74.
4. Won R. Method for delivering an active ingredient by controlled time release utilizing a novel delivery vehicle which can be prepared by a process utilizing the active ingredient as a porogen, Patent No 4690825 US: 1987.
5. Mastrobattista E, Koning GA, Storm G. Immunoliposomes for the targeted delivery of antitumor drugs. Advance Drug Delivery Reviews. 1999;10:40(1-2):103–127.
6. Maeda H, Matsumura Y. Tumoritropic and lymphotropic principles of macromolecular drugs. Crit Rev Ther Drug Carrier Syst. 1989;6:193–210.
7. Gref R1, Minamitake Y, Peracchia MT, Trubetskoy V, Torchilin V, Langer R. Biodegradable long-circulating polymeric nanospheres. Science. 1994;263(5153):1600–1603.
8. Mansour AM, Drevs J, Esser N, et al. A new approach for the treatment of malignant melanoma: Enhanced antitumor efficacy of an albumin binding doxorubicin prodrug that is cleaved by matrix metalloproteinase 2. Cancer Res. 2003;63:4062–6.
9. Guo X, Szoka FC, Jr. Chemical approaches to triggerable lipid vesicles for drug and gene delivery. Acc Chem Res. 2003;36:335–41.
10. Yockman JW, Maheshwari A, Han SO, Kim SW. Tumor regression by repeated intratumoral delivery of water soluble lipopolymers/p2CMVmIL-12 complexes. J Control Release, 2003;87:177–86.
11. Nomura T, Saikawa A, Morita S, et al. Pharmacokinetic characteristics and therapeutic effects of mitomycin C-dextran conjugates after intratumoural injection. J Control Release. 1998;52:239–52.
12. Barker DD, Berk AJ. Adenovirus proteins from both E1B reading frames are required for transformation of rodent cells by viral infection and DNA transfection. Virology. 1987;156:107–21.
13. Khuri FR, Nemunaitis J, Ganly I, et al. A controlled trial of intratumoral ONYX-015, a selectively-replicating adenovirus, in combination with cisplatin and 5-fluorouracil in patients with recurrent head and neck cancer. Nat Med. 2000;6:879–85.
14. Hecht JR, Bedford R, Abbruzzese JL, et al. A phase I/II trial of intratumoral endoscopic ultrasound injection of ONYX-015 with intravenous gemcitabine in unresectable pancreatic carcinoma. Clin Cancer Res. 2003;9:555–61.
15. Reid T, Galanis E, Abbruzzese J, et al. Hepatic arterial infusion of a replication-selective oncolytic adenovirus (dl1520): Phase II viral, immunologic, and clinical endpoints. Cancer Res. 2002;62:6070–9.
16. Vasey PA, Shulman LN, Campos S, et al. Phase I trial of intraperitoneal injection of the E1B-55-kd-gene-deleted adenovirus ONYX-015 (dl1520) given on days 1 through 5 every 3 weeks in patients with recurrent/refractory epithelial ovarian cancer. J Clin Oncol. 2002;20:1562–9.

17. Galanis E, Okuno SH, Nascimento AG, et al. Phase I-II trial of ONYX-015 in combination with MAP chemotherapy in patients with advanced sarcomas. Gene Ther. 2005;12:437–45.
18. Lamprecht A, Yamamoto H, Takeuchi H, Kawashima Y. Nanoparticles enhance therapeutic efficiency by selectively increased local drug dose in experimental colitis in rats. J Pharmacol Exp Ther. 2005;315:196–202.
19. Beduneau A, Saulnier P, Hindre F, Clavreul A, Leroux JC, Benoit JP. Design of targeted lipid nanocapsules by conjugation of whole antibodies and antibody Fab' fragments. Biomaterials. 2007;28:4978–4990.
20. Deckert PM. Current constructs and targets in clinical development for antibody-based cancer therapy. Current Drug Targets. 2009;10:158–175.
21. Hong M, Zhu S, Jiang Y, Tang G, Pei Y. Efficient tumor targeting of hydroxycamptothecin loaded PEGylated niosomes modified with transferrin. J Control Release. 2009;133:96–102.
22. Zensi A, Begley D, Pontikis C, Legros C, Mihoreanu L, Wagner S, Büchel C, Briesen Hv, Kreuter J. Albumin nanoparticles targeted with ApoE enter the CNS by transcytosis and are delivered to neurons. J Control Release. 2009;137:78–86.
23. Canal F, Vicent MJ, Pasut G, Schiavon O. Relevance of folic acid/polymer ratio in targeted PEGepirubicin conjugates. J Control Release. 2010;146:388–399.
24. Pirollo KF, Chang EH. Does a targeting ligand influence nanoparticle tumor localization or uptake? Trends Biotechnol. 2008;26:552–558.
25. Kirpotin DB, Drummond DC, Shao Y, Shalaby MR, Hong K, Nielsen UB, Marks JD, Benz CC, Park JW. Antibody targeting of long-circulating lipidic nanoparticles does not increase tumor localization but does increase internalization in animal models. Cancer Res. 2006;66:6732–6740.
26. Mikhail AS, Allen C. Block copolymer micelles for delivery of cancer therapy: transport at the whole body, tissue and cellular levels. J Control Release. 2009;138:214–223.
27. Raz A, Meromsky L, Lotan R. Differential expression of endogenous lectins on the surface of nontumorigenic, tumorigenic, and metastatic cells. Cancer Res. 1986;46:3667–72.
28. Gorelik E, Galili U, Raz A. On the role of cell surface carbohydrates and their binding proteins (lectins) in tumor metastasis. Cancer Metastasis Rev. 2001;20:245–77.
29. Yamazaki N, Kojima S, Bovin NV, et al. Endogenous lectins as targets for drug delivery. Adv Drug Deliv Rev. 2000;43:225–44. 24.
30. Olsnes S, Sandvig K. How protein toxins enter and kill cells. Cancer Treat Res. 1988;37:39–73.
31. Stefanadis C, Chrysochoou C, Markou D, Petraki K, Panagiotakos DB, Fasoulakis C, Kyriakidis A, Papadimitriou C, Toutouzas PK. Increased temperature of malignant urinary bladder tumors *in vivo*: The application of a new method based on a catheter technique. J. Clin. Oncol. 2001;19(3):676–681.
32. Gerweck LE, Seetharaman K. Cellular pH gradient in tumor versus normal tissue: Potential exploitation for the treatment o cancer. Cancer Res. 1996;56(6):1194–1198.
33. Gao M, Jia XR, Li Y, Liang DH, Wei Y. Synthesis and thermo-/pH- dual-responsive properties of poly (amidoamine) dendronized poly (2-hydroxyethyl) Methacrylate. Macromolecules. 2010;43:4314–4323.
34. Pang Y, Zhu Q, Zhou DL, Liu JY, Chen Y, Su Y, Yan DY, Zhu XY, Zhu BS. Synthesis of backbone thermo and pH dual-responsive hyperbranched poly (amine-ether)s through proton-transfer polymerization. J. Polym. Sci. Part A: Polym. Chem. 2011:49:966–975.

35. Li F, Wu H, Fan L, Zhang HT, Zhang H, Gu CH. Study of dual responsive poly[(maleilated dextran)-graft-(Nisopropylacrylamide)] hydrogel nanoparticles: Preparation, characterization and biological evaluation. Polym. Int. 2009;58:1023–1033.

36. Ma LW, Liu MZ, Liu HL, Chen J, Gao CM, Cui DP. Dual crosslinked pH- and temperature-sensitive hydrogel beads for intestine-targeted controlled release. Polym. Adv. Technol. 2010;21:348–355.

37. Kim IS, Oh IJ. Drug release from the enzyme-degradable and pH-sensitive hydrogel composed of glycidyl methacrylate dextran and poly (acrylic acid). Arch. Pharm. Res. 2005:28(8):983–987.

38. Li YW, Tong R, Xia HS, Zhang HJ, Xuan J. High intensity focused ultrasound and redox dual responsive polymer micelles. Chem. Commun. 2010;46;7739–7741.

39. Deol P, Khuller GK. Lung specific stealth liposomes: Stability, biodistribution and toxicity of liposomal antitubercular drugs in mice. Biochimica Biophysi Acta. 1997;1334:161–72.

40. Koo OM, Rubinstein I, Onyuksel H. Role of nanotechnology in targeted drug delivery and imaging: A concise review. Nanomedicine. 2005 Sep;1(3):193–212.

41. Koren E, Apte A, Jani A, Torchilin VP. Multifunctional PEGylated 2C5-immunoliposomes containing pH-sensitive bonds and TAT peptide for enhanced tumor cell internalization and cytotoxicity. J Control Release. 2012 Jun 10;160(2):264–73. doi: 10.1016/j.jconrel.2011.12.002. Epub 2011 Dec 13.

42. Koshkaryev A, Piroyan A, Torchilin VP. Increased apoptosis in cancer cells in vitro and in vivo by ceramides in transferrin-modified liposomes. Cancer Biol Ther. 2012 Jan 1;13(1):50–60. doi: 10.4161/cbt.13.1.18871.

43. Etzerodt A, Maniecki MB, Graversen JH, Møller HJ, Torchilin VP, Moestrup SK. Efficient intracellular drug-targeting of macrophages using stealth liposomes directed to the hemoglobin scavenger receptor CD163. J Control Release. 2012 May 30;160(1):72–80. doi: 10.1016/j.jconrel.2012.01.034. Epub 2012 Jan 27.

44. Kang KW, Chun MK, Kim O, Subedi RK, Ahn SG, Yoon JH, Choi HK. Doxorubicin-loaded solid lipid nanoparticles to overcome multidrug resistance in cancer therapy. Nanomedicine. 2010 Apr;6(2):210–3. doi: 10.1016/j.nano.2009.12.006. Epub 2010 Jan 6.

45. Kedar U, Phutane P, Shidhaye S, Kadam V. Advances in polymeric micelles for drug delivery and tumor targeting. Nanomedicine. 2010 Dec;6(6):714–29. doi: 10.1016/j.nano.2010.05.005. Epub 2010 Jun 11.

46. Arukuusk P, Pärnaste L, Oskolkov N, Copolovici DM, Margus H, Padari K, Möll K, Maslovskaja J, Tegova R, Kivi G, Tover A, Pooga M, Ustav M, Langel U. New generation of efficient peptide-based vectors, NickFects, for the delivery ofnucleic acids. Biochim Biophys Acta. 2013 May;1828(5):1365–73. doi: 10.1016/j.bbamem.2013.01.011. Epub 2013 Jan 26.

47. Wu Y, Sadatmousavi P, Wang R, Lu S, Yuan YF, Chen P. Self-assembling peptide-based nanoparticles enhance anticancer effect of ellipticine in vitro and in vivo. Int J Nanomedicine. 2012;7:3221–33. doi: 10.2147/IJN.S31858. Epub 2012 Jun 28.

48. Crombez L, Morris MC, Deshayes S, Heitz F, Divita G. Peptide-based nanoparticle for ex vivo and in vivo drug delivery. Curr Pharm Des. 2008;14(34):3656–65.

49. Nasrolahi Shirazi A, Tiwari R, Chhikara BS, Mandal D, Parang K. Design and biological evaluation of cell-penetrating peptide-doxorubicin conjugates as prodrugs. Mol Pharm. 2013 Feb 4;10(2):488-99. doi: 10.1021/mp3004034. Epub 2013 Jan 15.

50. Yuan DM, Lv YL, Yao YW, Miao XH, Wang Q, Xiao XW, Song Y. Efficacy and safety of Abraxane in treatment of progressive and recurrent nonsmall cell lung cancer patients: A retrospective clinical study. Thoracic Cancer. 2012;3(4):341–347.

51. Yan Z, Xia L, Qiu H, Chen P, Zhang B. Short-term outcomes of albumin-bound paclitaxel (abraxane)-containing chemotherapy in patients with advanced gastric cancer: A report of 14 cases. The Chinese-German Journal of Clinical Oncology. 2013;12(1):30-34.

52. Paik PK, James LP, Riely GJ, Azzoli CG, Miller VA, Ng KK, Sima CS, Heelan RT, Kris MG, Moore E, Rizvi NA. A phase 2 study of weekly albumin-bound paclitaxel (Abraxane®) given as a two-hour infusion. Cancer Chemother Pharmacol. 2011 Nov;68(5):1331–7. doi: 10.1007/s00280-011-1621-0. Epub 2011 Apr 3.

53. Zhang H, Chen C, Hou L, Jin N, Shi J, Wang Z, Liu Y, Feng Q, Zhang Z. Targeting and hyperthermia of doxorubicin by the delivery of single-walled carbon nanotubes to EC-109 cells. Journal of Drug Targeting. 2013;21(3):312–319.

54. Mody N, Tekade RK, Mehra NK, Chopdey P, Jain NK. Dendrimer, liposomes, carbon nanotubes and PLGA nanoparticles: one platform assessment of drug delivery potential. AAPS PharmSciTech. 2014 Apr;15(2):388–99. doi: 10.1208/s12249-014-0073-3. Epub 2014 Jan 16.

55. Farah RA, Clinchy B, Herrera L, Vitetta ES. The development of monoclonal antibodies for the therapy of cancer. Crit Rev Eukaryot Gene Expr. 1998;8(3-4):321–56.

56. Kim GJ, Nie S. Targeted cancer nanotherapy. Materials Today. August 2005;8(8):28–33. ISSN: 1369-7021, http://dx.doi.org/10.1016/S1369-7021(05)71034-8.

57. Köhler G, Milstein C. Continuous cultures of fused cells secreting antibody of predefined specificity. Nature. 1975 Aug 7;256(5517):495–7.

58. Storm G, Daan J, Crommelin A. Liposomes: quo vadis? Pharmaceutical Science & Technology Today. 1 April 1998;1(1):19–31. ISSN: 1461-5347, http://dx.doi.org/10.1016/S1461-5347(98)00007-8.

59. Gupta U, Agashe HB, Asthana A, Jain NK. Dendrimers: Novel polymeric nanoarchitectures for solubility enhancement. Biomacromolecules. 2006 Mar;7(3):649–58.

60. Wen S, Liu H, Cai H, Shen M, Shi X. Targeted and pH-responsive delivery of doxorubicin to cancer cells using multifunctional dendrimer-modified multi-walled carbon nanotubes. Adv Healthc Mater. 2013 Sep;2(9):1267–76. doi: 10.1002/adhm.201200389. Epub 2013 Feb 28.

61. Foldvari M, Bagonluri M. Carbon nanotubes as functional excipients for nanomedicines: II. Drug delivery and biocompatibility issues. Nanomedicine. 2008 Sep;4(3):183–200. doi: 10.1016/j.nano.2008.04.003. Epub 2008 Jun 11.

62. Liu Z, Chen K, Davis C, Sherlock S, Cao Q, Chen X, Dai H. Drug delivery with carbon nanotubes for in vivo cancer treatment. Cancer Res. 2008 Aug 15;68(16):6652–60. doi: 10.1158/0008-5472.CAN-08-1468.

63. Liu Z, Fan AC, Rakhra K, Sherlock S, Goodwin A, Chen X, Yang Q, Felsher DW, Dai H. Supramolecular stacking of doxorubicin on carbon nanotubes for in vivo cancer therapy. Angew Chem Int Ed Engl. 2009;48(41):7668–72. doi: 10.1002/anie.200902612.

64. Wong Shi Kam N, Dai H. Single-walled carbon nanotubes for transport and delivery of biological cargos. 2006.

65. Kam NW, O'Connell M, Wisdom JA, Dai H. Carbon nanotubes as multifunctional biological transporters and near-infrared agents for selective cancer cell destruction. Proc Natl Acad Sci U S A. 2005 Aug 16;102(33):11600–5. Epub 2005 Aug 8.

66. Shi Kam NW, Jessop TC, Wender PA, Dai H. Nanotube molecular transporters: Internalization of carbon nanotube-protein conjugates into Mammalian cells. J Am Chem Soc. 2004 Jun 9;126(22):6850–1.

67. Liu Z, Tabakman S, Welsher K, Dai H. Carbon nanotubes in biology and medicine: In vitro and in vivo detection, imaging and drug delivery. Nano Res. 2009 Feb 1;2(2):85–120.

68. Liu Z, Tabakman SM, Chen Z, Dai H. Preparation of carbon nanotube bioconjugates for biomedical applications. Nat Protoc. 2009;4(9):1372–82. doi: 10.1038/nprot.2009.146. Epub 2009 Sep 3.

69. Firme CP 3rd, Bandaru PR. Toxicity issues in the application of carbon nanotubes to biological systems. Nanomedicine. 2010 Apr;6(2):245–56. doi: 10.1016/j.nano.2009.07.003. Epub 2009 Aug 20.

70. Jain AK, Dubey V, Mehra NK, Lodhi N, Nahar M, Mishra DK, Jain NK. Carbohydrate-conjugated multiwalled carbon nanotubes: development and characterization. Nanomedicine. 2009 Dec;5(4):432–42. doi: 10.1016/j.nano.2009.03.001. Epub 2009 Mar 31.

71. Sandler J, Shaffer MSP, Prasse T, Bauhofer W, Schulte K, Windle A. Development of a dispersion process for carbon nanotubes in an epoxy matrix and the resulting electrical properties. Polymer. 1999;40(21):5967–5971. http://dx.doi.org/10.1016/S0032-3861(99)00166-4.

72. Silva LBD, Fagan SB, Mota R. Ab initio study of deformed carbon nanotube sensors for carbon monoxide molecules. Nano Letters. 2004;4(1):65–67. http://dx.doi.org/10.1021/nl034873d.

73. Guldi DM, Rahman GMA, Prato M, Jux NJ, Qin S, Ford W. Single-wall carbon nanotubes as integrative building blocks for solar energy conversion. General & Introductory Chemistry. 2005;44(13):2015-2018. http://dx.doi.org/10.1002/anie.200462416.

74. Chin KC, Gohel A, Chen WZ, Elim HI, Ji W, Chong GL, Sow CH, Wee ATS. Gold- and silver-coated carbon nanotubes: An improved broad-band optical limiter. Chemical Physics Letters. 2005;409(1-3):85–88. http://dx.doi.org/10.1016/j.cplett.2005.04.092.

75. Guo DJ, Li HL. Carbon. 2005;43:1259.

76. Wu HP, Wu XJ, Ge MY, Zhang GQ, Wang YW, Jiang J. Properties investigation on isotropical conductive adhesives filled with silver coated carbon nanotubes. Composites Science and Technology. 2007;67(6):1182–1186. http://dx.doi.org/10.1016/j.compscitech.2006.05.010.

77. Lee K, Lee H, Bae KH, Park TG. Heparin immobilized gold nanoparticles for targeted detection and apoptotic death of metastatic cancer cells. Biomater. 2010;31:6530–6536.

78. Tarnawski R, Ulbricht M. Amphiphilic gold nanoparticles: Synthesis, characterization and adsorption to PEGylated polymer surfaces. Colloid Surfac A: Physicochem Engineer Aspects. 2011;374:13–21.

79. Deb S, Patra HK, Lahiri P, Dasgupta AK, Chakrabarti K, Chaudhuri U. Multistability in platelets and their response to gold nanoparticles. Nanomed: Nanotechnol Biol Med. 2011;7376–384.

80. Nalawade P, Mukherjee T, Kapoor S. High-yield synthesis of multispiked gold nanoparticles: Characterization and catalytic reactions. Colloid Surfac A: Physicochem Engineer Aspects. 2012;396:336–340.

81. Benkovicova M, Vegso K, Siffalovic P, Jergel M, Luby S, Majkova E. Preparation of gold nanoparticles for plasmonic applications. Thin Solid Films. 2013;543:138–141.

82. Leamon CP, Reddy JA. Folate-targeted chemotherapy. Adv Drug Deliv Rev. 2004 Apr 29;56(8):1127–41.

83. Low PS, Henne WA, Doorneweerd DD. Discovery and development of folic-acid-based receptor targeting for imaging and therapy of cancer and inflammatory diseases. Acc Chem Res. 2008 Jan;41(1):120–9. Epub 2007 Jul 27.

84. Kamen BA, Capdevila A. Receptor-mediated folate accumulation is regulated by the cellular folate content. Proc Natl Acad Sci U S A. 1986 Aug;83(16):5983–7.

85. Sugapriya D, Biswal BK, Sumantran VN, Verma RS. Augmented sensitivity to methotrexate by curcumin induced overexpression of folate receptor in KG-1 Cells. Biochimie. 2013;95:1567–1573.

86. Shen Y, Zhou Z, Sui M, Tang J, Xu P, Van Kirk EA, Murdoch WJ, Fan M, Radosz M. Charge-reversal polyamidoamine dendrimer for cascade nuclear drug delivery. Nanomedicine (Lond). 2010 Oct;5(8):1205–17. doi: 10.2217/nnm.10.86.

87. Warenius HM, Galfre G, Bleehen NM, Milstein C. Attempted targeting of a monoclonal antibody in a human tumour xenograft system. Eur J Cancer Clin Oncol. 1981 Sep;17(9):1009–15.

88. James JS, Dubs G. FDA approves new kind of lymphoma treatment. Food and Drug Administration. AIDS Treat News. 1997 Dec 5;(284):2–3.

89. Albanell J, Baselga J. Trastuzumab, a humanized anti-HER2 monoclonal antibody, for the treatment of breast cancer. Drugs Today (Barc). 1999 Dec;35(12):931–46.

90. De Roock W, Piessevaux H, De Schutter J, Janssens M, De Hertogh G, Personeni N, Biesmans B, Van Laethem JL, Peeters M, Humblet Y, Van Cutsem E, Tejpar S. KRAS wild-type state predicts survival and is associated to early radiological response in metastatic colorectal cancer treated with cetuximab. Ann Oncol. 2008 Mar;19(3):508–15.

91. Ferrara N. VEGF as a therapeutic target in cancer. Oncology. 2005;69 Suppl 3:11–6. Epub 2005 Nov 21.

92. Matsumura Y, Kataoka K. Preclinical and clinical studies of anticancer agent-incorporating polymer micelles. Cancer Sci. 2009 Apr;100(4):572–9.

93. Nobs L, Buchegger F, Gurny R, Allémann E. Biodegradable nanoparticles for direct or two-step tumor immunotargeting. Bioconjug Chem. 2006 Jan-Feb;17(1):139–45.

94. Miyano T, Wijagkanalan W, Kawakami S, Yamashita F, Hashida M. Anionic amino acid dendrimer-trastuzumab conjugates for specific internalization in HER2-positive cancer cells. Mol Pharm. 2010 Aug 2;7(4):1318–27. doi: 10.1021/mp100105c.

95. Adams GP, Schier R, McCall AM, Simmons HH, Horak EM, Alpaugh RK, Marks JD, Weiner LM. High affinity restricts the localization and tumor penetration of single-chain fv antibody molecules. Cancer Res. 2001 Jun 15;61(12):4750–5.

96. Qian ZM, Tang PL. Mechanisms of iron uptake by mammalian cells. Biochim. Biophys. Acta. 1995;1269:205–214.

97. Prost AC, Menegaux F, Langlois P, Vidal JM, Koulibaly M, Jost JL, Duron JJ, Chigot JP, Vayre P, Aurengo A, Legrand JC, Rosselin G, Gespach C. Differential transferrin receptor density in human colorectal cancer: A potential probe for diagnosis and therapy. Int. J. Oncol. 1998;13(4):871–875.

98. Ishida O, Maruyama K, Tanahashi H, Iwatsuru M, Sasaki K, Eriguchi M, Yanagie H. Liposomes bearing polyethyleneglycol-coupled transferrin with intracellular targeting property to the solid tumors in vivo. Pharm Res. 2001 Jul;18(7):1042–8.

99. Sahoo SK, Labhasetwar V. Enhanced antiproliferative activity of transferrin-conjugated paclitaxel-loaded nanoparticles is mediated via sustained intracellular drug retention. Mol Pharm. 2005 Sep–Oct;2(5):373–83.

100. Han L, Huang R, Liu S, Huang S, Jiang C. Peptide-conjugated PAMAM for targeted doxorubicin delivery to transferrin receptor overexpressed tumors. Mol Pharm. 2010 Dec 6;7(6):2156–65. doi: 10.1021/mp100185f. Epub 2010 Oct 14.

101. Ekblom P, Thesleff I, Lehto VP, Virtanen I. Distribution of the transferrin receptor in normal human fibroblasts and fibrosarcoma cells. Int J Cancer. 1983 Jan 15;31(1):111–7.

102. Bartlett DW, Su H, Hildebrandt IJ, Weber WA, Davis ME. Impact of tumor-specific targeting on the biodistribution and efficacy of siRNA nanoparticles measured by multimodality in vivo imaging. Proc Natl Acad Sci U S A. 2007 Sep 25;104(39):15549–54. Epub 2007 Sep 17.

103. Joyce GF. Amplification, mutation and selection of catalytic RNA. Gene. 1989 Oct 15;82(1):83–7.

104. Jayasena SD. Aptamers: An emerging class of molecules that rival antibodies in diagnostics. Clin Chem. 1999 Sep;45(9):1628–50.

105. Michel F, Ellington AD, Couture S, Szostak JW. Phylogenetic and genetic evidence for base-triples in the catalytic domain of group I introns. Nature. 1990 Oct 11;347(6293):578–80.

106. Lupold SE, Hicke BJ, Lin Y, Coffey DS. Identification and characterization of nuclease-stabilized RNA molecules that bind human prostate cancer cells via the prostate-specific membrane antigen. Cancer Res. 2002 Jul 15;62(14):4029–33. Erratum in: Cancer Res. 2012 Aug 1;72(15):3887.

107. Bagalkot V, Farokhzad OC, Langer R, Jon S. An aptamer-doxorubicin physical conjugate as a novel targeted drug-delivery platform. Angew Chem Int Ed Engl. 2006 Dec 11;45(48):8149–52.

108. Brooks PC, Montgomery AM, Rosenfeld M, Reisfeld RA, Hu T, Klier G, Cheresh DA. Integrin alpha v beta 3 antagonists promote tumor regression by inducing apoptosis of angiogenic blood vessels. Cell. 1994 Dec 30;79(7):1157–64.

109. Erdreich-Epstein A, Shimada H, Groshen S, Liu M, Metelitsa LS, Kim KS, Stins MF, Seeger RC, Durden DL. Integrins alpha(v)beta3 and alpha(v)beta5 are expressed by endothelium of high-risk neuroblastoma and their inhibition is associated with increased endogenous ceramide. Cancer Res. 2000 Feb 1;60(3):712–21.

110. Yu MK, Park J, Jeong YY, Moon WK, Jon S. Integrin-targeting thermally cross-linked superparamagnetic iron oxide nanoparticles for combined cancer imaging and drug delivery. Nanotechnology. 2010 Oct 15;21(41):415102. doi: 10.1088/0957-4484/21/41/415102. Epub 2010 Sep 17.

111. Meng S, Su B, Li W, Ding Y, Tang L, Zhou W, Song Y, Li H, Zhou C. Enhanced antitumor effect of novel dual-targeted paclitaxel liposomes. Nanotechnology. 2010 Oct 15;21(41):415103. doi: 10.1088/0957-4484/21/41/415103. Epub 2010 Sep 17.

112. Yin J, Li Z, Yang T, Wang J, Zhang X, Zhang Q. Cyclic RGDyK conjugation facilitates intracellular drug delivery of polymeric micelles to integrin-overexpressing tumor cells and neovasculature. J Drug Target. 2011 Jan;19(1):25–36. doi: 10.3109/10611861003663531. Epub 2010 Mar 16.

113. Bibby DC, Talmadge JE, Dalal MK, Kurz SG, Chytil KM, Barry SE, Shand DG, Steiert M. Pharmacokinetics and biodistribution of RGD-targeted doxorubicin-loaded nanoparticles in tumor-bearing mice. Int J Pharm. 2005 Apr 11;293(1–2):281–90.

114. Cirillo G, Hampel S, Spizzirri UG, Parisi OI, Picci N, Iemma F. Carbon nanotubes hybrid hydrogels in drug delivery: A perspective review. Biomed Res Int. 2014;2014:825017. doi: 10.1155/2014/825017. Epub 2014 Jan 21.

115. Sahoo SK, Parveen S, Panda JJ. The present and future of nanotechnology in human health care. Nanomedicine. 2007 Mar;3(1):20–31.

116. Kim KY. Nanotechnology platforms and physiological challenges for cancertherapeutics. Nanomedicine. 2007 Jun;3(2):103–10. Epub 2007 Apr 17.

117. Parveen S, Misra R, Sahoo SK. Nanoparticles: A boon to drug delivery, therapeutics, diagnostics and imaging. Nanomedicine. 2012 Feb;8(2):147–66. doi:10.1016/j.nano.2011.05.016. Epub 2011 Jun 7.

118. Chouhan R, Bajpai AK. Release dynamics of ciprofloxacin from swellable nanocarriers of poly(2-hydroxyethyl methacrylate): An in vitro study. Nanomedicine. 2010 Jun;6(3):453–62. doi: 10.1016/j.nano.2009.11.006. Epub 2010 Jan 4.

119. Mishra B, Patel BB, Tiwari S. Colloidal nanocarriers: A review on formulation technology, types and applications toward targeted drug delivery. Nanomedicine. 2010 Feb;6(1):9–24. doi: 10.1016/j.nano.2009.04.008. Epub 2009 May 15.

120. Bertrand N, Wu J, Xu X, Kamaly N, Farokhzad OC. Cancer nanotechnology: The impact of passive and active targeting in the era of modern cancer biology. Adv Drug Deliv Rev. 2014 Feb;66:2–25. doi: 10.1016/j.addr.2013.11.009. Epub 2013 Nov 22.

121. Liu Y, Miyoshi H, Nakamura M. Nanomedicine for drug delivery and imaging: A promising avenue for cancer therapy and diagnosis using targeted functional nanoparticles. Int J Cancer. 2007 Jun 15;120(12):2527–37.

122. Mehra NK, Mishra V, Jain NK. A review of ligand tethered surface engineered carbon nanotubes. Biomaterials. 2014 Jan;35(4):1267–83. doi: 10.1016/j.biomaterials.2013.10.032. Epub 2013 Nov 7.

123. Torchilin VP. Multifunctional nanocarriers. Adv Drug Deliv Rev. 2006 Dec 1;58(14):1532–55. Epub 2006 Sep 28.

124. Minotti G, Menna P, Salvatorelli E, Cairo G, Gianni L. Anthracyclines: Molecular advances and pharmacologic developments in antitumor activity and cardiotoxicity. Pharmacol Rev. 2004 Jun;56(2):185–229.

125. Verweij J, Clavel M, Chevalier B. Paclitaxel (Taxol) and docetaxel (Taxotere): Not simply two of a kind. Ann Oncol. 1994 Jul;5(6):495–505.

126. Samorì C, Ali-Boucetta H, Sainz R, Guo C, Toma FM, Fabbro C, da Ros T, Prato M, Kostarelos K, Bianco A. Enhanced anticancer activity of multi-walled carbon nanotube-methotrexate conjugates using cleavable linkers. Chem Commun (Camb). 2010 Mar 7;46(9):1494–6. doi: 10.1039/b923560d. Epub 2009 Dec 23.

127. Ren Y, Pastorin G. Incorporation of hexamethylmelamine inside capped carbon nanotubes. Advanced Materials. 2008;20(11):2031–2036.

128. Aryal S, Hu CM, Zhang L. Combinatorial drug conjugation enables nanoparticle dual-drug delivery. Small. 2010 Jul 5;6(13):1442–8. doi: 10.1002/smll.201000631.

129. Oberoi HS, Nukolova NV, Kabanov AV, Bronich TK. Nanocarriers for delivery of platinum anticancer drugs. Adv Drug Deliv Rev. 2013 Nov;65(13–14):1667–85. doi: 10.1016/j.addr.2013.09.014. Epub 2013 Oct 8.

130. Agnihotri J, Saraf S, Khale A. Targeting: New potential carriers for targeted drug delivery system. International Journal of Pharmaceutical Sciences Review and Research. 2011;8(2):117–123.

3 Chapter

INTELLIGENT DRUG DELIVERY APPROACHES UTILIZING POROUS NANOSTRUCTURED MATERIALS

1. INTRODUCTION: AN OVERVIEW

In recent years, nanomaterials and nanotechnology have been utilized in the medical domain for disease diagnosis and treatment. Investigations into medication delivery and targeting systems utilizing nanoparticles are conducted in nanomedicine to develop drug delivery systems [1]. The systems facilitate the identification of diseased tissues and the administration of therapy at the necessary site.

Drug carriers comprised micro- or nano-particles constructed from biodegradable, natural or synthetic polymers, microcapsules, lipoproteins, micelles, TNTs, nanoporous aluminum oxide, among others. Biodegradable organic/inorganic micro/nano-particles have been extensively researched due to their regulated size, shape, release characteristics, and superior biocompatibility [2–5]. Stimuli-responsive systems can enable drug release to target environments. Stimuli-responsive elements exhibit functionality that maintains an energy alteration in response to pH, temperature, magnetism, sound, and light [6–18].

Fabricating particles from stimulus-responsive polymers enables them to respond to certain pH levels and temperatures, facilitating controlled release. The pH-responsive polymer was investigated as a delivery mechanism for medicinal agents and was confirmed to extend drug release circulation in vivo. Magnetic nanoparticles, owing to their unique magnetic and optical properties, have significant potential in medication release and have been utilized in illness diagnostics and therapy. Consequently, medication delivery devices were developed utilizing magnetic targeting. Furthermore, micellar solutions, vesicular and liquid crystal dispersions exhibit significant promise, along with nanoparticle dispersions [22–23]. Colloidal drug carrier-based delivery systems can achieve targeted therapy through efficient drug loading and release mechanisms, together with reduced toxicity.

Recent advancements in the regulation of drug release from nanotube and nanopore materials encompass TNT arrays and anodic aluminum oxide nanopores, among others [24–26]. TNT arrays have been utilized in drug release for therapeutic applications due to their exceptional qualities, and it has been established that TNT arrays significantly transform localized drug delivery therapies. Moreover, the technique for fabricating TNT arrays establishes a novel nano-engineering approach to address the constraints of drug delivery systems. Ordered nanoporous materials were investigated to circumvent the constraints of traditional medication therapy, particularly in implanted drug delivery systems. Moreover, porous anodic aluminum oxides (AAOs) can replicate the dimensions of real bone, and AAO films are regarded as potential coatings for the medical sector. Consequently, AAO has been employed as a novel nano-platform for drug release.

2. ENERGETIC CHANGES OF SUBSTANCES FOR PHARMACEUTICAL DELIVERY

It is essential for the chemical functions to demonstrate stimuli-responsive activity. In certain instances, the eliciting cues are near the internal physiological milieu of the drug delivery system [27]. It is envisioned that various stimuli-responsive systems functioning concurrently integrate into a medication delivery system [28]. A temperature alteration in a thermo-responsive system may be triggered by a magnetic system.

2.1. pH-sensitive Drug Delivery

Polymer materials own structures with ionizable functionalities that become ionized at a specific pH where they acquire a positive or negative charge [29]. The transition of the functional group from one of water insolubility to one of water solubility under the effect of the ionization is called polyelectrolytes because of the presence of electrostatic charges in the water-soluble polymer structure.

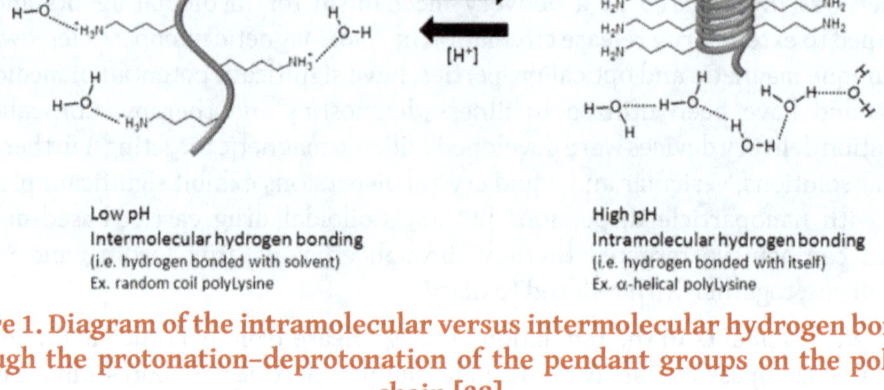

Figure 1. Diagram of the intramolecular versus intermolecular hydrogen bonding through the protonation–deprotonation of the pendant groups on the polymer chain [32].

There is a significant difference in the behavior of polymeric-charged functionalities and their uncharged counterparts in terms of their intermolecular effects on the surrounding environment and intramolecular effects within their own polymer molecules. The two types of interaction can be segregated into a polyelectrolyte and a solvent [29], and those between a polyelectrolyte and a surface [30]. In terms of the interaction between a polyelectrolyte and a solvent, there is a transition of the Gibbs free energy of mixing shifts from negative (-ΔG) in solubility to positive (+ΔG), where it is insoluble because the transition from an intermolecular hydrogen-bonded species to an intramolecular hydrogen-bonded species causes poor entropy of mixing [31]. The function is easily seen in the change in the secondary structure of polypeptides or proteins where there is a transition from an α-helical to a random coil secondary structure as a result of deprotonation or protonation, as is shown in Fig. 1 [32].

en the polyelectrolyte and the surface can be seen. If a surface owns an oppositely charged energy, the polyelectrolyte is proposed to interact in a number of different ways. If there is a long-range of electrostatic interaction, it is possible that the rearrangement of the polyelectrolyte chain expresses charged functionalities at the surface [33]. This rearrangement would change based on the pH, the charge density, the composition and distribution of charges along the polymer chain and the ionic strength of the solvent and so on. For the purposes of our discussion in this section, we focus on the pH and ionic strength.

We know that the introduction of salt will screen the electrostatic forces between the polyelectrolyte and the surface, as well as reduce both the intermolecular and intramolecular electrostatic repulsions. There is also a non-electrostatic affinity under certain conditions in the case of interactions between polyelectrolytes and charged surfaces [34]. Any increase in the ionic strength under the presence of salts would decrease the electrostatic affinity of the polyelectrolyte to the charged surface when the adsorption of polyelectrolyte on a charged surface is driven by only electrostatic forces, and the adsorption increases to an upper limit when the non-electrostatic affinity is high enough.

The responsiveness of a molecule to pH presents an interesting target for stimulated drug delivery. As we know, when an encapsulated drug species is internalized by a cell, it will enter the lysosome at some point within the process. The lysosome cell has a pH of 4.5–5.0 [35], which is exclusively different from other intracellular vesicle species. Therefore, a collapse or dissociation of the self-assembled species is triggered by pH and will result in the release of the encapsulant.

We know the role of the hydrophobic domain in the self-assembly of micellar systems is to minimize the interfacial free energy between incompatible phases. The hydrophobicity could be adjusted by increasing the molecular weight into the entanglement regime, which more effectively stabilizes both the hydrophobic domain and the self-assembled species. If we begin to change the composition of the hydrophobic domain, it will destabilize the condensed, self-assembled structure [36].

The pH-responsive vesicle or micellar systems would not be orally relevant if the stimuli range is ~5 since the premature release of drug cargo would occur in the acidic environment of the stomach (pH 1–3) [37]. The hydrogel particles are designed such that the cross-linked domains are a combination of covalent bonds and the collapse of multiple hydrophobic domains. In these cases, a change in the pH of the environment surrounding leads to a nonpolar, collapsed hydrophobic species to turn into a charged species. The change to charged groups also leads to the electrostatic repulsion of polyelectrolyte chains within close proximity to one another, which further drives the expansion of the gel network pore structure [38]. The design is typically used in drug applications where the drug needs to be delivered within the immediate proximity of a desired cell and does not require the system to facilitate the cellular internalization response. In either of these cases, systems can be designed with negative charges as well, which shifts the operable pH range to more basic stimuli. One can envision tuning their respective systems by compositionally shifting their ratios of cationic to anionic stimuli-responsive groups to allow for a specific release window (Fig. 2) [38].

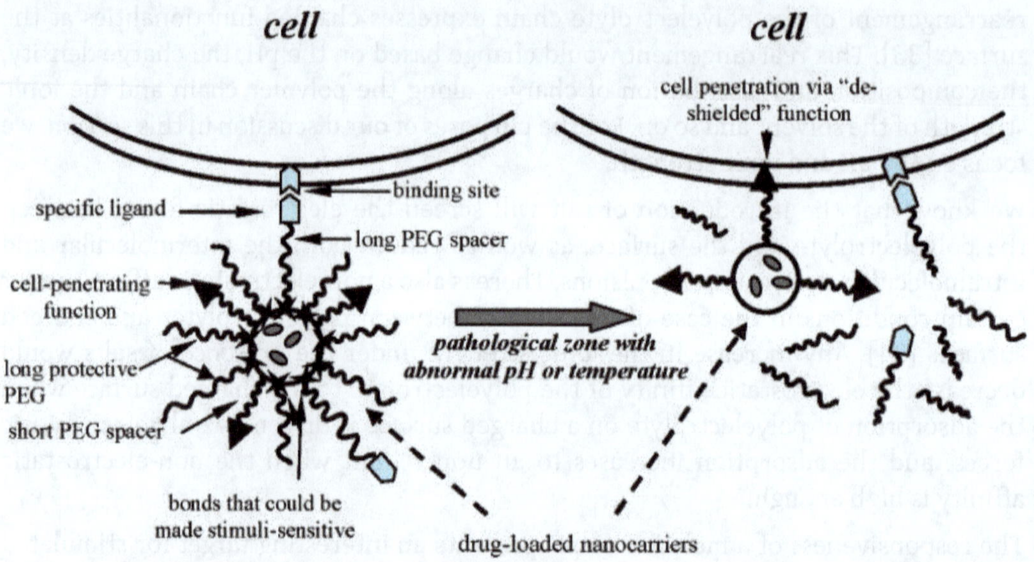

Figure 2. Interaction of the multifunctional pH-responsive pharmaceutical nanocarrier with the target cell. Local stimuli-dependent removal of protecting PEG chains or mAb-PEG moieties allows for the direct interaction of the CPP moiety with the cell membrane [38].

2.2. Temperature-responsive pharmaceutical administration

The combination of a polymer with a solvent in a binary mixture involves a series of phases of varying degrees of stability primarily in relation to its composition and temperature. Within some compositional range, a material can reach a minimum energy equilibrium state known as the binodal curve that describes a critical limit at which two phases can be either stable on one side or unstable on the other side, representing the limits of solvent interaction between two phases [39]. Plus, a curve known as the spinodal curve describes the limit of absolute instability between phases. A complete decomposition of the system is produced when it is changed to composition within the spinodal curve [40].

The point at which the spinodal and binodal curves meet is known as the lower critical solution temperature (LCST) [41]. The LCST represents a point below which the material becomes miscible, where the Gibbs free energy of mixing is negative (-ΔG) and above which it is completely immiscible, and where the Gibbs free energy of mixing is positive (+ΔG) due to poor entropy of mixing [42]. The degree of polymerization and the polydispersity of the polymer chains can be a strong influence on the energetics of mixing and therefore can shift the values for the LCST. Typically, polymer chains with higher degrees of polymerization lead to higher values for the LCST. Polymers that exhibit an LCST behavior can have their solubility tuned based on temperature change.

We have known that the self-assembly of vesicle and micellar species is controlled by several factors, such as chemical composition, shape, charge, and so on, and species with specific size, shape, stability, and delivery efficiency are assembled under the effect of these factors [43]. For a vesicle species comprised of amphiphilic copolymers, there is much focus about their design. The chemical functionality tells us the rigidity of the system and the way hydrophobic or hydrophilic are, as well as whether a charged species is present [44].

The bond rotation of rigid species require a higher number of polymer repeats, and there are limitations in the modes of bending, so higher molecular weights is required in order to reach the entanglement regime for the more rigid systems. The closer the molecular weight is to the entanglement molecular weight, the more stable the assembled species [45]. The chemical composition will tell us the ratio of the hydrophilic and hydrophobic components, as well as the degree of polymerization of the collapsed hydrophobic domain.

Yatvin and Weinstein pioneered the concept of temperature-triggered local drug delivery using temperature-sensitive liposomes (TSLs) [46–47]. Here, a chemotherapeutic drug is encapsulated in a heat-sensitive nanovesicle that prevents extravasation of the drug into healthy tissues at physiological temperature. The experiment about temperature-induced drug delivery was performed in small rodents with a subcutaneous tumor on the hind limb where hyperthermia was realized through putting the leg into a water bath [48]. Both tumor tissue and the whole hind limb were found with temperature-induced drug delivery phenomenon. The control of the temperature remained demanding when temperatures were monitored with thermocouples inserted into the tumor. The concept of temperature-triggered drug delivery has been extended to magnetic resonance (MR) image-guided drug delivery by the co-encapsulation of a paramagnetic magnetic resonance imaging (MRI) contrast agent in the lumen of TSLs (Fig. 3) [49].

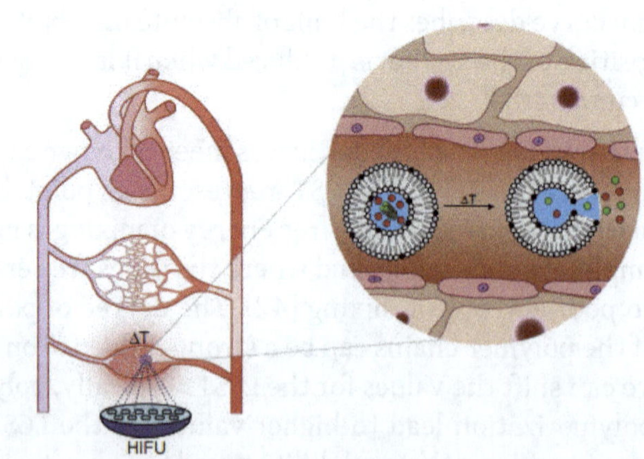

Figure 3. MR image-guided drug delivery illustration of the release of temperature-triggered drug using temperature-sensitive liposomes and HIFU. The co-release of MRI contrast agents from the liposome loaded with temperature-sensitive drug allows to non-invasively visualize and quantify the drug release process [49].

It has been revealed that the external aqueous medium was separated from the liposomal aqueous lumen by a single continuous bilayer of phospholipids that is from the self-assembly of phospholipids into liposomes [50]. These self-assembled structures have been investigated as molecular MRI contrast agents for drug delivery systems. Temperature-sensitive liposomes release encapsulated drugs at the melting phase transition temperature (Tm) of the lipid bilayer (Fig. 3). Structural changes in the lipid membrane occur as it transfers from a gel to the liquid-crystalline phase at transition temperature [51]. In comparison to the liquid-crystalline phase, liposomal membranes in the gel phase are less permeable to water and drugs.

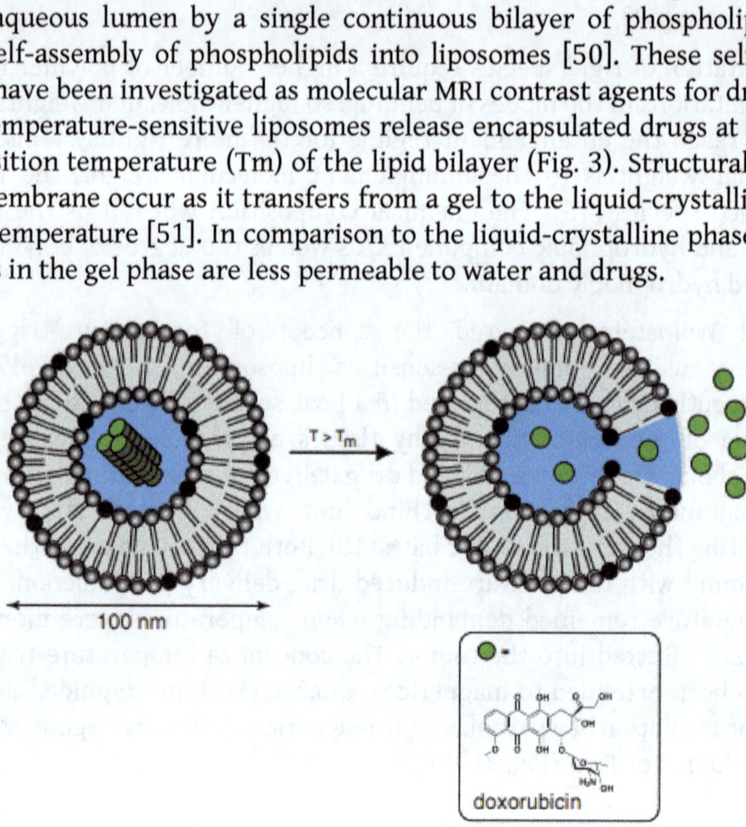

Figure 4. Schematic representation of heat-triggered dox release from TSLs [49].

Various other thermo-responsive functions can be included inside the polymer domain to induce porosity or swelling in a system, alongside NIPAAm, with each system exhibiting a distinct LCST, or in certain instances, an adjustable LCST [52]. The suitable choice of thermo-responsive functionality to achieve the intended behavior is essential. The selection of responsive functionality must ensure that the system is, at a minimum, bioinert to qualify as a contender for a medication delivery system.

2.3. Magnetic-sensitive drug delivery

The stimuli-responsive behavior is dependent on the local physiological environment, such as in both cases of pH and temperature. We could direct the stimuli toward the targeted area of delivery instead of the stimuli-responsive behavior depending on a localized environment. We will adjust the chemical functionality to allow for a relevant response if there is fine control over sources that induce a direct movement including a magnetic field, light, and sound. The response is an attractive or repulsive force relative to the field direction in the case of magnetic materials. Both the material chemical functionality and the viscosity properties of the particle within a physiological system are critical in determining the extent of the response to a magnetic field (Fig. 5) [53–54]. Magnetic particles are typically divided based on size into single-domain and multi-domain particles [55]. The single-domain particles fall in a small size regime, where decreases in size correspond to an increase in coercivity to a peak level before dropping to zero. The zero point identifies a superparamagnetic material, which is one whose magnetic moment is induced in the direction of the applied magnetic field and in the absence of a magnetic field returns to an unaligned state [56].

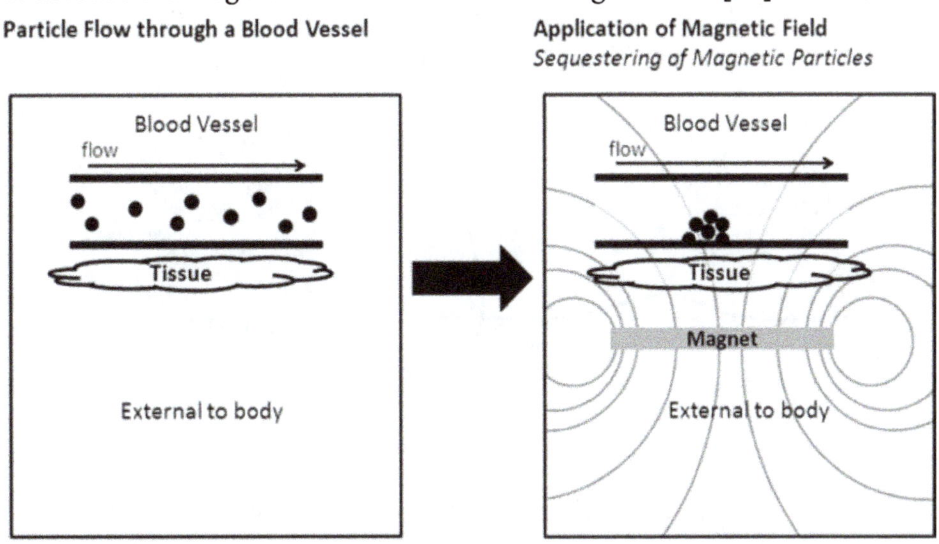

Figure 5. Diagram of the basic forces involved in the sequestration of magnetic nanoparticles in the bloodstream [53].

Similar to thermo-responsive and pH-responsive systems, magneto-responsive materials are systems that respond to an applied stimulus rather than a naturally occurring one. Light and sound are appropriate stimuli for responsive materials [57]. The stimulus is an externally applied magnetic field capable of immobilizing a particle in flow concerning magnetic materials [58]. The design of magnetic materials encompasses various parameters, including particle size, stabilizing agents, atomic composition, and others [59]. Larger magnetic particles have more susceptibility to manipulation by a magnetic field. The stabilizing function of the particle surface is essential for the particle to operate well as a physiological system. The atomic identity pertains to the metallic atoms utilized in the composition of the particles. In the implementation of a magnetic field, emphasis must be given to a single-domain magnetic particle approach for the immobilization of pharmacological entities [60]. The system relies on a diminutive particle system to operate within the superparamagnetic regime. For instance, iron oxide (Fe3O4) systems are employed in which drug species are conjugated to the surface. A larger silica particle system serves as the matrix for these ferromagnetic particles, which are subsequently surface-functionalized with chemically inert groups [60]. Figure 6 presents a schematic representation of the production process for drug-loaded magnetic and fluorescent chitosan nanoparticles [61]. The amino groups of chitosan, including cationic linear polysaccharide molecules, maintain a positive charge under weakly acidic circumstances, resulting in a lengthy and interwoven chain with positive charges along its backbone. The negatively charged aqueous quantum dots, Fe3O4 nanoparticles, and ionized COO- groups of cefradine (pKa = 2.5 and 7.3) along the positive backbone are electrostatically attracted under mildly acidic circumstances [61].

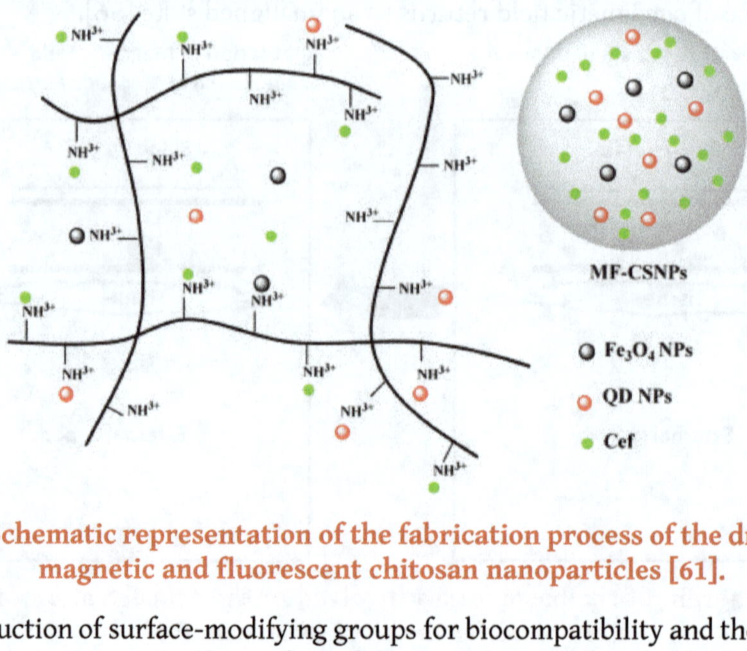

Figure 6. Schematic representation of the fabrication process of the drug-loading magnetic and fluorescent chitosan nanoparticles [61].

The introduction of surface-modifying groups for biocompatibility and the magnitude of the magnetic moment at the surface of the particle are reduced, which may limit its physiological application. Therefore, the design of these immobilized magnetic systems involves three basic factors: particle size (<10 nm), bioinert surface functionalities, and mode of drug incorporation (conjugated or dispersed within matrix) [62]. Magnetic drug delivery systems formed using this design strategy have shown promise for clinical evaluation and treatment of brain tumor patients using a tandem approach involving acoustic and magnetic targeting of tissue across the blood–brain barrier.

The domain choices allow tunable size and magnetic susceptibility for the drug delivery system. This degree of versatility allows for a multitude of surface functionalizations in order to present a drug delivery system that is physiologically bioinert.

2.4. Ultrasound-sensitive drug delivery

Ultrasound technology can induce a self-assembled species to serve as a nucleation location for pore creation in a membrane barrier, hence improving delivery [63]. The process of acoustic droplet vaporization propels a superheated droplet through a phase transition, resulting in the creation of gas micro-bubbles, which then induces membrane pore development by sonoporation [64]. Ultrasound's permeabilizing effects have been utilized in transdermal drug administration for several therapies, including diabetes [65]. Ultrasound has been utilized for the precise disruption of drug carrier vessels, including contrast or acoustically active liposomes, facilitating the release of their therapeutic payload for absorption by target cells (Fig. 7) [66]. Moreover, sonoporation has been linked to gene therapy for the delivery of nonviral plasmid DNA into target cells.

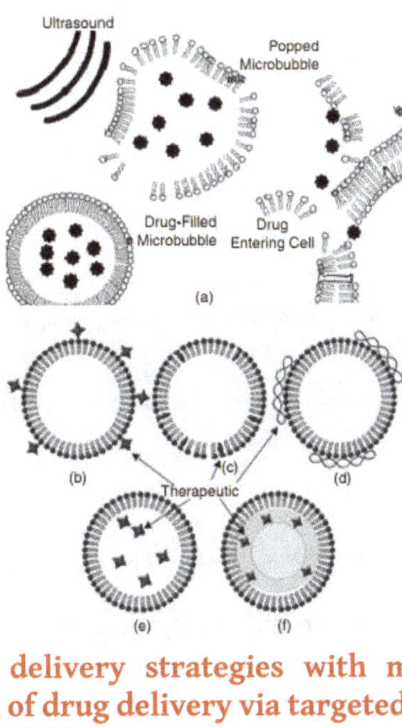

Figure 7. Various drug delivery strategies with micro-bubble carriers. (a) Schematic representation of drug delivery via targeted micro-bubble destruction with ultrasound. Models of different therapeutic agents loading styles, such as the (b) attaching to the micro-bubble membrane, (c) imbedding in the membrane, (d) bonding noncovalently to the micro-bubble surface, (e) packing in the interior of the micro-bubble, and (f) incorporating into an oily film surrounding the micro-bubble [66].

In the case of ultrasound responsive systems, it is required for the stabilization of acoustic cavitation's gas–liquid interface and the compatibility with liquid interface to generate gas bubbles. The primary requirements of the stabilized system are extended circulation lifetime, effective size range, and efficient stimulated release of encapsulated drug via the application of ultrasound [67–68].

The circulation lifetime of the gas microbubbles is associated with the amphiphilic component that stabilizes the interface. We have known that lipid bilayer systems have a significantly short thickness, which offers little stability of microbubbles in vivo in the case of gas–liquid interfaces. Amphiphilic copolymer systems offer a significant improvement to the interfacial membrane stability, while maintaining tunability to drive membrane curvature [69].

It is known that the targeted size of allowing for tumor membrane permeability and gas microbubble stabilization is less than 750 nm. The curvature can be further tuned to form nanobubbles as a preform to merge into microbubble systems at the cell membrane interface. It is an example of improving the stability of the microbubble with no discernible effect to the biological delivery. The energy of the applied ultrasound stimulus can adjust the size regimes and stabilize the desired interfacial curvature effectively (Fig. 8) [70].

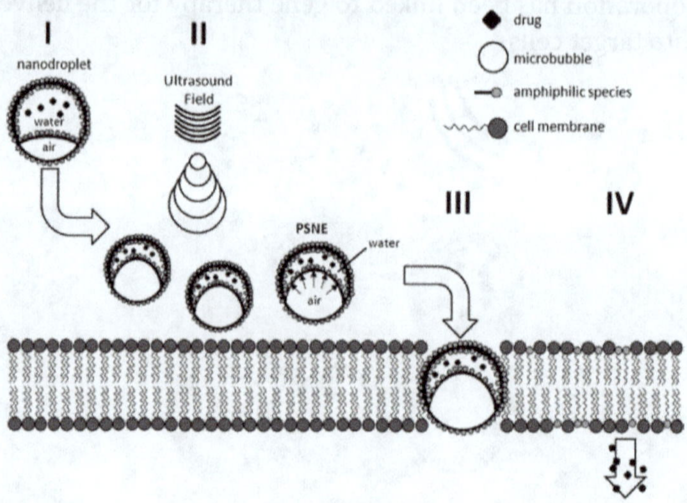

Figure 8. Diagram of the cavitation of PSNE (Phase-Shift Nanoemulsion) nanodroplets from ultrasound [70].

The efficient administration of the adhering medicine is pertinent to echogenicity, defined as the capacity to reflect a signal based on the oscillation, expansion, and contraction of the microbubble system [71]. The echogenicity is influenced by the selection of component mixes, including water and PFP, the surfactant, and the dimensions of the microbubble system. The tendency indicates that enhancing impedance between components and stabilizing high-curvature systems may optimize drug release characteristics in vivo [72].

2.5. Light-sensitive drug delivery

The materials species is influenced by the presence of a specific energy wavelength of light as well as the particle species is influenced by the direction of the magnetic field in magnetic systems. The chemical structure of the drug delivery system destabilizes or changes conformation in response to the absorbed energy input when visible, ultraviolet (UV), or infrared (IR) light is directed at a desired target region. TiO_2 photocatalysts have been mostly used for the purification of air and water by UV light irradiation. However, the limited photocatalytic activity of TiO_2 within the UV range presents difficulties in biomedical and tissue engineering applications owing to the potential harmful effects of UV light. In this part, we focused on the extension of the photocatalytic activity of TiO_2 to the visible light region by doping nitrogen into the TiO_2 crystal structure, which would allow remote control of antibiotic elution by visible light irradiation [73].

A new delivery system that affords control of the time of drug elution and accurate dosing of antibiotics to the target area is required. TiO_2 nanotubes have been studied predominantly in the field of photocatalysis [74–76], solar cells [77], and biomedical engineering [78–80], because of their excellent photocatalytic activity and biocompatibility. In addition, the high surface area and unique shape of TiO_2 nanotubes make them a promising option for application in drug delivery systems. TiO_2 nanotubes arrays fabricated by electrochemical anodization can be described as a layer of tightly packed, vertically aligned and ordered nanotube structures with hexagonal arrangement, which grow perpendicularly to the Ti surface [81]. Fig. 9A and 9B show illustrations of the chemical cell and the fabrication process of TNTs by electrochemical anodization of Ti. Typical scanning electron microscopy images of prepared TNTs are shown in Fig. 9c, with the top and the cross-sectional views showing nanotubes separated into individual entities featuring closed ends at the bottom side [82].

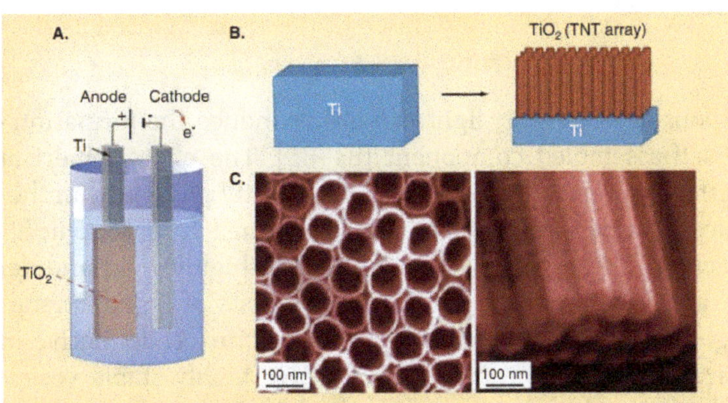

Figure 9. Schematic illustration of TNTs synthesis process and corresponding SEM images of typical morphology and structure. (a) Preparation of TNTs layer by electrochemical cell and anodization process. (b) Formation of self-organized and vertically aligned TNTs on Ti substrate. (c) SEM images of the typical morphology of TNT structures [82].

Kyung-Suk Moon et al. [83] immobilized Gold nanorods (GNR) at the surface of TiO_2 nanotubes via a grafting technique and investigated on-off drug release triggered by near-IR laser irradiation. In addition, antimicrobial activity was monitored to assess the effectiveness of GNR-grafted TiO_2 nanotubes in allowing remotely controlled drug release by IR laser irradiation. The elution concentrations of tetracycline loaded at the surface of GNR-grafted TiO_2 nanotubes were evaluated after 30 s of IR light irradiation with a near-IR laser. The release concentrations of tetracycline from GNR-grafted TiO_2 nanotubes with IR light irradiation (674.52 ± 169.58 μ μg/mL) were significantly higher than those from other experimental conditions, such as TiO_2 nanotubes with or without IR light irradiation and GNR-grafted TiO_2 nanotubes without IR laser irradiation (Fig. 10) [83].

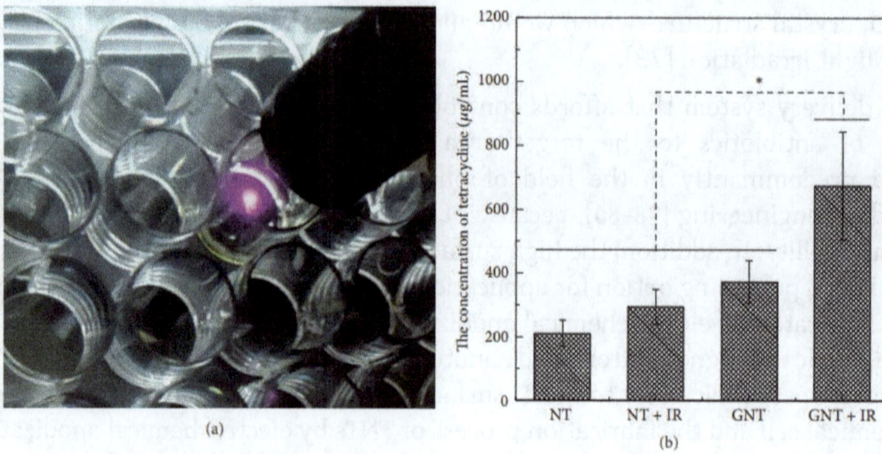

Figure 10. a) Near-IR laser and IR light irradiation and (b) the concentration of tetracycline released by IR light irradiation (NT, NT + IR, GNT, and GNT + IR in the graph designate TiO_2 nanotubes only, near-IR laser irradiated TiO_2 nanotubes, GNR-grafted TiO_2 nanotubes, and near-IR laser irradiated GNR grafted TiO_2 nanotubes, resp.) [83].

For photo-responsive materials, light can either induce the formation of an isomer or degrade a self-assembled component [84–85]. The photoisomerization strategy relies on the effective destabilization of a liquid crystal phase within the hydrophobic domain of micelle or vesicle species that are formed from amphiphilic molecules or macromolecules. The aggregated region will be highly rigid and densely packed in the trans state if the hydrophobic domain consists of liquid crystal groups [86]. The visible light or heat is used to return the structure to its native initial state in photo-isomerization-induced systems that involve highly stable vesicle or micellar self-assembled systems that rapidly reform their densely packed domains.

2.6. Nanoporous engineered drug delivery

Recently, nanoporous anodic alumina (NAA) has become one of the most popular self-ordered periodic, porous templates. In general the highly developed, superior ordering of nanopores in NAA templates is obtained by using a two-step anodization process. NAA has been of great interest due to its outstanding material properties, including electrical insulation, optical transparency, and chemical stability, and most recently, because of its biologically inert and biologically compatibility properties [87]. The use of NAA as a drug delivery platform has been explored in several fields, such as biomedical devices for dental and bone implants, vectors, or carriers for cells transplantion. The suitability of NAA loaded with catalase, endostatin, and vitamin C as sustainable, quasi-linear drug-releasing platform for ophthalmic applications has been demonstrated by Orosz et al. [88].

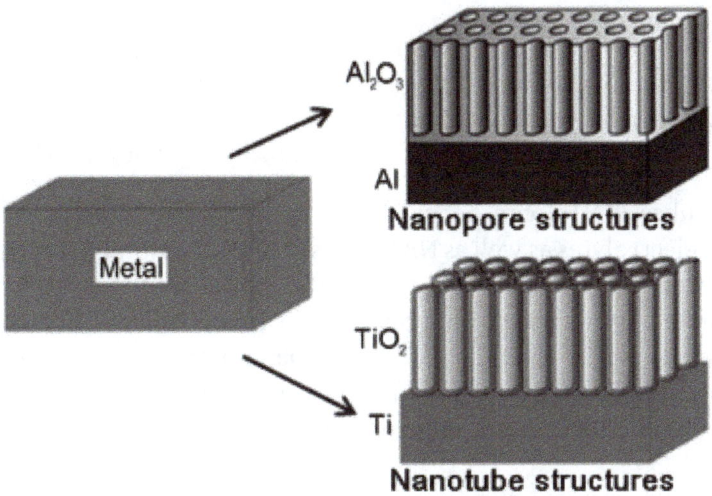

Figure 11. Schematic diagram showing the self-ordering anodization on selected metals (Al and Ti) to produce nanoporous and nanotube metal oxides (Al_2O_3 and TiO_2) with highly-ordered and self-aligning uniform structures. These two materials were explored as non-eroding drug-releasing implants for LDD applications [89].

Depending on the metal type, electrolyte, current, and voltage, two different oxide growth morphologies, such as nanoporous aluminum oxide (Al_2O_3) and nanotube titanium dioxide (TiO_2), can be obtained by a self-ordering electrochemical anodization process as shown in Fig. 11 [89]. The structural features of NAA can be controlled by the anodization parameters, so the functionalities of NAA in terms of pore geometry is an advantage for developing drug-releasing implants as the diffusion of molecules from the nanopores can be tuned by geometry [90]. Jeonet et al. [91] developed a sophisticated system by combining NAA chips with electrically responsive polymers, in which the pore mouths of NAA were modified with polypyrrole doped with dodecylbenzenesulfonate anion (PPy/dB) by electro-polymerization on the upper surface of NAA platforms. The large volume change of that polymeric blend was used to achieve pore mouth actuation by an external electrical stimulus (Fig. 12) [90].

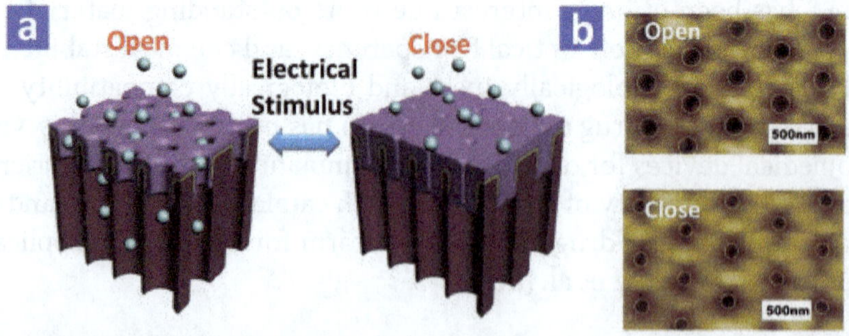

Figure 12. Electrically responsive drug-releasing NAA chip. (a) The mechanism of an electrically responsive drug-releasing chip based on NAA and PPy-DBS (reversible cycle). (b) AFM images of NAA chips before and after the application of electrical stimulus (pore mouth reduction) [90].

Titania nanotubes (TNTs) can be produced by anodizing metallic titanium (Ti) in different acid electrolytes as well as NAA; TNTs feature a nanotube structure during the anodization process (Fig. 13a and b) [92]. Different electrochemical approaches have made it possible to engineer the nanoporous structure of TNTs. TNT-based implants are recognized as one of the most promising nanomaterials to address the inherent drawbacks of conventional systemic drug administration due to their capability to localize the release of drugs over affected bones sites in a controllable manner [91].

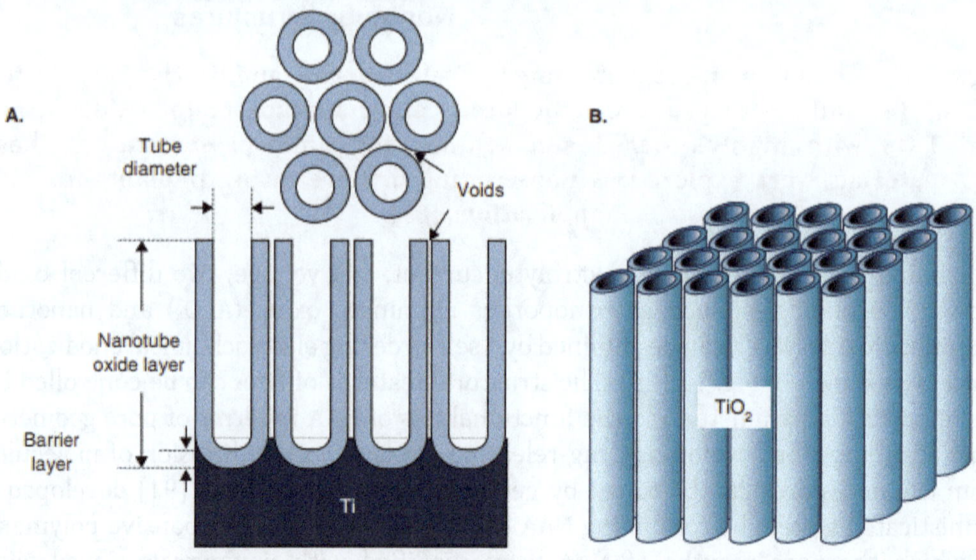

Figure 13. (a) Typical structures of nanotube titania fabricated by electrochemical anodization of titanium, (b) TiO_2 nanotube structures fabricated by electrochemical anodization in NH_4F/ethylene glycol electrolyte showing the cross-sectional image of self-supporting TiO_2 nanotube layer and the entire structure (nanotube film) not detached from Ti substrate (inset) [92].

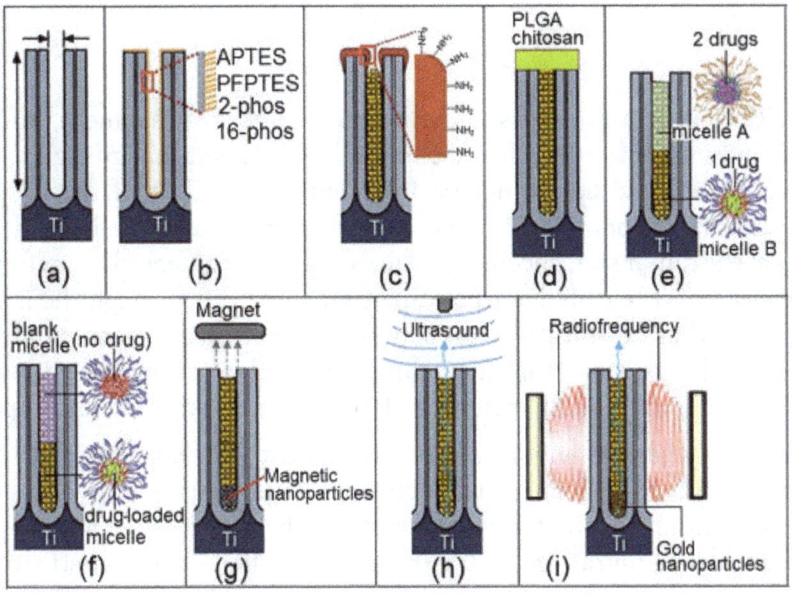

Figure 14. Schematic diagram showing different strategies developed by our group for controlling drug release from drug-releasing implants based on TNTs [90].

In terms of the drug loading and release properties and capabilities of TNTs layers, the drug release from nanotubes is governed by a diffusion process when TNTs come into contact with the physiological milieu inside the host body, as schematically presented in Fig. 14 [90]. The release process is established by the mass transfer of drug molecules from the nanotubes, considering that the drug is completely soluble in the physiological solution without precipitation at particular concentrations. This diffusion-controlled process can be described by Fick's first law, which is governed by a number of factors such as the molecular size and charge of drugs, the diameter and length of nanotubes, their charge and surface chemistry, interfacial interaction between drug molecules and nanotube surface, dissolution rate of drugs, diffusion coefficient, pH, and so on [82].

In addition, the surface charges of TNTs can be rendered hydrophobic or hydrophilic to accommodate a variety of drug molecules should be mentioned. In vitro drug release with the aid of polymeric micelles as drug nano-carriers [93–94] and targeted drug release by means of gold nanoparticles stimulated by radiofrequency field [95] and magnetic nanoparticles under the influence of a magnetic nanoparticles that are under the influence of a magnetic field [96].

Properties of NAA and TNTs that can control drug release but non-degrade in vivo are not suitable for some specific applications, such as drug-releasing implants for treating eye-related diseases [90]. Other nanostructure materials including porous silicon can also be applied to develop biodegradable drug-releasing implants with improved capabilities for definite requirement of clinical applications [91].

3. APPLICATIONS

3.1. Smart micelles for cancer

The methods of utilizing increased permeability, ligand attachment, and selective receptor-ligand interactions could enable micelles to target malignancies. Enhancing drug bioavailability and achieving the intended lethal effect of the drug released from micelle carriers upon reaching the tumor site is crucial. To achieve drug release specifically at the tumor site, micelle structures must be engineered as environmentally responsive systems, typically incorporating functionalities through the introduction of temperature/thermo-sensitive, pH-sensitive, or ultrasound-activated polymers. Micelles, referred to as "smart micelles," can dynamically alter their physical properties in response to external stimuli, including pH, temperature, and chemical species.

The micelle copolymer has an ionizable component, and its stability is pH-dependent due to the sensitivity of the micelles to pH changes. The medication is liberated from the micelle upon exposure to an acidic environment. The pH-sensitive micelles exhibited prolonged residence duration and enhanced half-life characteristic of micellar nanoparticles in animal models. In comparison to non-pH-sensitive micelles, the pH-sensitive micelles demonstrated a favorable effect in malignancies [97]. The potential of pH-sensitive micelles may enhance medication delivery to neoplastic tumors.

A different method for creating environmentally responsive micelles involves including temperature sensitivity into their structure. Localized hyperthermia is therapeutically employed to treat malignancies, as the vasculature of tumors is more susceptible to hyperthermia than that of normal tissue [98]. Temperature-sensitive micelles may be incorporated into a synergistic regimen, wherein elevated temperatures trigger localized medication release and directly eliminate tumor cells. A prevalent technique employs a thermo-sensitive polymer exhibiting LCST behavior to produce temperature-responsive micelles. An elevation in temperature beyond the LCST renders the entire system hydrophobic, resulting in precipitation from the solution.

Ultrasound activation is a crucial approach for site-specific medication release from smart micelles. Various processes may facilitate drug transport, such as localized temperature elevation in tissues, the generation of highly reactive free radical species that can expedite polymer degradation, and cavitation that enhances cell membrane permeability [99]. Ultrasound was used to improve the antitumor efficacy of both free doxorubicin and micelle-encapsulated doxorubicin in which micelles with ultrasound broke tumor growth an additional several days over micelles without ultrasound. Bio-distribution studies revealed that ultrasound not only increased the level of drug accumulation in the tumor, but also lowered the level of drug accumulation in the kidneys and heart [100–101]. Ultrasound-sensitive micelles may reduce adverse effects and enhance the efficacy of chemotherapy in tumor treatment.In summary, micelles can be activated by altering temperature, pH, ultrasound, and light exposure. Optimally engineered micellar biomaterials for medication delivery may reduce cancer mortality.

3.2. Ultrasound-sensitive drug delivery for theranostics

Ultrasound is an exceptionally valuable technique for advanced therapies that is already extensively utilized in clinical practice. Furthermore, ultrasound-activated drug delivery systems can be integrated with ultrasound contrast agents or microbubbles to develop "theranostics," which merge diagnostic imaging with therapeutic drug delivery [102]. Ultrasound-activated theranostics can enhance the identification and management of malignant tumors and cardiovascular conditions, including atherosclerotic plaque [102].

Ultrasound-triggered theranostics has been shown to be an effective method for cancer treatment. Doxorubicin-loaded micelles and doxorubicin-loaded microbubbles were intravenously administered to mice with breast cancer tumors, allowing visualization of the agents at the tumor site via ultrasound, followed by degradation through ultrasound to release doxorubicin at the tumor location. Ultrasound augmented the intracellular absorption of doxorubicin by neoplastic cells, leading to the regression of breast tumors in a murine model. These findings may substantially influence the treatment of additional malignant tumors by ultrasound-assisted imaging and pharmacological administration.

Ultrasound-activated medication delivery systems can concurrently identify regions necessitating treatment and direct drug administration to these locations. Smart materials are at the nascent phase of development but possess the potential to facilitate rational disease treatment, enhance clinical results, and improve the quality of life for patients with complex chronic conditions.

3.3. Nanoporous implants for localized pharmacological administration

TNTs are an alternative technology capable of resolving some issues in dentistry, as it is a cost-effective solution that can be readily integrated into dental implants [82]. The application of TNT-based delivery systems can also be broadened to encompass regenerative medicine and dentistry, as well as preventive therapy. A comprehensive examination of various factors pertinent to TNT applications in dentistry, encompassing investigations of osteoblast adhesion to TNT surfaces, biocompatibility, the release of specific drugs and silver nanoparticles, and periodontium regeneration through the administration of multiple growth factors that promote osteogenesis (Fig. 15) [82]. TNTs can function as carriers for genes and drug delivery, including growth factors and stem cells, thereby promoting osseointegration and bone regeneration associated with dental implants [103].

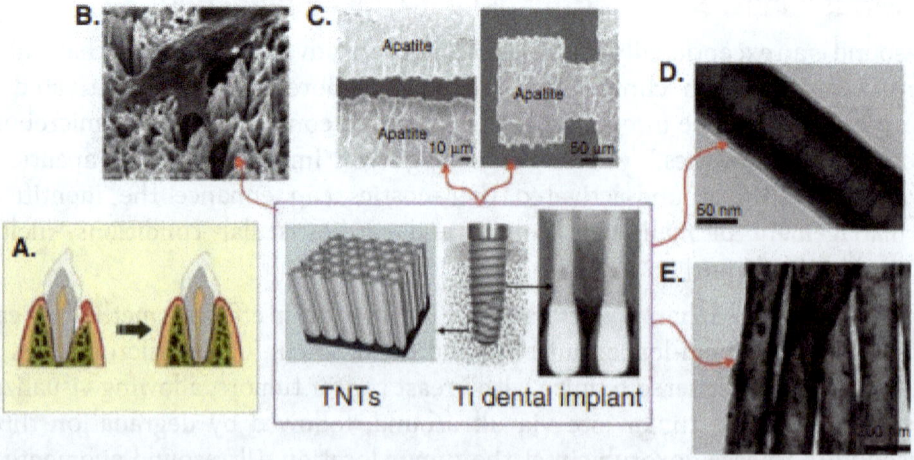

Figure 15. Schematic diagram summarizing the applications of TNTs in dentistry. (a) Periodontium problem and proposed regeneration by delivery of multiple growth factors inducing osteogenesis, (b) the adhesion of osteoblast cells to TNTs surface, (c) the growth of hydroxyapatite on TNTs, (d) the cross-sectional view of a single TNT revealing the drug sodium naproxen on the inside, and (e) anti-bacterial silver nanoparticles incorporated within TNT [82].

The encapsulation of sensitive pharmaceuticals in nano-carriers, such as polymer micelles, was conducted within TNTs. Aw et al. proposed a possible approach to safeguard sensitive medicines and proteins from degradation while designing TNT-based drug-releasing systems with enhanced release capabilities [93]. Moreover, utilizing multi-drug payloads, polymeric micelles containing various pharmaceuticals were incorporated into the TNTs, which are constructed from two or more immiscible layers of drug carriers exhibiting contrasting interfacial properties of hydrophobicity and hydrophilicity, designed to facilitate a series of temporally controlled sequential releases [104].

The aforementioned studies corroborated that NAAs and TNTs are capable of loading and releasing a diverse array of medicines, with the potential to modulate their drug release properties and facilitate the simultaneous release of several medications in various manners. These methodologies are designed to attain optimal drug dosage, release rate, and duration required for a wide array of specialized therapy. The design of triggered drug release from NAAs and TNTs utilizing diverse external signaling sources (thermal, magnetic, electromagnetic, acoustic, or mechanical activation) is a remarkable attribute that presents significant prospects for integrating NAAs and TNTs with sensing capabilities. NAAs and TNTs demonstrate significant versatility in biomedical applications, serving as innovative smart implants and drug-delivery systems.

4. CONCISE SUMMARY

The utilization of smart materials for targeted medication release in specific physiological environments is a highly advantageous strategy for effective therapeutic treatment. We have examined the essential characteristics and materials design pertinent to five stimuli-responsive systems: pH, temperature, magnetism, sound, and light. Stimuli-responsive systems are categorized as "smart" materials, each incorporating two primary principles for material design. Drawing from our prior understanding of degradation, release, and self-assembly, we propose novel ideas of excitation, cavitation, and magnetophoresis for material design techniques. The chapter delineated a collaborative approach using magnetophoresis, thermal phase transition, and certain conceptual methodologies for light excitation. Numerous smart material systems are presently undergoing clinical development, including ultrasound and magnetic hyperthermia systems, for cancer treatment. Research has demonstrated that drug-releasing systems exhibit superior capabilities and efficacy compared to traditional therapies, presenting alternative methods for the effective delivery of therapeutics throughout various regions of the host body while minimizing the adverse effects linked to high dosages of highly toxic medications. Notwithstanding the aforementioned results, further comprehensive study is necessary to render drug-releasing implants viable for clinical applications. It is essential to emphasize that integrating localized drug-releasing systems with conventional treatments like surgery, radiation, and systemic chemotherapy may yield more effective clinical therapies for addressing the most formidable and resilient diseases, such as cancer, while minimizing adverse effects. Furthermore, the anticipated integration of TNT implants with sensors, microchips, and the advancement of sophisticated triggered medication release mechanisms is predicted to materialize in the future. In conclusion, the utilization of smart materials to investigate the drug delivery system is appropriate, and the design of these materials encompasses many stimuli-responsive systems, including pH, temperature, magnetic, light, and sound. Furthermore, smart material systems are presently undergoing diverse phases of clinical development utilizing ultrasound and magnetic hyperthermia technologies for cancer treatment.

REFERENCES

1. L. Li, D. Chen, Y. Zhang, Z. Deng, X. Ren, X. Meng, F. Tang, J. Ren, L. Zhang, Magnetic and fluorescent multifunctional chitosan nanoparticles as a smart drug delivery system, Nanotechnology, 2007, 18(40): 405012.
2. N. Doshi, S. Mitragotri, Designer biomaterials for nanomedicine, Advanced Functional Materials, 2009, 19(24): 3843–3854.
3. V. Thiviyanathan, A. D. Somasunderam, D. G. Gorenstein, Combinatorial selection and delivery of thioaptamers, Biochemical Society Transactions, 2007, 35(1): 50–52.
4. Y. Y. Song, F. Schmidt-Stein, S. Bauer, P. Schmuki, Amphiphilic TiO2 nanotube arrays: An actively controllable drug delivery system, Journal of the American Chemical Society, 131(12): 4230–4232.
5. S. Ghosh, C. Yang, T. Cai, Z. Hu, A. Neogi, Oscillating magnetic field-actuated microvalves for micro- and nanofluidics, Journal of Physics D: Applied Physics, 2009, 42(13): 135501.

6. M. Hrubý, C. Konák, K. Ulbrich, Polymeric micellar pH-sensitive drug delivery system for doxorubicin, Journal of Controlled Release, 2005, 103(1): 137–148.
7. A. Yudina, M. de Smet, M. Lepetit-Coiffé, S. Langereis, L. Van Ruijssevelt, P. Smirnov, V. Bouchaud, P. Voisin, H. Grüll, C. T. Moonen, Ultrasound-mediated intracellular drug delivery using microbubbles and temperature-sensitive liposomes, Journal of Controlled Release, 2011, 155(3): 442–448.
8. X. Y. Li, X. L. Zheng, X. W. Wei, G. Guo, M. L. Gou, C. Y. Gong, X. Huo, D. M. Wang, L. J. Chen, Y. Q. Wei, Z. Y. Qian, A novel composite drug delivery system: Honokiol nanoparticles in thermosensitive hydrogel based on chitosan, Journal of Nanoscience and Nanotechnology, 2009, 9(7): 4586–4592.
9. J. L. Zhang, R. S. Srivastava, R. D. K. Misra, Core-shell magnetite nanoparticles surface encapsulated with smart stimuli-responsive polymer: Synthesis, characterization, and LCST of viable drug-targeting delivery system, Langmuir, 2007, 23(11): 6342–6351.
10. A. Ito, M. Shinkai, H. Honda, T. Kobayashi, Medical application of functionalized magnetic nanoparticles, Journal of Fermentation Technology, 2005, 100(1): 1–11.
11. M. Shinkai, Functional magnetic particles for medical application, Journal of Bioscience and Bioengineering, 2002, 94: 600–613.
12. A. K. Gupta, M. Gupta, Synthesis and surface engineering of iron oxide nanoparticles for biomedical applications, Biomaterials, 2005, 26(18): 3995–4021.
13. S. Mornet, S. Vasseur, F. Grasset, P. Veverka, G. Goglio, A. Demourgues, J. Portier, E. Pollert, E. Duguet, Magnetic nanoparticle design for medical applications, Progress in Solid State Chemistry, 2006, 34(2–4): 237–247.
14. J. Zhang, R. D. K. Misra, Magnetic drug-targeting carrier encapsulated with thermosensitive smart polymer: Core-shell nanoparticle carrier and drug release response, Acta Biomaterialia, 2007, 3(6): 838–850.
15. S. Mornet, S. Vasseur, F. Grasset, E. Duguet, Magnetic nanoparticle design for medical diagnosis and therapy, Journal of Materials Chemistry, 2004, 14(14): 2161–2175.
16. K. D. Harris, R. Cuypers, P. Scheibe, C. L. van Oosten, C. W. M. Bastiaansen, J. Lub, D. J. Broer, Large amplitude light-induced motion in high elastic modulus polymer actuators, Journal of Materials Chemistry, 2005, 15(47): 5043–5048.
17. S. Juodkazis, N. Mukai, R. Wakaki, A. Yamaguchi, S. Matsuo, H. Misawa, Reversible phase transitions in polymer gels induced by radiation forces, Nature, 2000, 408(6809): 178–181.
18. C. S. Kwok, P. D. Mourad, L. A. Crum, B. D. Ratner, Self-assembled molecular structures as ultrasonically-responsive barrier membranes for pulsatile drug delivery, Journal of Biomedical Materials Research, 2001, 57(2): 151–164.
19. R. Fernández-Urrusuno, P. Calvo, C. Remuñán-López, J. L. Vila-Jato, M. J. Alonso, Enhancement of nasal absorption of insulin using chitosan nanoparticles, Pharmaceutical Research, 1999, 16(10): 1576–1581.
20. O. Kayser, A. Lemke, N. Hernandez-Trejo, The impact of nanobiotechnology on the development of new drug delivery systems, Current Pharmaceutical Biotechnology, 2005, 6(1): 3–5.
21. V. L. Colvin, M. C. Schlamp, A. P. Alivisatos, Light-emitting diodes made from cadmium selenide nanocrystals and a semiconducting polymer, Nature, 1994, 370(6488): 354–357.
22. C. C. Müller-Goymann, Physicochemical characterization of colloidal drug delivery systems such as reverse micelles, vesicles, liquid crystals and nanoparticles for topical administration, European Journal of Pharmaceutics & Biopharmaceutics, 2004, 58(2): 343–356.

23. R. Haag, Supramolecular drug-delivery systems based on polymeric core-shell architectures, Angewandte Chemie International Edition, 2004, 43(3): 278–282.
24. D. Losic, S. Simovic, Self-ordered nanopore and nanotube platforms for drug delivery applications, Expert Opinion on Drug Delivery, 2009, 6(12): 1363–1381.
25. D. Losic, M. S. Aw, A. Santos, K. Gulati, M. Bariana, Titania nanotube arrays for local drug delivery: Recent advances and perspectives, Expert Opinion on Drug Delivery, 2015, 12(1): 103–127.
26. K. Noh, K. S. Brammer, C. Choi, S. H. Kim, C. J. Frandsen, S. Jin, A new nano-platform for drug release via nanotubular aluminum oxide, Journal of Biomaterials and Nanobiotechnology, 2011, 2(3): 226–233.
27. K. Shimizu, H. Fujita, E. Nagamori, Oxygen plasma-treated thermoresponsive polymer surfaces for cell sheet engineering, Biotechnology and Bioengineering, 2010, 106(2): 303–310.
28. J. F. Mano, Stimuli-responsive polymeric systems for biomedical applications, Advanced Engineering Materials, 2008, 10(6): 515–527.
29. J. F. Joanny, L. Leibler, Weakly charged polyelectrolytes in a poor solvent, Journal de Physique, 1990, 51(6): 545–557.
30. D. Andelman, J. F. Joanny, Polyelectrolyte adsorption, Comptes Rendus de l'Académie des Sciences-Series IV-Physics, 2000, 1(9): 1153–1162.
31. J. L. Zhang, R. S. Srivastava, R. D. K. Misra, Core-Shell Magnetite Nanoparticles Surface Encapsulated with Smart Stimuli-Responsive Polymer: Synthesis, Characterization, and LCST of Viable Drug-Targeting Delivery System, Langmuir, 2007, 23(11): 6342–6351.
32. Y. Goto, L. J. Calciano, A. L. Fink, Acid-induced folding of proteins, Proceedings of the National Academy of Sciences, 1990, 87(2): 573–577.
33. M. Schmidt (Ed.), Polyelectrolytes with defined molecular architecture II (Google eBook) (p. 231), Springer: Heidelberg, 2004.
34. M. R. Bohmer, O. A. Evers, J. M. H. M. Scheutjens, Weak polyelectrolytes between two surfaces: Adsorption and stabilization, Macromolecules, 1990, 23(8): 2288–2301.
35. G. M. Cooper, The cell: A molecular approach (2nd ed.), Sunderland, MA: Sinauer Associates, 2000.
36. E. G. Bellomo, M. D. Wyrsta, L. Pakstis, D. J. Pochan, T. J. Deming, Stimuli-responsive polypeptide vesicles by conformation-specific assembly, Nature Materials, 2004, 3(4): 244–248.
37. S. K. De, N. R. Aluru, B. Johnson, W. C. Crone, D. J. Beebe, J. Moore, Equilibrium swelling and kinetics of pH-responsive hydrogels: Models, experiments, and simulations, Journal of Microelectromechanical Systems, 2002, 11(5): 544–555.
38. R. M. Sawant, J. P. Hurley, S. Salmaso, A. Kale, E. Tolcheva, T. S. Levchenko, V. P. Torchilin, "SMART" drug delivery systems: Double-targeted pH-responsive pharmaceutical nanocarriers, Bioconjugate Chemistry, 2006, 17(4): 943–949.
39. R. H. Kaul (Ed.), Aqueous two-phase systems: Methods and protocols, New York: Humana Press, 2000.
40. J. W. Cahn, On spinodal decomposition, Acta Metallurgica, 1961, 9(9): 795–801.
41. G. Charlet, G. Delmas, Thermodynamic properties of polyolefin solutions at high temperature: 1. Lower critical solubility temperatures of polyethylene, polypropylene and ethylene-propylene copolymers in hydrocarbon solvents, Polymer, 1981, 22(9): 1181–1189.

42. N. T. Southall, K. A. Dill, A. D. J. Haymet, A view of the hydrophobic effect, The Journal of Physical Chemistry B, 2002, 106(3): 521–533.
43. K. Kita-Tokarczyk, J. Grumelard, T. Haefele, W. Meier, Block copolymer Vesicles-Using concepts from polymer chemistry to mimic biomembranes, Polymer, 2005, 46(11): 3540–3563.
44. A. Shavit, R. A. Riggleman, Influence of backbone rigidity on nanoscale confinement effects in model glass-forming polymers, Macromolecules, 2013, 46(12): 5044–5052.
45. H. Aranda-Espinoza, H. Bermudez, F. S. Bates, D. E. Discher, Electromechanical limits of polymersomes, Physical Review Letters, 2001, 87(20): 208301.
46. M. B. Yatvin, J. N. Weinstein, W. H. Dennis, R. Blumenthal, Design of liposomes for enhanced local release of drugs by hyperthermia, Science, 1978, 202(4374): 1290–1293.
47. J. N. Weinstein, R. L. Magin, M. B. Yatvin, D. S. Zaharko, Liposomes and local hyperthermia-selective delivery of methotrexate to heated tumors, Science, 1979, 204(4389): 188–191.
48. G. Kong, G. Anyarambhatla, W.P. Petros, R.D. Braun, O.M. Colvin, D. Needham, M.W. Dewhirst, Efficacy of liposomes and hyperthermia in a human tumor xenograft model: Importance of triggered drug release, Cancer Research, 2000, 60(24): 6950–6957.
49. M. de Smet, E. Heijman, S. Langereis, N. M. Hijnen, H. Grüll, Magnetic resonance imaging of high intensity focused ultrasound mediated drug delivery from temperature-sensitive liposomes: An in vivo proof-of-concept study, Journal of Controlled Release, 2011, 150(1): 102–110.
50. A. D. Bangham, R. W. Horne, Negative staining of phospholipids and their structural modifications by surface active agents as observed in electron microscope, Journal of Molecular Biology, 1964, 8(5): 660–668.
51. E. Evans, D. Needham, Physical-properties of surfactant bilayer-membranes-thermal transitions, elasticity, rigidity, cohesion, and colloidal interactions, Journal of Physical Chemistry B, 1987, 91(16): 4219–4228.
52. M. A. Ward, T. K. Georgiou, Thermoresponsive polymers for biomedical applications, Polymers, 2011, 3(3): 1215–1242.
53. Y. Zhang, N. Kohler, M. Zhang, Surface modification of superparamagnetic magnetite nanoparticles and their intracellular uptake, Biomaterials, 2002, 23(7): 1553–1561.
54. P. A. Voltairas, D. I. Fotiadis, L. K. Michalis, Hydrodynamics of magnetic drug targeting, Journal of Biomechanics, 2002, 35(6): 813–821.
55. J. Gittleman, B. Abeles, S. Bozowski, Superparamagnetism and relaxation effects in granular Ni-SiO_2 and Ni-Al_2O_3 films, Physical Review B, 1974, 9(9): 3891–3897.
56. A. Aharoni, Introduction to the theory of ferromagnetism, Oxford: Oxford University Press, 2000.
57. K. Kataoka, C. Scholz, N. Rapoport, Physical stimuli-responsive polymeric micelles for anti-cancer drug delivery, Progress in Polymer Science, 2007, 32(8): 962–990.
58. A. Senyei, K. Widder, G. Czerlinski, Magnetic guidance of drug-carrying microspheres, Journal of Applied Physics, 1978, 49(6): 3578-3583.
59. G. P. Hatch, R. E. Stelter, Magnetic design considerations for devices and particles used for biological high-gradient magnetic separation (HGMS) systems, Journal of Magnetism and Magnetic Materials, 2001, 225(1): 262–276.
60. S. Gómez-Lopera, R. Plaza, A. Delgado, Synthesis and characterization of spherical magnetite/biodegradable polymer composite particles, Journal of Colloid and Interface Science, 2001, 240(1): 40–47.

61. L. Li, D. Chen, Y. Zhang, Z. Deng, X. Ren, X. Meng, F. Tang, J. Ren, L. Zhang, Magnetic and fluorescent multifunctional chitosan nanoparticles as a smart drug delivery system, Nanotechnology, 2007, 18(40): 405102.

62. M. Mitsumori, M. Hiraoka, T. Shibata, Y. Okuno, Y. Nagata, Y. Nishimura, Targeted hyperthermia using dextran magnetite complex: A new treatment modality for liver tumors, Hepato-gastroenterology, 1996, 43(12): 1431–1437.

63. C. X. Deng, F. Sieling, H. Pan, J. Cui, Ultrasound-induced cell membrane porosity, Ultrasound in Medicine & Biology, 2004, 30(4): 519–526.

64. H. Pan, Y. Zhou, F. Sieling, J. Shi, J. Cui, C. Deng, Sonoporation of cells for drug and gene delivery, In Proceedings of the Annual International Conference of the IEEE Engineering in Medicine and Biology Society. 2004, 5: 3531–3534.

65. P. Zhang, T. Porter, An in vitro study of a phase-shift nanoemulsion: A potential nucleation agent for bubble-enhanced HIFU tumor ablation, Ultrasound in Medicine & Biology, 2010, 36 (11): 1856–1866.

66. E. C. Pua, P. Zhong, Ultrasound-mediated drug delivery, IEEE Engineering in Medicine and Biology, 2009, 28(1): 64–75.

67. J. Du, R. K. O'Reilly, Advances and challenges in smart and functional polymer vesicles, Soft Matter, 2009, 5 (19): 3544–3550.

68. G. Bajic, L. Yatime, R. B. Sim, T. Vorup-Jensen, G. R. Andersen, Structural insight on the recognition of surface-bound opsonins by the integrin I domain of complement receptor 3, Proceedings of the National Academy of Sciences of the United States of America, 2013, 110(41): 16426-16431.

69. S. R. Sirsi, M. A. Borden, Microbubble compositions, properties and biomedical applications, Bubble Science Engineering and Technology, 2012, 1(1–2): 3–17.

70. E. Y. Lukianova-Hleb, X. Ren, J. A. Zasadzinski, X. Wu, D. O. Lapotko, Plasmonic nanobubbles enhance efficacy and selectivity of chemotherapy against drugresistant cancer cells, Advanced Materials, 2012, 24(28): 3831–3837.

71. S. D. Tiukinhoy-Laing, S. Huang, M. Klegerman, C. K. Holland, D. D. McPherson, Ultrasound-facilitated thrombolysis using tissue-plasminogen activator-loaded echogenic liposomes, Thrombosis Research, 2007, 119(6): 777–784.

72. A. Mueller, B. Bondurant, D. F. O'Brien, Visible-light-stimulated destabilization of PEG-liposomes, Macromolecules, 2000, 33(13): 4799–4804.

73. S. Oh, K. S. Moon, J. H. Moon, J. M. Bae, S. Jin, Visible light irradiation-mediated drug elution activity of nitrogen-doped TiO_2 nanotubes, Journal of Nanomaterials, 2013, 2013: 802318.

74. H. F. Zhuang, C. J. Lin, Y. K. Lai, L. Sun., J. Li, Some critical structure factors of titanium oxide nanotube array in its photocatalytic activity, Environmental Science & Technology, 2007, 41(13): 4735–4740.

75. M. Paulose, K. Shankar, S. Yoriya, H. E. Prakasam, O. K. Varghese, G. K. Mor, T. A. Latempa, A. Fitzgerald, C. A. Grimes, Anodic growth of highly ordered TiO2 nanotube arrays to 134μm in length, Journal of Physical Chemistry B, 2006, 110(33): 16179-16184.

76. Y. K. Lai, J. Y. Huang, H. F. Zhang, V. P. Subramaniam, Y. X. Tang, D. G. Gong, L. Sundar, L. Sun., Z. Chen, C. J. Lin, Nitrogen-doped TiO2 nanotube array films with enhanced photocatalytic activity under various light sources, Journal of Hazardous Materials, 2010, 184(1–3): 855–863.

77. M. D. Ye, J. J. Gong, Y. K. Lai, C. J. Lin, Z. Q. Lin, High-Efficiency Photoelectrocatalytic Hydrogen Generation Enabled by Palladium Quantum Dots-Sensitized TiO2 Nanotube Arrays, Journal of the American Chemical Society, 2012, 134(38): 15720-15723.

78. M. Bigerelle, K. Anselme, B. Noel, I. Ruderman, P. Hardouin, A. Iost, Improvement in the morphology of Ti-based surfaces: A new process to increase in vitro human osteoblast response, Biomaterials, 2002, 23(7): 1563–1577.

79. Y. K. Lai, L. X. Lin, F. Pan, J. Y. Huang, R. Song, Y. X. Huang, C. J. Lin, H. Fuchs, L. F. Chi, Bioinspired Patterning with Extreme Wettability Contrast on TiO_2 Nanotube Array Surface: A Versatile Platform for Biomedical Applications, Small, 2013, 9(17): 2945–2953.

80. C. G. Galbraith, M. P. Sheetz, Forces on adhesive contacts affect cell function, Current Opinion in Cell Biology, 1998, 10(5): 566–571.

81. A. Ghicov, P. Schmuki, Self-ordering electrochemistry: A review on growth and functionality of TiO2 nanotubes and other self-aligned MOx structures, Chemical Communication, 2009, 20(32): 2791–2808.

82. D. Losic, M. S. Aw, A. Santos, K. Gulati, M. Bariana, Titania nanotube arrays for local drug delivery: Recent advances and perspectives, Expert Opinion on Drug Delivery, 2015, 12(1): 103–127.

83. K. S. Moon, J. M. Bae, S. Jin, S. Oh. Infrared-Mediated Drug Elution Activity of Gold Nanorod-Grafted TiO2 Nanotubes, Journal of Nanomaterials, 2014, 2014: 750813.

84. W. Brown, Thermal fluctuations of a single-domain particle. Physical Review, 1963, 130(5): 1677–1686.

85. P. Shum, J. M. Kim, D. H. Thompson, Phototriggering of liposomal drug delivery systems. Advanced Drug Delivery Reviews, 2001, 53(3): 273–284.

86. K. A. K. Musa, L. A. Eriksson, Photodegradation mechanism of the common nonsteroid anti-inflammatory drug diclofenac and its carbazole photoproduct. Physical Chemistry Chemical Physics, 2009, 11(22): 4601–4610.

87. E. Gultepe, D. Nagesha, S. Sridhar, M. Amiji, Nanoporous inorganic membranes or coatings for sustained drug delivery in implantable devices, Advanced Drug Delivery, 2010, 62(3): 305–315.

88. K. E. Orosz, S. Gupta, M. Hassink, M. Abdel-Rahman, L. Moldovan, F. H. Davidorf, N. I. Moldovan, Delivery of antiangiogenic and antioxidant drugs of ophthalmic interest through a nanoporous inorganic filter, Molecule Vision, 2004, 10(68): 555–565.

89. M. S. Aw, M. Kurian, D. Losic, Non-eroding drug-releasing implants with ordered nanoporous and nanotubular structures: Concepts for controlling drug release, Biomaterials Science, 2014, 2: 10–34.

90. A. Santos, M. S. Aw, M. Bariana, T. Kumeria, Y. Wang, D. Losic. Drug-releasing implants: Current progress, challenges and perspectives, Journal of Materials Chemistry B, 2014, 2: 6157–6182.

91. G. Jeon, S. Y. Yang, J. Byun, J. K. Kim, Electrically actuatable smart nanoporous membrane for pulsatile drug release, Nano Letter, 2011, 11(3): 1284–1288.

92. D. Losic, S. Simovic, Self-ordered nanopore and nanotube platforms for drug delivery applications, Expert Opinion on Drug Delivery, 2009, 6(12):1363–1381.

93. M. S. Aw, S. Simovic, J. Addai-Mensah, D. Losic, Polymeric micelles in porous and nanotubular implants as a new system for extended delivery of poorly soluble drugs, Journal of Materials Chemistry, 2011, 21 (20): 7082–7089.

94. M. S. Aw, K. Gulati, D. Losic, Controlling drug release from titania nanotube arrays using polymer nanocarriers and biopolymer coating, Journal of Biomaterials & Nanobiotechnology, 2011, 2(5): 477–484.

95. M. Bariana, M. S. Aw, E. Moore, N. H. Voelcker and D. Losic, Radiofrequency-triggered release for on-demand delivery of therapeutics from titania nanotube drug-eluting implants, Nanomedicine, 2014, 9(8): 1263–1275.

96. M. S. Aw, J. Addai-Mensah and D. Losic, Magnetic-responsive delivery of drug-carriers using titania nanotube arrays, Journal of Materials Chemistry, 2012, 22(14): 6561–6563.

97. D. Shenoy, S. Little, R. Langer, M. Amiji, Poly(ethylene oxide)-modified poly(betaamino ester) nanoparticles as a pH-sensitive system for tumor-targeted delivery of hydrophobic drugs: Part 2. In vivo distribution and tumor localization studies. Pharmaceutical Research, 2005, 22(12): 2107–2114.

98. J. van der Zee, Heating the patient: A promising approach? Annals of Oncology, 2002, 13(8): 1173–1184.

99. S. Mitragotri, Healing sound: The use of ultrasound in drug delivery and other therapeutic applications, Nature Reviews Drug Discovery, 2005, 4(3): 255–260.

100. A. V. Kabanov, E. V. Batrakova, V. Y. Alakhov, Pluronic block copolymers for overcoming drug resistance in cancer, Advanced Drug Delivery Reviews, 2002, 54(5): 759–779.

101. Z. G. Gao, H. D. Fain, N. Rapoport, Controlled and targeted tumor chemotherapy by micellar-encapsulated drug and ultrasound. Journal of Controlled Release, 2005, 102(1): 203–222.

102. A. T. Nguyen, S. P. Wrenn, Acoustically active liposome-nanobubble complexes for enhanced ultrasonic imaging and ultrasound-triggered drug delivery. Wiley Interdisciplinary Reviews in Nanomedicine and Nanobiotechnology, 2014, 6(3): 316–325.

103. Y. H. Lee, G. Bhattarai, I. S. Park, G. R. Kim, G. E. Kim, M. H. Lee, H. K. Yi, Bone regeneration around N-acetyl cysteine-loaded nanotube titanium dental implant in rat mandible, Biomaterials, 2013, 34(38): 10199–10208.

104. M. S. Aw, J. Addai-Mensah, D. Losic, A multi-drug delivery system with sequential release using titania nanotube arrays, Chemical Communications, 2012, 48(27): 3348–3350.

4 Chapter

ACTIVE-TARGETED NANOTHERAPY AS AN INTELLIGENT CANCER TREATMENT

1. INTRODUCTION: AN OVERVIEW

The primary objective of pharmaceutical scientists and physicians is to optimize the safety and efficacy of pharmacological therapy. Consequently, drug targeting represents the optimal strategy. This topic is essential for certain disorders, such as cancer treatments, which necessitate a delicate equilibrium between the eradication of malignant and healthy tissues, encompassing harm to the immune system and rapidly proliferating cells. Recently developed nanotechnological approaches as active targeted carriers in medical therapy have garnered considerable attention [1–4]. Active targeting entails the conjugation of various ligands, including antibodies, biological proteins, peptides, sugars, and vitamins, or a specific ligand to the medication or drug delivery system, facilitating interaction with cell receptors and promoting drug accumulation within target cells.

Specifically, "targeting" can be categorized into three levels:

- First-order targeting: When the delivery is to a specific organ, for example, drugs may be targeted to the liver because of its leaky or fenestrated vasculature or loose junctions; the drug is not released in other tissues because of their nonleaky vasculature.
- Second-order targeting or cellular targeting: When a drug delivery system releases the drug to a particular cell within an organ or a tissue.
- Third-order or subcellular targeting: When the delivery is to distinct cell types with biological barrier transport, for example, epithelial cells or cells of the lung-associated lymphatic tissue. A good example is the delivery of genes. The delivery system carries the gene, enters specific cells and releases the gene intracellularly. This is the third order and the most sophisticated type of targeting.

Conventional targeting actions can be categorized as passive and active targeting. Drug delivery methods designed as targeted carriers encompass micelles, nanoparticles, polymeric conjugates, and liposomes. Nanoparticles safeguard the pharmaceutical compound against early degradation, inhibit interactions with the biological milieu, and augment the absorption of medications into targeted tissues. Nanoparticle technologies have the potential to augment the therapeutic index of pharmaceuticals by improving their efficacy and/or strengthening their tolerance within the organism. Nanoparticles may enhance the bioavailability of water-insoluble pharmaceuticals, transport substantial payloads, and facilitate the creation of innovative classes of bioactive macromolecules (e.g., DNA and siRNA) [4–8]. To date, more than twenty nanotechnology products have received approval from the US Food and Drug Administration (FDA) for clinical application, with numerous others in clinical and preclinical research.

Our research concentrated on targeted medicine delivery systems derived from nanobiotechnology. Nanoparticles can augment the intracellular concentration of medications in malignant cells by active targeting techniques, including folate, monoclonal antibodies (mAbs), and aptamer ligands, while minimizing toxicity in normal cells. Nanoparticles in bioscience are being actively developed for in vivo tumor imaging, biomolecular profiling of cancer biomarkers, and targeted medication administration. Nanoparticles persist in the bloodstream for an extended duration and might passively concentrate at target locations following systemic delivery due to the permeable tumor vasculature and inadequately developed lymphatic outflow, known as the increased permeation and retention (EPR) effect.In this chapter, we focus on explaining anticancer agents loaded in different nanoparticles and how they could be targeted to different tissues especially to solid tumors by attaching specific ligands [6–8].

2. NANO DRUG DELIVERY

Drug delivery systems such as lipid-, polymer-, liposome-, dendrimeric-, or biomacromolecule-based nanoparticles can be designed to improve the pharmacological and therapeutic properties of drugs administered parenterally or by other routes of administration. There is significant interest in utilizing the benefits of DDS for in vivo administration of novel pharmaceuticals and for their application in targeted therapies. Drug targeting enhances therapeutic efficacy and diminishes the adverse effects linked to pharmaceuticals and therapeutic agents [10–12]. Various carriers can be used to deliver a drug in a stable and protective form for conventional or targeted shape (Figure 1); however, it is nanotechnology that offers the most unique and intriguing approach in the field of nanomedicine.

Nanobiotechnology, characterized by the biomedical applications of nanoscale biomacromolecular systems or nano-sized materials integrated with biomaterials, is an expeditiously advancing field within nanoscience. Nanomedicines are defined as delivery systems inside the nanometer size range (ideally 1–100 nm) that incorporate encapsulated, disseminated, adsorbed, or conjugated pharmaceuticals and imaging agents. They can also promote significant progress in the detection, diagnosis, and treatment of illnesses, human malignancies, and vaccine administration, hence giving rise to a new discipline of nanobiotechnology [13–16]. Nanoparticles are currently under active development for in vivo tumor imaging, biomolecular profiling of cancer biomarkers, and targeted medication administration. Nanotechnology-based approaches can be extensively utilized in the management of several malignant disorders [17, 18].

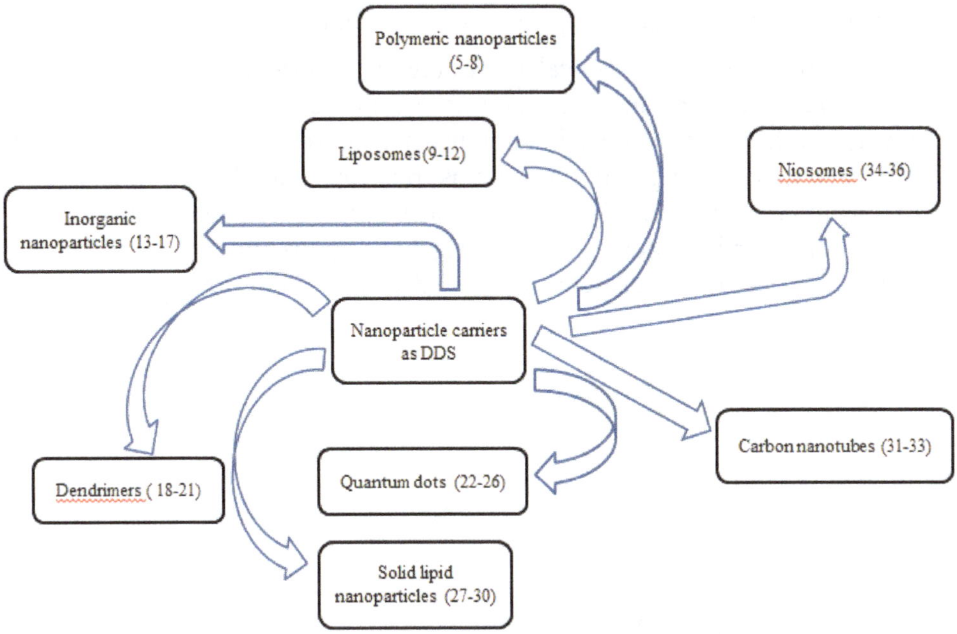

Figure 1. The different types of nanocarriers

Nanocarriers possess various advantages compared to free medicines. They safeguard labile medicines from degradation in biological settings, augment drug uptake in specific tissues such as solid tumors, enable adjustment of pharmacokinetics and biodistribution, and improve intracellular penetration.

Nanotechnology applications in medicine, known as nanomedicine, have integrated many nanoparticles with diverse chemistry and architecture into targeted drug delivery systems. Nanotechnology encompasses the engineering of multifunctional devices at the nanoscale, comparable in size to massive biological molecules, viruses, and other synthetic macromolecules. These devices can transport one or two detecting signals and/or therapeutic substances for targeted drug administration [19, 20]. Nanotechnology is well introduced in drug delivery technology for several advantages such as first passive drug delivery, increasing of drug solubility, increasing of drug half-life in the body, modification of the drug distribution pattern, and improvement of pharmacokinetics, which will result in improved efficacy. With these advantages, the future of drug delivery cannot be predicted and some problems exist such as site cytotoxicity [21–26].

Currently, the fundamental issue with cancer treatment is that they include an exercise in careful control between the destruction of malignant tissue and healthy tissues, such as damage to the immune system and profoundly replicating cells (gastrointestinal epithelia and hair follicles).

It is important to detect the revelation of malignant cells sufficiently early and in a stage that is sensible for convenient treatment. Recently, created nanotechnology drug delivery systems are promising approaches for oncologists.

The use of nanoparticles in medical treatment has increased in recent years. For example, micro- and nanoparticles, such as polymeric nanoparticles (synthetic or natural polymers), polymeric micelles, dendrimer, and solid lipid nanoparticles (SLN) have long been used as drug delivery systems to encapsulate drugs and protect them from extracellular enzymatic degradation, providing vehicles for delivering drugs to the target area, and are now being investigated as powerful platforms for vaccine delivery [27–33]. Figure 2 represents some kind of nanocarrier in drug delivery.

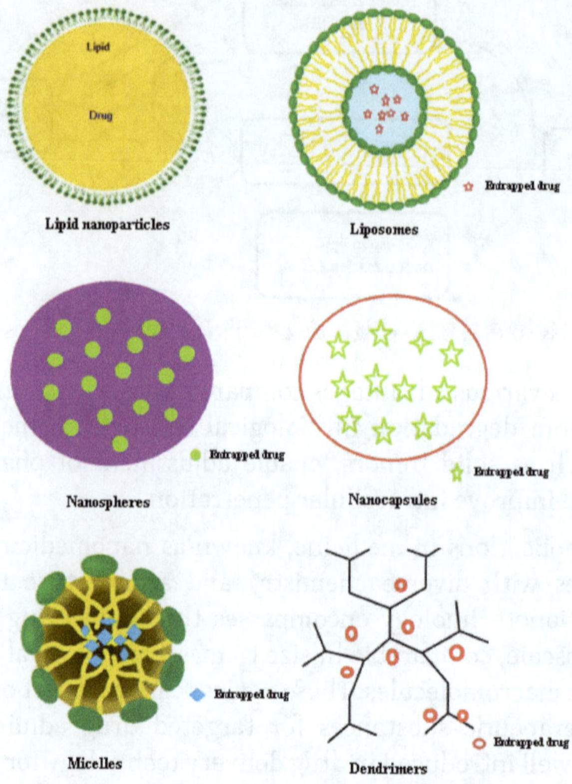

Figure 2. Basic structure of nanoparticles

Being inspired by physiologically existing nanomachines, nanoparticles are designed to safely reach their target and specifically release their therapeutic agent at the site of the disease, thus increasing the drug's tissue bioavailability. Nanoparticles used in this manner for enhanced permeation and retention effect of cancerous cells that are caused by leaky angiogenetic vessels and poor lymphatic drainage has been, in turn, used to explain why macromolecules and nanoparticles are found at higher ratios in tumors compared with normal tissues [29]. Carriers are associated with the drug in a covalent or noncovalent attached mode of targeting materials, and they have been used for the delivery of drug exactly on the target tissue.

In this study, we focus on important nanoparticles such as polymeric nanoparticles and liposomes and their recent results on targeting drug delivery systems for the purpose of biomaterial.

3. BIOCONJUGATION OF NANOCARRIERS FOR TARGET THERAPY

The conjugation of bioagents to nanocarriers is one of the most important functions of the targeted drug delivery system. For this purpose, several methods and works have been performed until now [34–36].

One of the usual methods for attaching biomolecular ligands to nanoparticle's surface is diimide-activated amidation by direct coupling of carboxylic acid to legends using N-ethyl- N-(3-dimethyl aminopropyl) carbodiimide hydrochloride (EDAC) or N,N-dicyclohexyl carbodiimide (DCC) as a coupling agent. The schematic perspective of the connection of proteins to carbon nanotubes (CNTs) by means of diimide-activated amidation is presented in Figure 3. Functionalization of carbon nanotubes was likewise completed using 1-pyrenebutanoic acid, succinimidyl ester for the immobilization of biomolecules, anti-fullerene IgG monoclonal antibody bound to single-wall carbon nanotubes. Proteins and DNA have also been used to modify multiwall carbon nanotubes (MWCNT) [36].

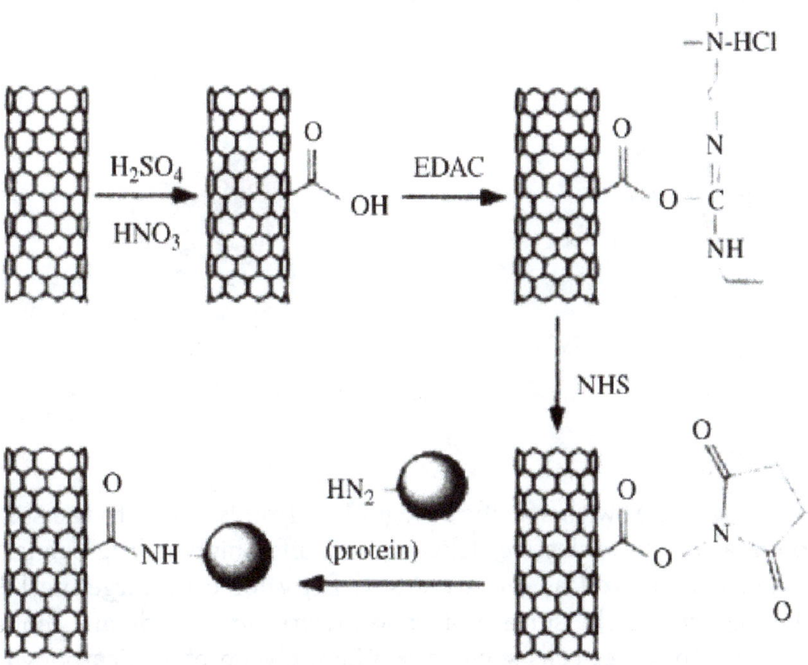

Figure 3. Schematic view of the attachment of proteins to CNTs via diimide activated amidation [51]

Recently, the ubiquitous alkyne–azide Huisgen "click" reaction has been used to attach proteins to NPs (Figure 4). A variety of proteins have been attached in functional form using this method, including lipase, horseradish peroxidase, and luciferase [34]. Hapuarachchige et al. [37] investigated the click reaction for specific internalization of nanotherapeutics. In this study, the pretargeting component, anti-HER2 humanized monoclonal antibody, functionalized with azide groups, labels cancer cells. This group demonstrated high efficacy for targeted nanotherapeutics using the click reaction.

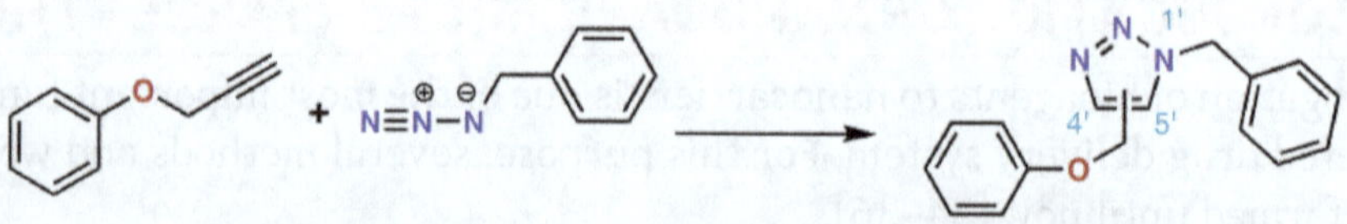

Figure 4. Azide-alkyne Huisgen cycloaddition "click" reaction

The biotin- streptavidin interaction (Figure 5) is widely used for the conjugation of NP systems. The formation of avidin (or streptavidin)–biotin complexes is useful in a wide variety of applications. This specific binding is largely used to immobilize enzymes, antibodies, or DNA. Biotin is a small molecule, which could bind to avidin or streptavidin binding sites with very high affinity (Ka = 10^{15} M^{-1}).

In addition, avidin and streptavidin are tetrameric proteins that have four known binding sites for biotin (Figure 5). Streptavidin with an isoelectric point equivalent to 5 is accordingly ideally utilized over avidin, which has a PI of 10.5, to maintain a strategic distance from nonspecific interactions [35, 38].

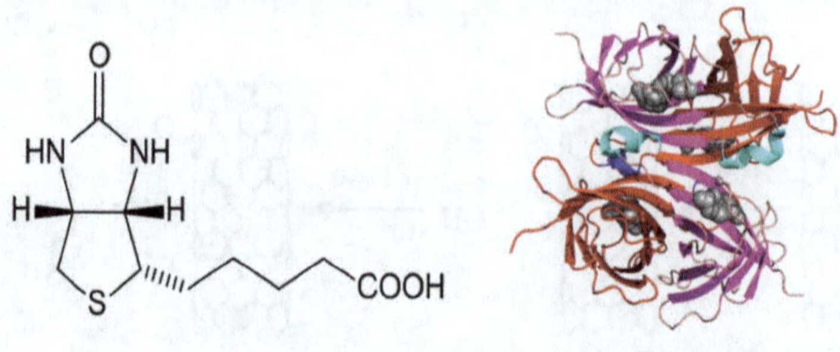

(a) (b)

Figure 5. Biotin structure (a) and the simple graph for biotin-avidine binding (b)

4. ACTIVE TARGETING USING POLYMERIC NANOCARRIER

Polymeric nanoparticles with specific recognition ligands bound to the surface have a good potential for site-selective delivery, and offer higher drug carrier capacity than bioconjugates, as well as improved specificity for drug targeting [1, 39–41]. The attached ligands to the surface of nanocarriers can include any molecule that specifically binds to target cells such as peptides, glycoproteins, carbohydrates and polymers, and monoclonal antibodies, which have been the most broadly studied [20, 24].

Kocbek and coworkers developed new active-targeted poly (D,L-lactic-co-glycolic acid) (PLGA) nanoparticles by attaching mAb, which have the ability to target specific antigens on breast epithelial cancer cell lines. Attempts to attach mAb to nanoparticles by covalent bonding were less successful, since the natural action of the bound mAb was inactivated. The specificity of the immunonanoparticles was shown from their selective distribution in a co-culture of MCF-10A neoT and Caco-2 cells, resulting in their final internalization by the former cells [42].

A novel, nonviral, polyethylenimine (PEI)-based, HER2-targeted gene transfer vector has been investigated. The anti-HER2 humanized antibody, trastuzumab (HerceptinR), was used as the targeting moiety to the HER2 overexpressing cancer cells. Subsequently, trastuzumab conjugation of PEI may render PEI a much more selective gene delivery carrier for anticancer gene therapy. The opinion of attaching a targeting ligand, with intrinsic antitumor activity, to a gene transfer vector may be beneficial for further investigations [43].

Recently, poly (butyl cyanoacrylate) (PBCA) NPs coated with polysorbate-80 have been proposed as suitable drug carriers for brain drug delivery. Nerve growth factor (NGF) is important for the survival of peripheral ganglion cells and central cholinergic neurons of the basal forebrain. In spite of its inability to cross the blood–brain barrier (BBB), the NGF activity on these neuronal populaces and its adequacy in avoiding neurodegeneration recommended its potential utilization in the treatment of neurological pathologies, for example, diabetic neuropathies and Huntington's disease. Systemic administration of NGF loaded in P80-coated PBCA NPs successfully reversed scopolamine-induced amnesia and improved recognition and memory in acute amnesia rat model [44].

Yang and coworkers synthesized doxorubicin magnetic PLGA nanoparticles conjugated with well-tailored antibodies for the detection and therapy of breast cancer. They suggested that magnetic nanocrystals embedded in polymeric nanoparticles did not inhibit the nanoparticle formulation or drug release kinetics. The multimodal nanoparticles demonstrated remarkable cancer cell affinity and ultrasensitivity via magnetic resonance imaging. However, the in vivo effects of the NPs were not evaluated [45].

Due to the overexpression of the folate receptor on tumor surface, the folate has been popularly used as a targeting moiety for various anticancer agents to avoid their nonspecific attacks on normal tissues and also to increase their cellular uptake within target cells [46–48]. Derakhshandeh et al. prepared the folate-decorated biodegradable PLGA nanoparticles for tumor targeting. In this study, folate-conjugated PLGA was synthesized and then PLGA-Fol nanoparticles were prepared by nanoprecipitation method, adopting PLGA as a drug carrier, folic acid (FA) as a targeting ligand, and 9-nitrocampthotecin (9-NC) as an anticancer drug model. The in vitro intracellular uptake of nanoparticles showed that the PLGA-Fol nanoparticles have been more efficiently taken up by MCF-7 cells compared with nonfolate-mediated carriers, and also showed greater cytotoxicity than other treated groups [49].

Active-targeted nanocarriers to the special sites and cellular uptake are especially important to therapeutics that is not taken up easily by cells, and they require facilitation by fusion, endocytosis, or other processes to access their cellular active sites. They can also enhance the penetration and distribution of nanomedicine within the tumor interstitium and resistant cancer cells. Active targeting nanocarriers have various points of interest over targeting ligand–drug conjugates [47].

Recently, Wu et al. [50] investigated polymeric nanoparticles for the treatment of metastases. This group studied the ability of micellar nanocarriers incorporating (1,2-diaminocyclohexane) platinum(II) for liver metastases of bioluminescent murine colon adenocarcinoma C-26 treatment, during overt and preangiogenic metastatic stages and thus obtained a novel approach for early diagnosis and treatment of metastases.

5. INORGANIC NANOPARTICLES FOR TARGETED DRUG DELIVERY

Porous inorganic nanoparticles with high specific surface area have recently emerged as attractive material for the development of delivery systems, where various guest molecules could be absorbed into the pores and later released into various solutions [51, 52].

Inorganic nanoparticles, for example, gold and iron oxide, are usually conjugated with the drug, polyethylene glycol (PEG), and the targeting ligands. It gives the idea that the PEG coating and ligand design are common constituents in most types of nanoparticles for anticancer delivery. These carriers have several applications in cancer diagnosis and treatment, and large portions of them have quickly moved into clinical trials. Overall, there is still a space for optimization in the field of nanoparticle pharmacokinetics such as enhanced plasma retention time and tumor bioavailability and understanding the effectiveness of targeting ligands in the cancer treatment. The need to add to a novel and productive legand has never been more noteworthy, and the use of proper conjugation chemistry is essential [20].

Recently, Zhou et al. prepared a surface engineered of NaGd F4:Ce/Tb hybrid nanoparticles with DNA for new type of pH-responsive therapeutic platform to enhance the therapeutic efficiency while minimizing side effects. The introduction of the layer of aptamer molecule on the surface facilitated the cellular uptake of the resulting nanocomposite into specific target cells via receptor-mediated endocytosis. This group proved that the hybrid nanocarrier may serve as a practical and multifunctional probe for cancer therapy [53].

6. LIPOSOMES IN TARGETED MEDICATION DELIVERY

The dispersion of neutral phospholipids or amphiphilic lipids (such as cholesterol and glycolipids) in an aqueous solution results in the creation of closed vesicular structures that morphologically resemble cells. These enclosed vesicles are referred to as "Liposomes" [54] (fat bodies) and are composed of hydrated bilayers. Liposomes can replicate cell membrane structures and have the capacity to encapsulate hydrophilic substances in the aqueous core or to include lipophilic substances within the lipid bilayer. Preliminary investigations on the behavior of liposomes and encapsulated substances commenced around 1970 [55].

In 1974, Gregoriadis advocated for the use of liposomes as drug carriers in cancer chemotherapy, and subsequently, interest in liposomes has surged, with significant focus on their application as drug carriers. Three essential criteria must be satisfied for liposomes to be effective in drug delivery to neoplastic tissues: (i) extended blood circulation, (ii) sufficient tumor accumulation, and (iii) regulated drug release and absorption by tumor cells, with a release profile aligned with the pharmacodynamics of the drug [56–60].

Stealth liposomes are proposed to transport the drug within the aqueous core and are typically adorned with recognition molecules, receiving much research and application [61]. The unsatisfactory results of existing medicines perpetually drive the quest for novel therapeutic techniques. This encompasses the activation of standard vasculature to generate tumor blood vessels and the participation of immune response components in tumor formation and proliferation. The impediment of these procedures presents a compelling therapeutic strategy and a novel category of anticancer agents, including angiogenesis inhibitors and anti-inflammatory medications [62].

Tumor-associated inflammation is recognized as a significant promoter of tumor growth and so constitutes a compelling target for anticancer therapy. Glucocorticoids (GCs), a powerful category of anti-inflammatory medications, demonstrated anticancer effects at elevated daily dosages. This dosage results in significant side effects, including morbidity and mortality, due to strong immunosuppression. Recently, researchers have enhanced this adverse therapeutic index by utilizing long-circulating liposomes as the glucocorticoid delivery nanocarrier. This vehicle may significantly impede tumor growth following the delivery of a single weekly dose [63].

The efficacy of the liposomal formulation was ascribed to alterations in drug pharmacokinetics, including augmented blood circulation and glucocorticoid accumulation within the tumor, as well as the enhanced permeability and retention impact.

Recent data indicate that a primary mechanism of the anticancer effect of GC inside the tumor microenvironment is the reduction of macrophage activity and the downregulation of pro-angiogenic factors produced by functional tumor-associated macrophages. Furthermore, in vitro data indicated a direct cytotoxic and antiproliferative effect on both endothelium and tumor cells [64].

Kluza et al. created paramagnetic and fluorescent liposomes that encapsulate prednisolone phosphate to assess its anticancer efficacy and treatment response. This study evaluated the cytotoxicity of novel multifunctional liposomes (120 nm in diameter) administered at a dosage of 20 mg/kg/week in C57BL/6 mice implanted with B16F10 melanoma, comparing the results to those of the free drug formulation. It was observed to strongly limit tumor growth in comparison to untreated mice, similarly to the free form [63].

PEGylated liposomal doxorubicin (DOX) is authorized for the treatment of refractory ovarian cancer and Kaposi sarcoma in the United States. In this carrier, the drug's effectiveness was maintained, and the cardiac toxic impact was markedly reduced [18].

Albumin nanoparticle-bound paclitaxel, licensed in the United States for metastatic breast cancer treatment, demonstrates superior performance relative to the traditional castor oil-based formulation and exhibits reduced side effects [18].

Liposomes may serve as a non-viral vector for the delivery of siRNA to target cells in gene therapy. Mokhtarieh and his colleagues devised an innovative technique for generating asymmetric liposome particles (ALPs) with highly effective siRNA encapsulation. In their study, liposomes were synthesized using the solvent evaporation and dialysis technique, consisting of ionizable cationic 1,2-dioleoyl-3-dimethylammonium-propane and 1,2-dioleoyl-sn-glycero-3-phosphoethanolamine (DOPE) to encapsulate siRNA, while the outer layer comprised 1,2-distearoyl-sn-glycero-3-phosphocholine, DOPE, polyethylene glycol-1,2-distearoyl-sn-glycero-3-phosphatidylethanolamine (PEG–PE), and cholesterol. Ninety percent of siRNA was encapsulated into liposomes with a negatively charged surface. The surface-modified ALPs with a polyarginine peptide (R12) facilitated nonspecific cellular penetration, but unmodified liposomes exhibited no cellular uptake. The alteration of ALP's surface by the antihuman epidermal growth factor receptor antibody (anti-EGFR) facilitates EGFR-mediated uptake in nonsmall cell lung cancer cell lines, but the NIH-3T3 cell line, lacking the receptor, does not exhibit uptake [65].

The induced release of pH-sensitive liposomes is likely the most biocompatible approach for delivering medications directly into the cytoplasm of cells. Upon internalization into endosomes, liposomes are subjected to an acidic milieu. Reddy and Low formulated a pH-sensitive lipid composition using DOPE and citraconic anhydride to create liposomes. The resultant liposomes were noted to be stable at neutral pH although fusogenic at pH 5 [66]. Figure 6 illustrates the schematic representation of the liposome in targeted medication delivery.

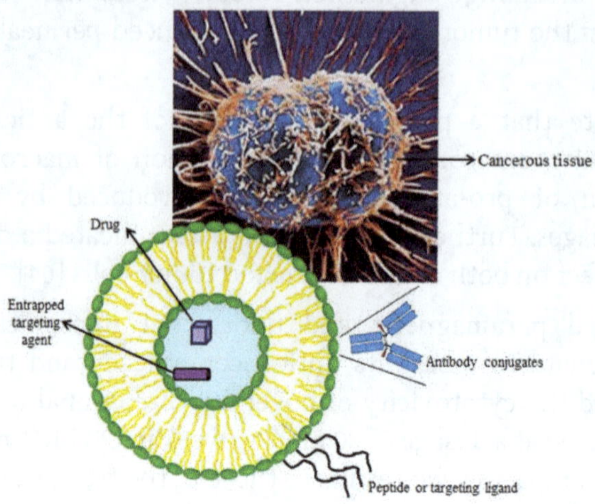

Figure 6. Liposome in target drug delivery

Choi and colleagues produced an amphiphilic DNA hybrid duplex utilizing Watson-Crick base pairing and DNA bioconjugation with cholesterol or the tLyp-1 tumor-homing peptide. The resulting amphiphilic DNA hybrid duplexes may self-assemble in an aqueous solution into nanoliposomes using tLyp-1 peptides as the outside ligand. This nanocarrier can effectively encapsulate doxorubicin and possesses a pH-sensitive shape that facilitates drug release in the acidic milieu of tumor cell cytoplasm [67]. These findings present a novel method for the targeted delivery of doxorubicin to specific cells in cancer treatment, while also regulating drug release in acidic environments such endosomes or lysosomes. Chiang et al. examined the amalgamation of polymer and liposome in the formulation of carriers. This group developed pH-responsive polymer-liposomes for intracellular medication delivery and targeted cancer treatment. This study indicates that the mix of carriers holds promise for targeted medication administration in the future, particularly when integrated with biotechnology.

7. SOLID LIPID NANOPARTICLES AS A TARGETED DRUG DELIVERY SYSTEM

In the late 1990s, SLNs were proposed for brain drug targeting application independently by two research groups, although the first proof of lipid particle transport across the BBB had already been provided. SLNs are colloidal carrier systems, which provide controlled-release profiles for many substances [68–72]. Kashanian et al. prepared aqueous dispersions of lipid nanoparticles using a modified, pH-sensitive derivative of phosphatidyl ethanolamine loaded with triamcinolone acetonide as a drug. The SLNs prepared in this study were able to control the release of drug under acidic conditions. This group showed that with increasing pH, the amount of releasing drug is increased due to the burst effect in this condition as well [30].

Studying the pharmacokinetics of two anticancer agents, namely camptothecin and doxorubicin, drug accumulation in the brain was observed after both oral and i.v. administration when loaded into SLN. As previously shown in PACA NPs, better results in brain targeting were achieved when SLN surface characteristics were modified by means of PEG derivatives or PEG-containing surfactants [73].

8. GOLD NANOPARTICLES IN TARGET DRUG DELIVERY

The bactericidal activity of gold nanoparticles (GNPs) coupled with ampicillin, streptomycin, and kanamycin was assessed. Gold nanoparticles were conjugated with antibiotics and medicines during their manufacture by functionalizing the gold particles with linkers such as amino acids, glutathione, and polyethylene glycol. The conjugated gold nanoparticles exhibited enhanced antibacterial efficacy and reduced minimum inhibitory concentration (MIC) relative to the free drug against three bacterial strains: Escherichia coli DH5a, Micrococcus luteus, and Staphylococcus aureus. In addition, nanoconjugate could increase their heat stability [80,81].

Bergen and colleagues developed nanoparticle formulations of gold nanoparticles (GNPs) with differing particle sizes, surface charges, and surface hydrophilicity. This study involves the attachment of galactose to the surface of nanoparticles through the conjugation of PEG-thiol and galactose-PEG-thiol to gold colloids. This approach was utilized to identify NP formulations that exhibit hepatocyte-targeted delivery in vivo. This group observed that the presence of galactose ligands greatly influenced targeting efficiency [82].

9. NIOSOMES

Nonionic surfactant vesicles (niosomes), are biodegradable, relatively nontoxic, more stable, and inexpensive, and therefore could be an alternative to liposomes [83]. Due to the encapsulation of a wide range of toxic drugs such as antiviral, anticancer, and anti-AIDS drugs in niosomes, this carrier is so valuable in the delivery of proteins and biological medications. Niosome is a promising carrier system in comparison with ionic drug carriers, which are relatively toxic and moderately harmful [84].

Bragagni and coworkers developed a stable and safe niosomal formulation to effectively encapsulate DOX. The developed formulation, in virtue of its relatively high efficiency of drug encapsulation and good stability, could find useful applications as an effective tool for achieving DOX brain delivery, exploiting the brain uptake properties of the glucose-targeted vesicles [85].

Preliminary in vivo studies involved the i.v. administration of a single dose of the developed niosome formulation with respect to the target tissue. This formulation gave rise to stable and nano-sized vesicles, which are able to improve doxorubicin brain delivery. Positive results of preliminary in vivo studies require future pharmacokinetic studies to gain more insight into the mechanism of drug transport of functionalized niosomes [86].

10. QUANTUM DOTS

Quantum dots (QDs), semiconductor fluorescent nanoparticles, ranging from 2 to 10 nm in size has a core of hundreds to thousands of atoms of group II and VI elements (e.g., cadmium, technetium, zinc, and selenide) or group III (e.g., tantalum) and V elements (e.g., indium). This carrier with a cadmium selenide core and a zinc sulfide shell, by a coating of an amphiphilic polymer, is ordinarily utilized for drug delivery systems [87]. QDs greatly expand the possibilities for fluorescence imaging of cells and living animals [88].

QDs have been conjugated to antibodies, allowing for simultaneous labeling and accurate quantification of these target proteins in one target section. Direct conjugation of targeted antibodies to the surface of QDs in a molar ration of four to ten, without the use of secondary antibodies, might be the best approach to achieve multiplex detection of molecular targets.

QDs can be bioconjugated to either the 3′ or 5′ end of an oligo sequence. Xiao and Barker have discussed the ability to control the number of attached oligonucleotides by the use of a streptavidin–biotin quantum dot system [89].

This bioconjugate has a high affinity to target cells and causes minimum nonspecific binding to normal cells. The quantum dot-based assay was developed that could quantitatively detect the estrogen receptor, progesterone receptor, and ERBB2 (e.g., MCF-7, BT474, and MDA-231 cells) in paraffin-embedded human breast cancer cells [90]. These cell lines were overexpressed by these receptors and were stained simultaneously with multiple quantum dots, which were directly bioconjugated to targeting antibodies for these three proteins [91].

Biotinylated DNA probes for labeled cells by streptavidin-coated quantum dots could identify of ERBB2, even at low levels of expression. This information recommends that the use of quantum dot-labeled oligonucleotides for detecting gene amplification especially at low levels of expression may offer points of interest over the standard fluorescence in situ hybridization (FISH) method [91].

11. TARGETING DRUG DELIVERY WITH MAGNETIC NANOPARTICLES

Magnetic nanoparticles (MNPs) offer several advantages when used as a drug carrier, including the large surface area, which can be properly modified to attach to drug molecules. Magnetic NPs can also be used with other carriers for drug delivery. Ensuring biocompatibility and nontoxicity, iron oxide-based particles (magnetite) with superparamagnetic characteristics are commonly used as magnetically responsive components, which can be manipulated by an external magnetic field gradient. Based on these properties, the superparamagnetic nanoparticles could be transported through the vascular system, concentrated in a specific part of the body with the aid of a magnetic field, and used as a carrier [92–94].

Iron oxide nanoparticles have found applications in the so-called magnetic drug targeting. Iron oxide nanoparticles in an external magnetic field are able to deliver particles to the desired target area [95, 96] and fix them there while the drug is released to exert a local effect [97]. Although magnetic targeting has been evaluated for a number of tumor-targeting studies, the most recent work is related to brain cancer.

It has been demonstrated that the release of drugs from magnetoliposomes could be controlled by an alternative current magnetic heating [98]. Although magnetoliposomes could be specifically heated to 42°C, the heating was mostly limited inside the thin lipid bi-layers [99].

Hsu and Su developed magnetic lipid nanoparticles with sizes ranging from 5 to 25 mm, composed of multiple drugs controlling their release in a desired pattern. The lipid matrices are solid at body temperature and melt around 45–55°C. In this study, the dissipated magnetic heat liquefied the encompassing lipid networks and resulted in an accelerated release of the encapsulated drugs.

Three accomplishments resulted: (1) Preparation of magnetic lipid nanoparticles with co-encapsulated drugs and heating components; (2) conjugation of surface-modified g-Fe_2O_3 particles that can be remotely energized to activate the heating and rapid drug release; and (3) designing a new nanocarrier, which can accomplish localized heating and pulsative release [99].

Zhu et al. prepared the chitosan-coated magnetic nanoparticles (CS MNPs) as carriers of 5-fluorouracil (CS–5-FuMNPs) through a reverse microemulsion method. It was found that the synthesized CS–5-Fu MNPs were spherical in shape with an average size of 100 ± 20 nm, low aggregation, and good magnetic responsivity. The result of CS–5-Fu MNPs cytotoxicity on K562 cancer cells showed that the nanoparticles have significant antitumor activities, and FITC-labeled nanoparticles could effectively enter into the cancer cells and induce cell apoptosis [74].

Gollavelli and Ling [75] investigated a novel magnetic and fluorescent graphene nanoparticles with a simple noncovalent approach. In this work, a hydrophobic silicon napthalocyanine bis (trihexylsilyloxide) (SiNc4) photosensitizer was adopted to immobilizing onto water-dispersible magnetic and fluorescent graphene (MFG) via pep stacking to yield MFGeSiNc4 functioned as a theranostic nanocarrier. The developed MFGeSiNc4 may thus be utilized as a potential theranostic nanocarrier for phototherapy of cancer cells with a single light source for less time-consuming and cost-effective treatments with a minimal therapy dose.

12. TARGETED DELIVERY FOR VACCINE

The unique properties of nanoparticles, which can be altered by planned application, make excellent approaches for immunization and treatment of different diseases. The use of nanoparticles as vaccine adjuvants and carriers has opened up an entire new field of research. Different materials in the viral (20-200 nm) or bacterial (200-5000 nm) size ranges introduced in vaccine formulations with a stable half-life prevent enzymatic degradation of antigen and increase antigen uptake by specifically targeting specialist antigen-presenting cells (APCs) [76,100]. Some nanoparticle-based vaccines are designed to include ligands that can target APC and hence help trigger immune responses. Some possess internal adjuvants, triggering toll-like receptor (TLR) ligation and local danger signals to potentiate the effective antigen presentation to T cells.

Different designs and compositions of nanoparticle-based vaccines allow for specific tailoring of antigen delivery to the target cell type or specific tissue. In addition, the size of the particles plays a major role in the mechanism of particle uptake by APCs, influencing the type of the resulting immune response [100].

More recently a synthetic nanoparticle vaccine platform that targets lymph node-resident dendritic cells (DCs) has been developed, capable of mounting an immune response to conjugated antigen. The cross-presentation by DCs was demonstrated by direct antibody staining and in vitro stimulation of $CD8^+$ T cells from OT-I mice and was indeed the most efficient with the reduction-sensitive conjugation.

Similarly, interferon (IFN) production by $CD4^{+}$ T cells from OT-II mice has been observed. Finally, immunization with OVA peptide-bearing nanoparticles resulted in in vivo proliferation and IFN production by adoptively transferred CD8+ OT-I T cells and was also the most efficient with reduction-sensitive linking of the peptide antigen. These results demonstrate the relevance of the poly (propylene sulfide) nanoparticle vaccine platform and antigen conjugation scheme for activating both cytotoxic and helper T-cell responses [101].

13. NONCOVALENT PROTEIN–NANOPARTICLE CONJUGATION USED FOR TARGETED DRUG DELIVERY

Some of the studies have investigated the thermodynamics of binding between proteins and nanomaterials, demonstrating that properly functionalized NPs interact with proteins in an analogous fashion to protein–protein interactions. The biophysical characteristics of these interactions, such as binding affinity, residence time, binding cooperatively of NP, and the common serum proteins such as albumin, have been quantitatively described in the buffer medium to determine the behavior of proteins on NP surfaces [34,102].

Carbon nanotubes have a high surface area for chemical interactions and conjugations. The nonspecific protein–nanotube conjugates contain electrostatic interactions and hydrogen bonding, especially when carbon nanotubes are pretreated with oxidative acids (Figure 7) [103,104].

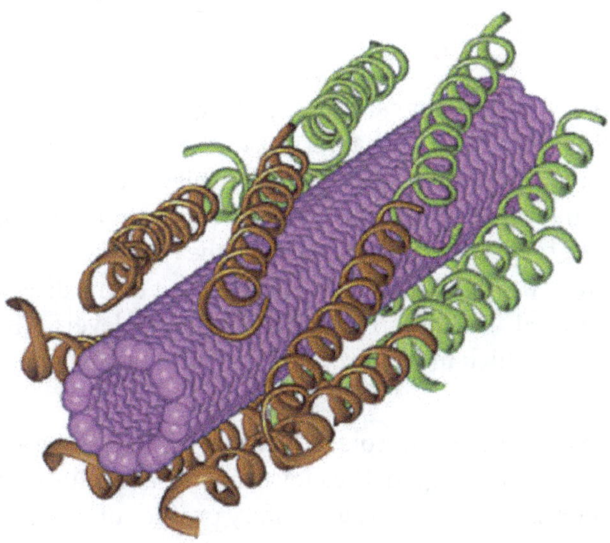

Figure 7. Immobilization of biomacromolecules on carbon nanotube surfaces

This conjugation technique employs specific chemical reagents with established chemistry to facilitate the controlled linkage of proteins to nanotubes. Amino groups on protein surfaces, particularly from residues like lysine and carboxylic acids attached to nanotubes, are exposed through oxidative acid treatments and play a significant role in specific conjugations, forming amide connections [35].

PEG was co-adsorbed onto single-wall nanotube (SWNT) devices alongside polyethylenimine in a separate publication. The pendant primary amine groups on PEI were accessible for subsequent biotin derivatization, facilitating streptavidin recognition (Figure 8) [105].

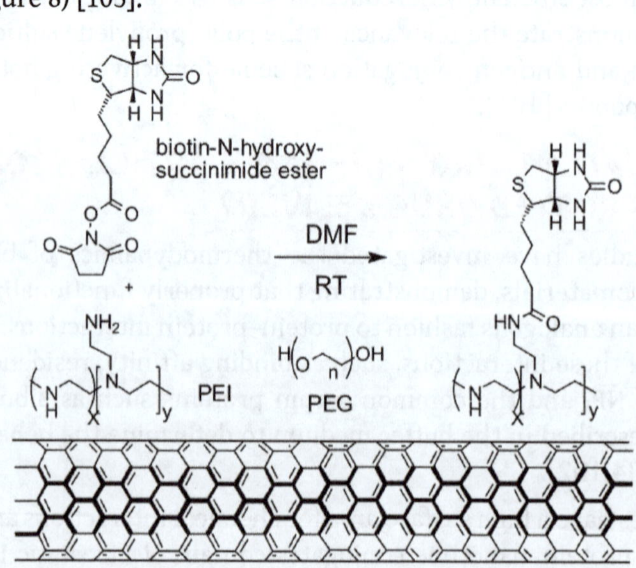

Figure 8. Absorption of polymer on the nanotube surface with the aid of PEG and PEI

14. CONCISE SUMMARY

Targeted drug delivery, sometimes called smart drug delivery, is a method of delivering medication to a patient in a manner that increases the concentration of the medication in infective organs or cells, relative to others. The objective of a targeted drug delivery system is to prolong, localize, and concentrate the drug in the target diseased tissue. The advantages of the targeted release system are the reduction in the frequency of the dose administration by the patient, more uniform effect of the drug, reduction of drug side effects, and reduced fluctuation in circulating drug levels. The disadvantage of the system is high cost, which makes profitability more troublesome and productivity difficult.

Nanotechnology plays an important role in therapies of the future as "nanomedicines" by enabling this situation to happen, thus lowering doses required for efficacy as well as expanding the therapeutic windows and safety profiles of new medicines.

Conventional chemotherapeutic agents are distributed nonspecifically in the body where they influence both cancerous and normal cells, thereby limiting the dose achievable within the tumor and also resulting in suboptimal treatment due to excessive toxicities. Molecularly targeted therapy has developed as one way to overcome the problem of nonspecifity of routine anticancer drugs. However, the development of resistance in cancer cells can avoid the cytotoxicity of ordinary chemotherapeutics as well as the more up-to-date targeted therapeutics [105].

Both passive- and active-targeted nanoparticles can enhance the intracellular concentration of drugs in cancer cells while avoiding toxicity in normal cells. Furthermore, when nanoparticles bind to specific receptors and then enter the cell, they are usually enveloped by endosomes via receptor-mediated endocytosis, thereby bypassing the recognition of P-glycoprotein, one of the main drug resistance mechanisms. However, although nanoparticles offer many advantages as drug carrier systems, there are still many limitations to be solved such as poor oral bioavailability, instability in circulation, inadequate tissue distribution, and toxicity.

15. NOMENCLATURE

Phrase	Abbreviation
Blood brain barrier 1,2-dioleoyl-sn-glycero-3-phosphoethanolamine	(BBB) DOPE
Antigen-presenting cell	APC
Carbon nanotubes	CNT
Dendritic cells N,N-dicyclohexyl carbodiimide	DC DCC
Doxorubicin	DOX
Drug delivery systems	DDS
N-ethyl-N-(3-dimethylaminopropyl) carbodiimide hydrochloride Epidermal growth factor receptor Enhanced permeation and retention Fluorescein isothiocyanate Folic acid	(EDAC) EGFR EPR FITC FA
Glucocorticoid	GC
Gold nanoparticles	GNP
Murine canin fibroblast Minimum inhibition concentration Magnetic nanoparticles	MCF-7 MIC MNP
Monoclonal antibodies	mAb
Multiwall carbon nanotubes	MWCNT
Poly (D, L-lactic-co-glycolic acid)	PLGA
Quantum dots	QD
Single-wall carbon nanotubes	SWCNT
Solid lipid nanoparticles	SLN
Triggering toll-like receptor	TLR

REFERENCES

1. Allen TM, Cullis PR 2004 Drug delivery systems: entering the mainstream. Science 303: 1818–1822
2. Farokhzad OC, Langer R 2009 Impact of nanotechnology on drug delivery. ACS Nano 3(1): 16–20
3. Petros RA, DeSimone JM 2010. Strategies in the design of nanoparticles for therapeutic applications. Nat Rev Drug Discov 9(8): 615–627

4. Shi J, Votruba AR, Farokhzad OC, Langer R 2010 Nanotechnology in drug delivery and tissue engineering: from discovery to applications. Nano Lett 10(9): 3223–3236.
5. Dawar S, Singh N, Kanwar RK, Kennedy RL, Veedu RN, Zhou SF, Krishnakumar S, Hazra S, Sasidharan S, Duan W, Kanwar JR 2013 Multifunctional and multitargeted nanoparticles for drug delivery to overcome barriers of drug resistance in human cancers. Drug Discov Today 18: 1292–1300.
6. Derakhshandeh K, Erfan M, Dadashzadeh S 2007. Encapsulation of 9-nitrocamptothecin, a novel anticancer drug, in biodegradable nanoparticles: factorial design, characterization and release kinetics. Euro J Pharm Biopharm 66: 34-41.
7. Afshari M, Derakhshandeh K and Hosseinzadeh L 2014 Characterization, cytotoxicity and apoptosis studies of methotrexate-loaded PLGA and PLGA-PEG nanoparticles. J Microencapsul 31: 239–245.
8. Derakhshandeh K, Fathi S 2012 Role of chitosan nanoparticles in the oral absorption of Gemcitabine. Int J Pharm. 437(1-2): 172–177.
9. Davis ME, Chen Z, Shin DM 2008 Nanoparticle therapeutics: an emerging treatment modality for cancer. Nat Rev Drug Discov 7(9): 771–782
10. Xu Q, Kambhampati SP, Kannan RM 2013 Nanotechnology approaches for ocular drug delivery. Middle East Afr J Ophthalmol 20: 26– 37.
11. Prokop A, Davidson JM2008. Nanovehicular intracellular delivery systems. J Pharm Sci 97: 3518–3590.
12. Kluza E, Yeo SY, Schmid S, van der Schaft DW.J, Boekhoven RW, Schiffelers RM, Storm G, Strijkers GJ, Nicolay K 2011 Anti-tumor activity of liposomal glucocorticoids: the relevance of liposome-mediated drug delivery, intratumoral localization and systemic activity. J Control Release 151: 10–17.
13. Ferrari M 2005 Cancer nanotechnology: opportunities and challenges. Nat Rev Cancer 5: 161–171.
14. Jain K 2005 Nanotechnology in clinical laboratory diagnostics. Clin Chim Acta 358: 37–54.
15. Sutton D, Nasongkla N, Blanco E, Gao J 2007 Functionalized micellar systems for cancer targeted drug delivery. Pharm Res 24: 1029–1046.
16. Xiang SD, Wilson K, Day S, Fuchsberger M, Plebanski M 2013 Methods of effective conjugation of antigens to nanoparticles as non-inflammatory vaccine carriers. Methods 60: 232–241.
17. Gao Z, Zhang L, Sun Y 2012 Nanotechnology applied to overcome tumor drug resistance. J Control Release 162: 45–55.
18. Yezhelyev MV, Gao X, Xing Y, Al-Hajj A, Nie S, O'Regan RM 2006 Emerging use of nanoparticles in diagnosis and treatment of breast cancer. Lancet Oncol 7: 657–667.
19. Vasir JK, Reddy MK, Labhasetwar VD 2005 Nanosystems in drug targeting: opportunities and challenges. Curren Nanosci 1: 47–64.
20. Wang M, Thanou M 2010 Targeting nanoparticles to cancer. Pharmacol Res 62: 90–99.
21. Au JL, Jang SH, Zheng J, Chen CT, Song S, Hu L 2001 Determinants of drug delivery and transport to solid tumors. J Control Release 74: 31–46.
22. Fetterly GJ, Straubinger RM 2003 Pharmacokinetics of paclitaxel containing liposomes in rats. AAPS Pharm Sci 5: E32.
23. Hoarau D, Delmas P, David S, Roux E, Leroux JC 2004 Novel long circulating lipid nanocapsules. Pharm Res 21: 1783–1789.

24. Moghimi SM, Szebeni J 2003 Stealth liposomes and long circulating nanoparticles: critical issues in pharmacokinetics, opsonization and protein-binding properties. Prog Lipid Res 42: 463–478.

25. Wang T, Kievit FM, Veiseh O, Arami H, Stephen ZR, Fang C, Liu Y, Ellenbogen RG, Zhang M 2013 Targeted cell uptake of a noninternalizing antibody through conjugation to iron oxide nanoparticles in primary central nervous system lymphoma. World Neurosurg 80: 134–141.

26. Pissuwan D, Niidome T, CortieMB 2011 The forthcoming applications of gold nanoparticles in drug and gene delivery systems. J Control Release 149: 65–71.

27. Derakhshandeh K, Soheili M, Dadashzadeh S, Saghiri R 2010 Preparation and in vitro characterization of 9-nitrocamptothecin-loaded long circulating nanoparticles for delivery in cancer patients. Int J Nanomed 5: 463–471.

28. Derakhshandeh K, Hochhaus G, Dadashzadeh S 2011 In-vitro cellular uptake and transport study of 9-nitrocamptothecin PLGA nanoparticles across caco-2 cell monolayer model. Iran J Pharm Res 10: 425–434.

29. Parveen S, Misra R, Sahoo SK 2012 Nanoparticles: a boon to drug delivery, therapeutics, diagnostics and imaging. Nanomed Nanotechnol Biol Med 8: 147–166.

30. Kashanian S, Azandaryani AH, Derakhshandeh K 2011 New surface-modified solid lipid nanoparticles using N-glutarylphosphatidylethanolamine as the outer shell. Int J Nanomed 6: 2393–2401.

31. Afshari M, Derakhshandeh K, Hosseinzadeh L 2014 Characterisation, cytotoxicity and apoptosis studies of methotrexate-loaded PLGA and PLGA-PEG nanoparticles. J Microencapsul 31: 239–245.

32. Ramana LN, Sharma S, Sethuraman S, Ranga U, Krishnan UM 2014 Evaluation of chitosan nanoformulations as potent anti-HIV therapeutic systems. Biochimica et Biophysica Acta 1840: 476–484.

33. Shi C, Guo X, Qu Q, Tang Z, Wang Y, Zhou S 2014 Actively targeted delivery of anticancer drug to tumor cells by redox-responsive star-shaped micelles. Biomaterials: 1–12.

34. Rana S, YehYC, Rotello VM 2010 Engineering the nanoparticle–protein interface: applications and possibilities. Curr Opin Chem Biol 14: 828–834.

35. Kumar C 2005 Biofunctionalization of Nanomaterials. Copyright 8. WILEY-VCH Verlag GmbH & Co. KGaA, Weinheim. ISBN: 3-527-31381-8

36. Daniel S, Rao TP, Rao KS, Rani SU, Naidu GRK, Lee HY, Kawai T 2007 A review of DNA functionalized/grafted carbon nanotubes and their characterization. Sens Actuators B 122: 672–682.

37. Hapuarachchige S, Zhu W, Kato Y, Artemov D 2014 Bioorthogonal, two-component delivery systems based on antibody and drug-loaded nanocarriers for enhanced internalization of nanotherapeutics. Biomaterials 35: 2346–2354.

38. Olejnik M, Krajnik B, Kowalska D, Lin G, Mackowski S 2013 Spectroscopic studies of plasmon coupling between photosynthetic complexes and metallic quantum dots. J Phy Condens Matter 25: 1–12.

39. Yokoyama M 2005 Drug targeting with nano-sized carrier systems. J Artif Organs 8: 77–84.

40. Jia H, Zhu J, Wang X, Cheng H, Chen G, Zhao Y, Zeng X, Feng J, Zhang X, Zhuo R 2014 A boronate-linked linear-hyperbranched polymeric nanovehicle for pH-dependent tumor-targeted drug delivery. Biomaterials 35: 5240e–5249e

41. Kulhari H, Pooja D, Shrivastav S, Mc Naidu VG, Sistla R 2014 Peptide conjugated polymeric nanoparticles as a carrier for targeted delivery of docetaxel. Colloid Surf B 117: 166–173.
42. Kocbek P, Obermajer N, Cegnar M, Kos J, Kristl J 2007 Targeting cancer cells using PLGA nanoparticles surface modified with monoclonal antibody. J Control Release 120: 18–26.
43. Chiu SJ, Ueno NT, Lee RJ 2004 Tumor-targeted gene delivery via anti-HER2 antibody (trastuzumab, HerceptinR) conjugated polyethylenimine. J Control Release 97: 357–369.
44. Abdel Wahab BA, Evgenivetch PV, Alyautdin RN 2005 Brain targeting of nerve growth factor using poly(butylcyanoacrylate) nanoparticles. Internet J Pharmacol 3.
45. Yang J, Lee CH, Park J, Seo S, Lim EK, Song YJ, Suh JS, Yoon HG, Huh YM, Haam S 2007 Antibody conjugated magnetic PLGA nanoparticles for diagnosis and treatment of breast cancer. J Mater Chem 17: 2695–2699.
46. Sudimack J, Lee RJ 2000 Targeted drug delivery via the folate receptor. Adv Drug Deliv Rev 41: 147–162.
47. Koo OM, Rubinstein I, Onyuksel H 2005 Role of nanotechnology in targeted drug delivery and imaging: a concise review. Nanomedicine 1: 193–212.
48. Kim JS, Oh MH, Park JY, Park TG, Nam YS 2013 Protein-resistant, reductively dissociable polyplexes for in vivo systemic delivery and tumor-targeting of siRNA. Biomaterials 34: 2370–2379.
49. Heidarian S 2012 Folate targeted nanoparticles: preparation, physicochemical characterization and in vitro cytotoxicity effect. PhD thesis. Kermanshah University of Medical Science.
50. Wu H, Cabral H, Toh K, Mi P, Chen YC, Matsumoto Y, Yamada N, Liu X, Kinoh H, Miura Y, Kano MR, Nishihara H, Nishiyama N, Kataoka K 2014 Polymeric micelles loaded with platinum anticancer drugs target preangiogenic micrometastatic niches associated with inflammation. J Control Release 189: 1–10.
51. Tarn D, Ashley CE, Xue M, Carnes EC, Zink JI, Brinker CJ 2013 Mesoporous silica nanoparticle nanocarriers: biofunctionality and biocompatibility. Acc Chem Res 46: 792–801.
52. Chen C, Geng J, Pu F, Yang X, Ren J, Qu X 2011 Polyvalent nucleic acid/mesoporous silica nanoparticle conjugates: dual stimuli-responsive vehicles for intracellular drug delivery. Angew Chem Int Ed 50: 882–886.
53. Zhou L, Chen Z, Dong K, Yin M, Ren J, Qu X 2014 DNA-mediated biomineralization of rare-earth nanoparticles for simultaneous imaging and stimuli-responsive drug delivery. Biomaterials 35(30):8694-6702.
54. Hong JS, Vreeland WN, DePaoli Lacerda SH, Locascio LE, Gaitan Mi, Raghavan SR 2008 Liposome-templated supramolecular assembly of responsive alginate nanogels. Langmuir 24: 4092–4096.
55. Gregoriadis G, Ryman BE 1972 Fate of protein-containing liposomes injected into rats. An approach to the treatment of storage diseases. Eur J Biochem 24: 485–491.
56. Andresen TL, Jensen SS, Jorgensen K 2005 Advanced strategies in liposomal cancer therapy: problems and prospects of active and tumor specific drug release. Prog Lipid Res 44: 68–97.
57. Lim SB, Banerjee A, Önyüksel H 2012 Improvement of drug safety by the use of lipid-based nanocarriers. J Control Release 163: 34–45.
58. Kraft JC, Freeling JP, Wang Z, HO RJY 2014 Emerging research and clinical development trends of liposome and lipid nanoparticle drug delivery systems. J Pharm Sci 103: 29–52.

59. Howard MD, Greineder CF, Hood ED, Muzykanto VR 2014 Endothelial targeting of liposomes encapsulating SOD/catalase mimetic EUK-134 alleviates acute pulmonary inflammation. J Control Release 177: 34–41.

60. Ninomiya K, Yamashita T, Kawabata S, Shimizu N 2014 Targeted and ultrasound-triggered drug delivery using liposomes co-modified with cancer cell-targeting aptamers and a thermosensitive polymer. Ultrason Sonochem 21: 1482–1488

61. Yuan F, Leunig M, Huang SK, Berk DA, Papahadjopoulos D, Jain RK 1994 Microvascular permeability and interstitial penetration of sterically stabilized (stealth) liposomes in a human tumor xenograft. Cancer Res 54: 3352–3356.

62. Immordino ML, Dosio F, Cattel L 2006 Stealth liposomes: review of the basic science, rationale, and clinical applications, existing and potential. Int J Nanomed 1: 297–315.

63. Kluza E, Yeo SY, Schmid S, van der Schaft DWJ, Boekhoven RW, Schiffelers RM, Storm G, Strijkers GJ, Nicolay K 2011 Anti-tumor activity of liposomal glucocorticoids: the relevance of liposome-mediated drug delivery, intratumoral localization and systemic activity. J Control Release 151: 10–17.

64. Cho K, Wang X, Nie S, Chen Z, Shin DM 2008 Therapeutic nanoparticles for drug delivery in cancer. Clinical Cancer Res 14: 1310–1316.

65. Mokhtarieh AA, Cheong S, Kim S, Chung BH, Lee MK 2012 Asymmetric liposome particles with highly efficient encapsulation of siRNA and without nonspecific cell penetration suitable for target-specific delivery. Biochim Biophys Acta 1818: 1633–1641.

66. Reddy JA, Low PS 2000 Enhanced folate receptor mediated gene therapy using a novel pH-sensitive lipid formulation. J Control Release 64: 27–37.

67. Choi K, Kwon IC, Ahn HJ 2013 Self-assembled amphiphilic DNA-cholesterol/DNA-peptide hybrid duplexes with liposome-like structure for doxorubicin delivery. Biomaterials 34: 4183–4190

68. Muller RH, Mader K, Gohla S 2000 Solid lipid nanoparticles (SLN) for controlled drug delivery – a review of the state of the art. Eur J Pharm Biopharm 50: 161–177.

69. Rostami E, Kashanian S, Hemati Azandaryani A 2014 Preparation of solid lipid nanoparticles as drug carriers for levothyroxine sodium with in vitro drug delivery kinetic characterization. Mol Biol Rep. 41(5): 3521-3527.

70. Rostami E, Kashanian S, Hemati Azandaryani A, Faramarzi H, Ezzati J, Omidfar K 2014 Drug targeting using solid lipid nanoparticles. Chemis Phys Lipids 181: 56–61.

71. Bondi ML, Craparo EF 2010 Solid lipid nanoparticles for applications in gene therapy: a review of the state of the art. Expert Opin Drug Del 7: 7–18.

72. Mehnert W, Maeder K 2012 Solid lipid nanoparticles: production, characterization and applications, Adv Drug Deliv Rev 64: 83–101.

73. Jin SE, Kim CK 2012 Long-term stable cationic solid lipid nanoparticles for the enhanced intracellular delivery of SMAD3 antisense oligonucleotides in activated murine macrophages. J Pharm Pharm Sci 15: 467–482.

74. Zhu L, Ma J, Jia N, Zhao Y, Shen H 2009 Chitosan-coated magnetic nanoparticles as carriers of 5-fluorouracil: preparation, characterization and cytotoxicity studies. Colloids Surf B Biointerfaces 68: 1–6.

75. Gollavelli G, Ling YC 2014 Magnetic and fluorescent graphene for dual modal imaging and single light induced photothermal and photodynamic therapy of cancer cells. Biomaterials 35: 4499–4507.

76. Mishra D, Mishra H, Mishra PK, Nahar M, Dubey V, Jain NK 2010 Evaluation of solid lipid nanoparticles as carriers for delivery of hepatitis B surface antigen for vaccination using subcutaneous route. J Pharm Pharm Sci 13: 495–509.

77. Groneberg DA, Giersig M, Welte T, Pison U 2006 Nanoparticle-based diagnosis and therapy. Curr Drug Targets. 7: 643–648.

78. Gu YJ, Cheng J, Man CW, Wong WT, Cheng SH 2012 Gold-doxorubicin nanoconjugates for overcoming multidrug resistance. Nanomed 8: 204–211.

79. Bhattacharya D, Saha B, Mukherjee A, Ranjan Santra C, Karmakar P 2012 Gold nanoparticles conjugated antibiotics: stability and functional evaluation. Nanosci Nanotechnol 2: 14–21.

80. Paciotti GF, Kingston DGI, Tamarkin L 2006 Colloidal gold nanoparticles: a novel nanoparticle platform for developing multifunctional tumor-targeted drug delivery vectors. Drug Develop Res 67: 47–54.

81. Saha B, Bhattacharya J, Mukherjee A, Ghosh AK, Santra CR, Dasgupta AK, Karmakar P 2007 In vitro structural and functional evaluation of gold nanoparticles conjugated antibiotics. Nanoscale Res Lett 2: 614–622.

82. Bergen JM, von Recum HA, Goodman TT, Massey AP, Pun SH 2006 Gold nanoparticles as a versatile platform for optimizing physicochemical parameters for targeted drug delivery. Macromolecular Biosci 6: 506–516.

83. Uchegbu IF, Vyas SP 1998 Non-ionic surfactant based vesicles (niosomes) in drug delivery. Int J Pharm 172: 33–70.

84. Dufes C, Schatzlein AG, Tetley L, Gray AI, Watson DG, Olivier JC, Couet W, Uchegbu IF 2000 Niosomes and polymeric chitosan based vesicles bearing transferrin and glucose ligands for drug targeting. Pharm Res 17: 1251–1258.

85. Bragagni M, Mennini N, Ghelardini C, Mura P 2012 Development and characterization of niosomal formulations of doxorubicin aimed at brain targeting. J Pharm Pharm Sci 15: 94–102.

86. Bragagnia M, Menninia N, Ghelardinib C, Muraa P 2012 Development and characterization of niosomal formulations of doxorubicin aimed at brain targeting. J Pharm Pharm Sci 15: 184–196.

87. Medintz IL, Uyeda HT, Goldman ER, Mattoussi H 2005 Quantum dot bioconjugates for imaging, labelling and sensing. Nature Mater 4: 435–446.

88. Howarth M, Takao K, Hayashi Y, Ting A 2005 Targeting quantum dots to surface proteins in living cells with biotin ligase. Proc Natl Acad Sci U S A 102: 7583–7588.

89. Xiao Y, Telford WG, Ball JC, Locascio LE, Barker PE 2005 Semiconductor nanocrystal conjugates, FISH and pH. Nature Methods 2: 723–732.

90. Yezhelyev M, Morris C, Gao X 2005 Simultaneous and quantitative detection of multiple biomarkers in human breast cancers using semiconductor multicolor quantum dots breast cancer research and treatment. Breast Cancer Res Treat 94: 48–57.

91. Yezhelyev M, Gao X, Markus A 2005 Multiplex molecular diagnostic of tumor tissue using quantum dots. Am Soc Clin Oncol 23: 843–849.

92. Neuberger T, Schopf B, Hofmann H, Hofmann M, Rechenberg B 2005 Superparamagnetic nanoparticles for biomedical applications: possibilities and limitations of a new drug delivery system. J Magn Magn Mater 293: 483–496.

93. Chen JP, Yang PC, Ma YH, Wu T 2011 Characterization of chitosan magnetic nanoparticles for in situ delivery of tissue plasminogen activator. Carbohydr Polym 84: 364–372.

94. Cole AJ, Yang VC, David AE 2011 Cancer theranostics: the rise of targeted magnetic nanoparticles. Trends Biotechnol 29: 323–332.

95. Alexiou C, Jurgons R, Schmid R. Hilpert A, Bergemann C, Parak F, Iro H 2005 In vitro and in vivo investigations of targeted chemotherapy with magnetic nanoparticles. J Magn Magn Mate 293: 389–393.

96. Mahmoudi M, Sant S, Wang B, Laurent S, Sen T2011 Superparamagnetic iron oxide nanoparticles (SPIONs): development, surface modification and applications in chemotherapy. Adv Drug Deliv Rev 63: 24–46.

97. Liu X, Guan Y, Liu H, Ma Z, Yang Y, Wu X 2005 Preparation and characterization of magnetic polymer nanospheres with high protein binding capacity. J Magn Magn Mate 293: 111–118.

98. Babincova M, Cicmanec P, Altanerova V, Altaner C, Babinec P 2002 AC-magnetic field controlled drug release from magnetoliposomes: design of a method for site-specific chemotherapy. Bioelectro Chem 55: 17–25.

99. Hsu MH, Su YC 2008 Iron-oxide embedded solid lipid nanoparticles for magnetically controlled heating and drug delivery. Biomed Microdevices 10: 785–793.

100. Xiang SD, Wilson K, Day S, Fuchsberger M, Plebanski M 2013 Methods of effective conjugation of antigens to nanoparticles as non-inflammatory vaccine carriers. Methods 60: 232–241.

101. Hirosue S, Kourtis IC, van der Vlies AJ, Hubbell JA, Swartz MA 2010 Antigen delivery to dendritic cells by poly(propylene sulfide) nanoparticles with disulfide conjugated peptides: cross-presentation and T cell activation. Vaccine 28: 7897–7906.

102. Fu K, Huang W, Lin Y, Zhang D, Hanks TW, Rao AM, Sun YP 2002 Functionalization of carbon nanotubes with bovine serum albumin in homogeneous aqueous solution. J Nanosci Nanotechnol 2: 457–461.

103. Monteiro-Riviere, NA, Nemanich RJ, Inman AO, Wang YY, Riviere JE 2005 Multi-walled carbon nanotube interactions with human epidermal keratinocytes. Toxicol Lett 155: 377–384.

104. Chengqun Chen, Huijuan Zhang, Lin Hou, Jinjin Shi, Lei Wang, Chaofeng Zhang, Mingyue Zhang, Hongling Zhang, Xiufang Shi, Huixiang Li, Zhenzhong Zhang 2013 Single-walled carbon nanotubes mediated neovascularity targeted antitumor drug delivery system. J Pharm Pharm Sci 16(1):40-51.

105. Star, A, Gabriel JCP, Bradley K, Gruner G 2003 Electronic detection of specific protein binding using nanotube FET device. Nano Lett 3: 459–463.

106. Xiao Y, Barker PE 2004 Semiconductor nanocrystal probes for human metaphase chromosomes. Nucleic Acids Res 32: 28–33.

5 Chapter CANCER STEM CELLS: PERSPECTIVES AND TARGETING STRATEGIES

1. INTRODUCTION: AN OVERVIEW

Cancer continues to be a predominant cause of mortality in humans, and despite significant investments and endeavors, clinical trials aimed at eradicating or managing cancer progression have largely yielded unsatisfactory results [1, 2]. Cancer originates from normal cells due to the accumulation of several genetic changes that ultimately result in malignant phenotypes [3, 4]. Despite an enhanced comprehension of cancer biology and evolutionary genetic traits, the translation of these advancements into viable and effective treatment outcomes remains a challenge [5]. A compelling notion now under investigation in cancer research is the concept of cancer stem cells (CSCs), which may provide a solution [6]. This chapter delineates the principal attributes of cancer stem cells (CSCs) and underscores many essential methodologies employed in CSC research, emphasizing their potential utility in effective CSC-targeted therapy.

2. CSC: A PROGRESSIVE CONCEPT ADVANCING

2.1. The evolution of cancer genetics

Cancer biology and genetics have progressively confirmed cancer as a complex adaptive system. This seminal perspective was proposed by Peter Nowell in 1976, who saw cancer formation as an evolutionary process propelled by incremental mutations and sequential, subclonal selection at the nucleic acid level, a hypothesis analogous to Darwinian natural selection. This idea encompasses several fundamental characteristics. Genetic instability: cells have a variety of ways to maintain the structural integrity of their DNA. Cellular genetic structural variations (deletions, duplications, and rearrangements) or DNA point mutations can trigger biological alterations in cells that may result in tumorigenesis. The disruption of systems regulating genomic stability is accountable for neoplastic processes [8]. Defective repair mechanisms and genotoxic exposure may lead to specific mutational profiles in cancer cells, including those induced by cigarette carcinogens, UV radiation, and chemotherapy agents. Recurrent, mutation-specific characteristics in cancer may influence clonal selection [9]. Figure 1.

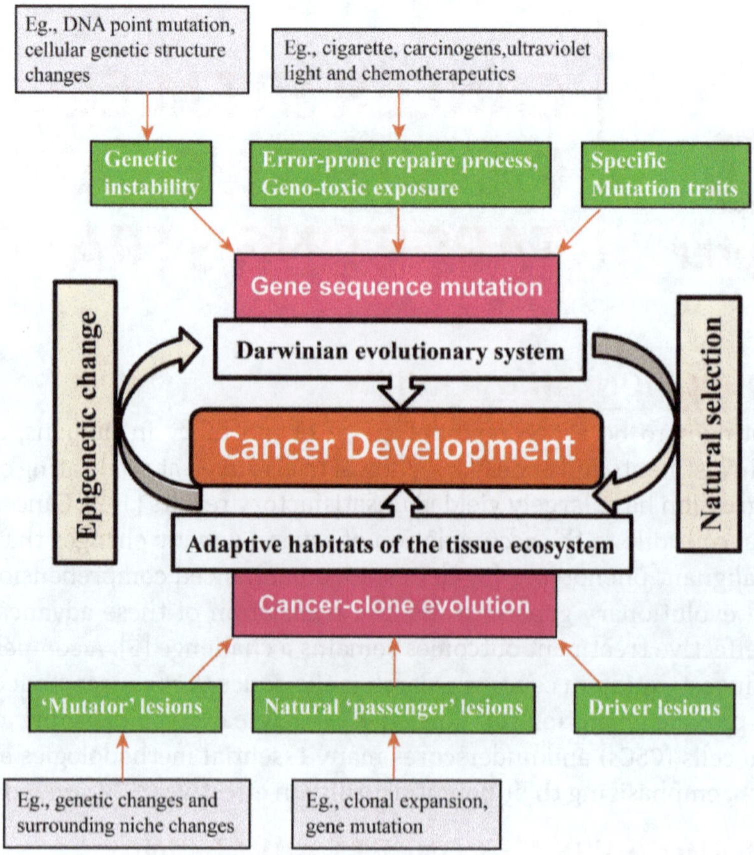

Figure 1. Genetic diversification and clonal dynamics of cancer development.

The tumor microenvironment comprises several cellular components that create an adaptable landscape and supply essential ingredients for the natural selection of cancer proliferation. The connection between cancer cells and their environment is reciprocal. Cancer cells can modify the extracellular environment to create specific niches that facilitate continued cancer proliferation and migration. The cancer microenvironment supplies external cues that facilitate the growth of cancer clones and the survival and proliferation of tumor cells. Spatial heterogeneity is essential for the evolution of cancer cells into a malignant phenotype and facilitates cell migration and distant invasion [12]. During cancer-clone growth, migratory cells infiltrate new environments where they encounter novel selective pressures, therefore accelerating the pace of additional cancer mutations [13]. The cancer niche is an open system. Besides the tissue locations and corresponding etiological environmental exposures of patients, the tissue microecosystem is influenced by many systemic or external factors [14]. Genotoxic exposures, including ultraviolet radiation, pathogenic infections, and prolonged dietary practices, can influence energy metabolism. They are believed to be the principal etiological factors in tumor initiation and the subsequent evolution of cancer clones [14]. The ecosystems of cancer cells can be modified after clinical therapy, during which the majority of cancer cells, along with healthy tissues, are eradicated through aggressive therapies. Nonetheless, certain specialized niches safeguard cells against cancer therapies, leading to the emergence of mutant or therapy-resistant cancer cells [15]. During cancer progression and tumor recurrence post-therapy, the basic unit of selection is a specialized cell, referred to as a cancer stem cell (CSC), which has significant self-renewal capability (Figure 2).

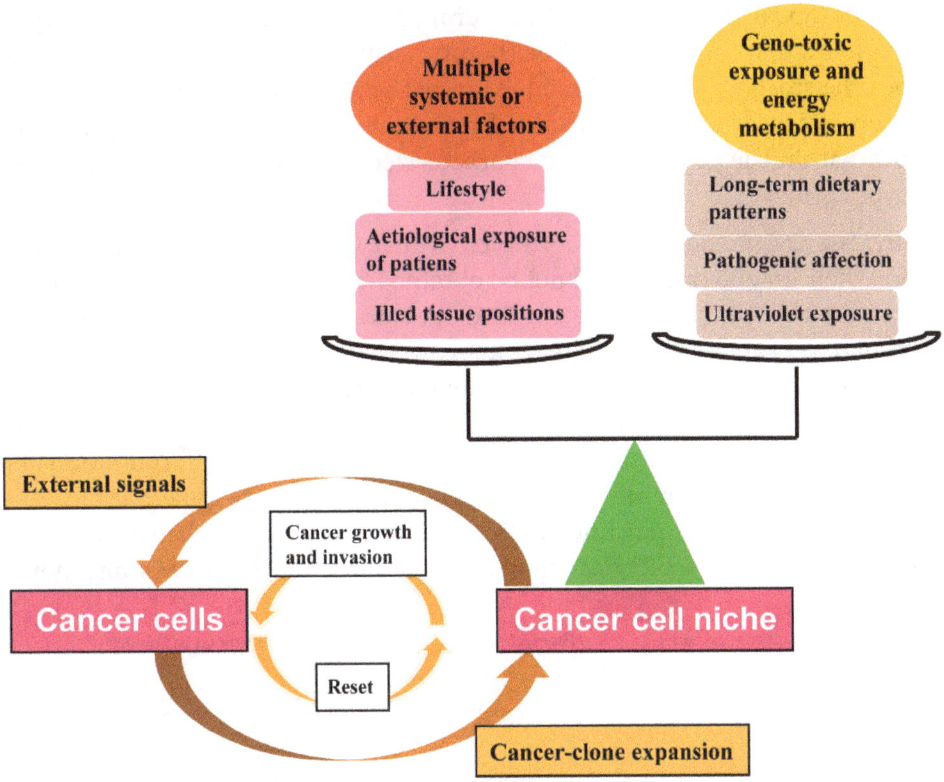

Figure 2. The cancer ecosystem.

2.2. Cancer Stem Cell Model

Cancer research was previously dominated by the clonal evolution model, also known as a conventional stochastic model, a concept whereby all cells within a tumor have equal potential to propagate and maintain a tumor following stepwise genetic and/or epigenetic changes, but they are hard to identify the tumorigenic subset [7, 16–19]. Recently, accumulated studies suggest cancers as hierarchical organizations, which is the basis of the hierarchical or CSC model [20]. In the CSC model, only a small subset of cancer cells possesses the ability to self-renew, differentiates, and reforms a tumor. CSCs, as "roots of cancer" operating in a hierarchical fashion, are defined by their abilities [20–24] (1) to form new tumors with high efficiency that histologically resembles the original tumors when xenotransplanted into immunodeficient mice, (2) to generate descendant cells possessing unlimited self-renewal (regeneration) potential but uncommitted differentiation options, and (3) to generate large populations of differentiated offspring and progenitor cells that exit the stem cell state and lose the ability to self-renew, thus no longer possessing tumorigenic potential. Such differentiated daughter cells can undergo limited rounds of cell division because they lack the intrinsic clonogenic characteristics that are essential for tumor initiation and long-term progression of the malignancy. The increasingly widespread attraction of the CSC model is due to the fact that it can provide a plausible account for poorly understood clinical phenomena, such as therapy resistance, as CSCs can resume growth and contribute to a new relapse after therapy suspension. It is critical to appreciate that both the stochastic and CSC models share the same conviction that only a small population of cancer cells are capable of maintaining cancer. The main difference is that CSCs within the CSC model are characterized with the help of distinct cellular phenotypes [20].

Critically, the CSC model stands on the basis that CSCs are reliable and stable over time, and their unique traits could not be obtained by differentiated descendants. It is worth to note that the persuading of CSC model has been accompanying with intense debates amongst cancer researchers. As evident from a new concept, the dynamic CSC model suggests that the CSC phenotype is much more fluid than previously predicted and can be regulated by external signals [25, 26]. Thus, not only can CSCs self-renew to create new progeny and differentiate to non-CSCs but the de-differentiation of non-CSCs to CSCs can also occur and thus return to the malignancy growth cycle [26–28]. This latest finding has significant implications for oncology in that future effective anticancer therapeutic strategies should aim at targeting both CSCs and non-CSCs (Figure 3).

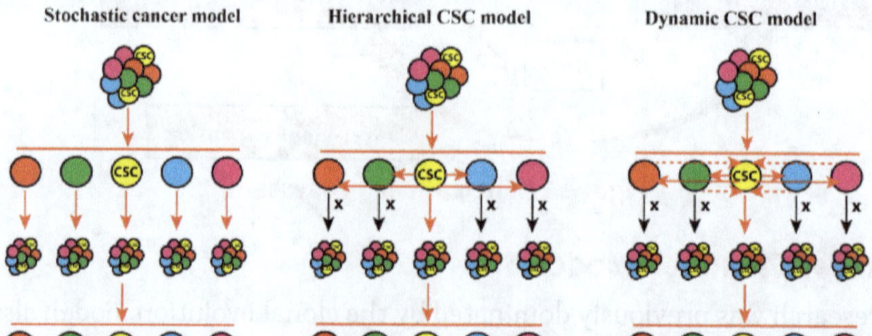

Figure 3. Stochastic cancer model versus hierarchical and dynamic CSC models of tumor heterogeneity.

3. CHALLENGES AND OPPORTUNITIES THE CSC THEORY FACES

Several challenges the CSC theory is now facing should be addressed before this concept can fetch benefits for the clinically relevant entity [29].

3.1. Frequency of CSCs

One challenge that is intensely debated is how many CSCs exist within a tumor. Some studies suggested that the frequency of CSCs is less than 1 in every 1000 cells in a tumor, which supports the hierarchical status between CSCs and non-CSCs [30, 31]. However, recent evidences reported that the number of cells that possess intrinsic tumorigenic potential is relatively higher [32, 33]. Hepatocytes possess the potential of self-renewal and unlimited proliferation under certain conditions [34, 35]. It is shown that various colorectal cancers do not follow the same hierarchy as their CSC frequencies vary [36]. More importantly, the prediction of the number of CSCs in a particular tumor type depends on multiple manual factors, including the experimental procedure designed, the choice of cell surface markers, and the types of immunodeficient mice into which the CSCs were injected. Chiba et al. used the technique of side population (SP) analysis to detect the subpopulations that act CSC functions and revealed that SP cells possess abilities of high proliferation and antiapoptosis in both Huh7 and PLC/PRF/5 cells with a percentage of 0.25% and 0.8%, respectively [37]. Kimura et al. determined the frequency of CSCs by analyzing cell surface markers and the percentage of CD133+ cells in Huh7 and PLC/PRF/5 were 2.7% and 23.5%, which is totally different with the number obtained on the base of EpCAM-positive cells, with a proportion of 89.1% and 40.7%, respectively [38]. However, Cao et al. found the CSC frequency of PLC/PRF/5 cells was 8.8% by using the sphere-forming assay [39]. Thus, considering a tumor as a hierarchical malignancy has intrinsic limitations, as a large population of cancer cells cooperate and contribute to tumor growth, which is consistent with the conventional nonhierarchical model of malignancies [40].

3.2. Therapy Resistance of CSCs

The failure of cancer initial treatment is normally explained due to the presence of a subset of resistant cancer cells. CSCs are supposed to be one of such cells; they are logically resistant to traditional chemotherapies owing to their "stem-like" features, including enhanced abilities of DNA damage repair and cellular detoxification capacity via elevated aldehyde dehydrogenase (ALDH) activity, increased expression of enhancement of ATP-binding cassette (ABC) surface transporters, and their nature quiescence [41–43]. CSCs with an up-regulation of antiapoptotic molecules or a high expression of drug efflux pumps respond quite differently when exposed to drugs; they can both survive after cancer treatment [44]. The rapid relapse of the malignancy suggests that the clonogenic core of the cancer was not effectively targeted, and this might be due to the de-differentiation of non-CSCs to CSCs [45]. Even though CSCs are believed to be the most promising candidates for overcoming chemoresistance and tumor recurrence, both CSCs and non-CSCs should be targeted eventually.

3.3. Isolation of CSCs

The isolation and subsequent assessment of CSCs are clearly a rapidly developing area in which diverse strategies were incorporated for obtaining higher CSC purities. One continual concern after isolation assays is that whether the proposed CSCs separated from the bulk of the tumor can still possess the intrinsic cellular properties. The selected CSCs require the distinct phenotypes that can generate a similar malignancy to the parental tumor when transplanted into immunodeficient mice [46]. The subsequent challenge is to optimize experimental procedures to allow xenotransplantation of viable single suspension cells into animals.

3.4. Targeting "confirmed" CSCs

Due to the relevance of cancer development, CSCs are ideal targets for molecular-directed therapies. The limitation is that CSCs are typically present at very low levels. In addition, CSC markers overlap with normal stem cells or between CSCs [47]. These drawbacks indicate that the identification of CSC markers for guiding molecular therapeutics is still in its infancy. Many CSC markers are not strictly CSC antigens since they present on normal cancer cells as well, but they are molecules that support CSCs in their niche.

The characterization of CSCs has led to some experimentally "confirmed" markers or markers involved in the process of targeting or interaction with CSCs. Epithelial cell adhesion molecule (EpCAM) is one of the most highly expressed tumor-associated markers, being found in a broad range of epithelial cancers. EpCAM has been "rediscovered" as a CSC antigen in breast, colon, prostate, and pancreatic cancers [48–50]. In studies on colon cancer tumorigenicity, EpCAMhighCD44+ was considered as a robust marker of more "stem-like" subpopulations. Also, recruiting effector cells to tumors using an anti-EpCAM/anti-CD3 bispecific antibody has been shown to be a promising strategy in the treatment of cancer [51].

In addition to cell-surface markers that are frequently utilized to identify CSCs, the high activity of signal transduction routes can also contribute to CSCs features [52]. The self-renewal capacity of CSCs leads to a long-term clonogenicity mutation, which might be effectively therapeutically targeted. The activation of intracellular signaling pathways associated with the self-renew of CSCs, including Wnt pathway, Hedgehog (Hh) pathway, and Notch pathway, can stimulate a more immature tumor phenotype, facilitate tumor invasion, and promote therapy resistance [53]. The interference of such pathways that promote CSC function might provide an effective therapeutic window for drugs in the war against cancer. These stem cell-associated surface marker proteins and pathways are promising targets for anticancer drug development

4. METHODS EMPLOYED FOR THE INVESTIGATION OF CANCER STEM CELLS

The principal problem in studying cancer stem cells (CSCs) is the capacity to detect and examine them in laboratory settings using both *in vitro* and *in vivo* testing. This section discusses the prevalent approaches employed for the isolation and characterisation of cancer stem cells (CSCs).

4.1. In vivo Xenotransplantation and Limiting Dilution Assay: The Gold Standard

Limiting dilution assays (LDAs) have been used in a broad variety of biological fields. LDA is an experimental technique that attempts to quantify the frequency of biological particles that perform a particular function within a larger mixed population [54]. The aim of LDA is to obtain highly precise data at the macro level. To achieve this goal, several conditions must be considered [55, 56]. First, the cells should be Poisson distributed. Second, the assay should be designed with maximum information containing both negative and positive cultures. Moreover, the conditions must be performed at the state that the response of a single limiting particle can be detected. Thus, the culture conditions should be uniform in all paralleled groups and wells [56].

The ability to determine the number of CSCs is a critical step for the success of in vivo transplantation. However, there has been little or no attempt to standardize this approach [57]. In all conditions tested, the statistical behavior of the system (Es) and changes in condition over time and statistical noise were the two major contributors to overall uncertainty [57]. However, as expected from statistical principles, Es declines with increasing number of replicates analyzed. Also, increasing the number of replicates beyond 96 is unlikely to provide substantial decreases in error, and fewer wells can be used to obtain results with similar precision. Another requirement that arises in stem cell research is the need to accommodate small numbers of replicates in a statistically consistent and defensible manner. Operator error, mouse-to-mouse error, and other errors appear to play minor roles. These findings establish parameters that contribute to the variability of LDA and provide strategies for the optimization and interpretation of the LDA-based CSC estimates. To this end, extreme limiting dilution analysis (ELDA) has emerged as the preferred method that is based on sound statistical principle and methodologies [58]. ELDA works well when the number of replicates is small.

The CSC concept brings essential predictions of cancer research including susceptibility to chemotherapy, aggressiveness of the disease, and the pace of recurrence that may largely be influenced by the functional properties of CSCs [48, 49, 59–61]. To functionally measure CSC potential, the operational assay of evaluating CSCs has been developed. The creation of an array of genetically modified immunodeficient mice enabling analogous xenograft experiments can be used to determine and quantify cells that obtain tumor-initiating activity in human tumors [48, 49, 59–61]. These xenograft models are considered the "gold standard" in CSC research; they are able to guide the biology and therapeutic responses of human CSCs.

The enumeration of CSCs has been performed using phenotypic markers in in vitro limiting dilution transplantation assays. Some key aspects should be considered [32]: (1) inefficient engraftment in mice may result in underestimation of the actual CSC frequency; (2) phenotypic characterization of CSCs may lead to different rates depending on the antibody combinations used, and the use of specific antibodies may induce immune-mediated clearance of CSCs [48]; (3) the approach of tumor implantation (e.g., intravenously, intrafemorally) critically defines engraftment and affects the export of stem cell frequency [62]; and (4) the kind of mouse strain used as tumor recipient and the degree of mouse immunodeficiency are other factors need to be considered [32]. It is reported that the use of adjuvants/culture supplementary (e.g., Matrigel or growth factors) influences not only the measured frequency of CSCs but their phenotypes as well [30, 32].

4.2. The Side Population Assay

In addition to the isolation and identification of CSCs through a set of cell surface markers (such as CD44+/CD24low/lin-/ALDH+, CD44+/CD24low, EpCAM+/CD44+/CD24–, or CD34+/CD38–). The SP discrimination assay is another flow cytometry method used to detect stem cells based on the properties of the Hoechst dye efflux via the ABC transporters [63]. The SP assay has been used to identify stem cell and progenitor populations in various tissues [64, 65]. However, several reports have stated that dye efflux is not a universal property of all stem cells although SPs are much abundant within stem cells [66]. SPs are not just restricted to the stem cell phenotypes as ABC transporters are also expressed by specialized cells in certain organs [67]. The ABC transporters are believed to play a key role in those tissues, protecting the cytotoxic effects of toxins [68]. However, the identification of CSCs has raised interests in the SP assay, and SP subpopulations isolated from some cancers possess capabilities of drug-resistant, self-renewal, and tumorigenicity when transplanted into immunocompromised mice [63]. The SP assay can play an extremely valuable role in the primary isolation and identification of potential stem/progenitor cells, when specific cell surface markers were absent.

4.3. Clonal Sphere Formation Assay and Proliferation (invasion assay) Assay

The clonal sphere formation assay is another functional method used for the identification of CSCs and their purification from the rest of neighboring cells [69, 70]. This assay begins with reliable single cell suspensions originating from primary tumors or established cancer cell lines. Serial dilutions of the single cancer cell suspensions are seeded on ultra-low attachment substrata in the presence of serum-free media with growth factors [71]. CSCs can grow into 3D nonadherent structures called spheres, while non-CSCs cannot survive in such culture conditions. The results of the assay may become more reliable if the spheres are serially passaged. The self-renewal capacity of sphere-generating cells can be estimated by evaluating the sphere formation frequency through LDA and measuring sphere size [72]. The sphere formation assay has been used to identify adult stem cells or CSCs from a number of tissues, including mammary gland, brain, skin, and human melanoma [73–76].

4.4. Enzymatic Assay of Cell-surface Markers

CSCs can be isolated by the enzymatic activities (ALDH activity) [77, 78]. The measurement of ALDH activity by ALDEFLUOR staining is useful to screen tumor cells for resistance to alkylating agents and to identify heterogeneity within tumor cells [79]. The ALDH+ population is consistent with CSC characteristics, generating tumors that recapitulate the phenotypic heterogeneity of the initial tumor. The measurement of ALDH populations revealed that the ALDH+ cells were capable of self-renewing into both ALDH+ and ALDH- cells [80]. A recent study in melanoma described both ALDH+ and ALDH- cells derived from patient biopsies (100 or 2000 cells, respectively) were able to efficiently form tumors. It is also reported that ALDH cells alone may not be sufficient for CSC selection [32]. Despite this, studies in breast cancer combining other CSC surface markers with Aldefluor have improved tumorigenic enrichment and this combination may prove to be a better strategy for enrichment of CSCs [32].

4.5. Slow-cycling Population Assay

The slow-cycling population assay differentiates cancer stem cells from progenitor cells by assessing the incorporation of tagged nucleotide precursors into cellular DNA synthesis [81]. Slow-cycling cells, such as cancer stem cells (CSCs), retain adequate labels for identification using anti-BrdU antibody staining or radioactive labeling [82]. Several technical challenges hinder the precision of BrdU detection: (1) demonstrating that cells exhibit comparable cycling in vitro and in vivo is difficult due to the invasive nature of the BrdU detection method, (2) it is unlikely that all stem cells can be uniformly labeled since BrdU incorporation occurs exclusively during the S phase of the cell cycle, and (3) label retention is contingent upon the duration of the cell cycle, with subsequent status seemingly changing as the organ matures [83]. Therefore, the quantification of stem cells by this assay necessitates additional validation through alternative approaches.

4.6. Lineage Labeling Assay

The lineage labeling assay was initially developed for understanding and tracing the biological developments of a cell, including the identification of cell origin, measuring lineage relationships, and determination of division patterns [84]. In this assay, cells are labeled (usually with a fluorescent dye or tag), followed by tracing in vitro and in vivo. There are several inherent limitations with this technique: (1) the experimental procedure can damage cells or some cells may have weak and/or transient expression of markers and unrestricted clonality [84] and (2) with whole-mount labeling, it is not possible to identify spatial relationships between stem cells and its transit amplifying progeny [85]. In this case, targeted cells are noninvasively labeled in their native environment, and the development of a progenitor cell and a composition of their lineages can be followed. It remains unclear whether the combination of these techniques can be extended to identify CSCs and metastatic initiating stem/progenitor cells.

While there has been a hot debate in recent years as to whether the CSC theory is correct, very recent lineage tracing studies have provided proof that a relatively small number of cells are capable of generating and maintaining a tumor. These studies used fluorescently labeled tumor cells and showed that the quiescent cells remained after further in vivo passages [86]. Furthermore, following treatment, these quiescent cells started to proliferate and generate proliferative progenitor cells that were capable of maintaining a tumor [87–89]. By eliminating these quiescent cells, tumor growth was impaired. These results link back to the theory that leaving a small population of CSCs after the conventional treatment lead to a recurrence of the tumor. Therefore, it is necessary to eliminate both populations of cells within a tumor to produce effective anticancer therapeutic strategies [90].

4.7. CSC Epigenome and Next-generation Sequencing

Whole genome sequencing has made tremendous contributions to cancer research, which enables researchers to discover and understand the rules of cancer development at the nucleic acid level [91, 92]. However, the genome instability and genetic variants limit to demonstrate cancer progression. It was speculated that there exist a senior layer of information, besides genome sequence for regulating differential gene expressions and thus determining cancer evolving. This concept was early prospected by Conrad Hal Waddington in 1942 and subsequently described as "epigenetic control system" by Nanney in 1958 [93, 94]. Epigenetics primarily refers to the study of chromosome variations that modulate gene transcription without alterations in the DNA sequences [95, 96]. Epigenome contains genetic information, not as stable as genome, representing the cellular epigenetic state varying with influence from external factors. Mechanisms produce such changes mainly include DNA methylation, histone modifications, nucleosome positioning, and chromatin remodeling [96]. These epigenetic regulation mechanisms are reported to be closely related with the gaining of stem cell-specific properties, whereby contributing to tumor inheterogeneous [97, 98]. Epigenetic alterations would offer survival benefits in CSC subpopulation which promotes the genetic expression to the self-renewal state, resulting in tumor initiation and further progression [99, 100]. The relevance of the DNA methylation and histone modifications in CSC regulation, subsequently with advancing tumor growth, were recently illustrated in various cancer models [97, 99, 101].

Next-generation sequencing (NGS), also known as high-throughput sequencing, has revolutionized the study of genomics and opened a new chapter of the epigenome research of cancer and stem cell [102, 103]. Four mainly NGS-based approaches have been developed to identify epigenome research, including methylated DNA immunoprecipitation sequencing (MeDIP-Seq), whole genome bisulfite sequencing (WGBS), reduced representation bisulfite sequencing (RRBS), and chromatin immunoprecipitation sequencing (ChIP-Seq). Compared with the previous approach, the innovative advantages of NGS have significantly accelerated the sequence of DNA and RNA and promoted the scientific sightings in CSC epigenome research.

5. THERAPEUTIC APPROACHES EMPLOYED FOR TARGETING CANCER STEM CELLS (CSCS)

Current failure of cancer treatment is normally due to the existence and functionalities of CSCs, which possess more chemoresistance than their non-CSC counterparts, to conventional treatments. Recently, multiple strategies have been developed for targeting and eradicating CSCs while sparing healthy tissues, thereby minimizing the patients to face therapy risks.

5.1. Targeting CSCs via Surface Markers

Since CSCs are attractive targets for anticancer treatment, the CSC-correlated cell surface proteins have been monitored extensively for identification, probable isolation and monitoring the variation of leukemic and solid CSCs in preclinical and clinical settings [104]. Studies using certain ligands or antibodies against CSC surface maker proteins, including EpCAM, CD47, CD44, CD90, CD133, IL-3R, immunoglobulin mucin TIM-3, ALDH+, and others, have advanced the therapeutic efficacy [105–108]. Limitations, such as the expression of such cell surface makers, may vary in different stages of cancer development; only a small subpopulation of CSCs standing in the summit among bunk of cancer cells, as well as overlapping of CSC-associated marker proteins with normal stem cells, impede the effectively targeting of CSCs [47]. For bench assays, it is recommended to employ functional studies such as in vivo LDA upon xenotransplantation to ascertain CSCs, rather than solely be dependent on the incidence of a single or a combination of multiple CSC markers. However, in case of in vivo CSC-based therapy, the CSC surface marker proteins present one of the very few feasible options for targeting CSCs in animals and patients, given the practical and ethical restrictions related with lineage tracing and xenotransplantation.

Accumulated attractions have been grasped in the development of aptamers (also known as chemical antibodies) and monoclonal antibodies for targeting CSCs via targeting surface marker proteins. Shigdar et al. have isolated two RNA aptamers using SELEX for targeting CSC surface markers, EpCAM, and CD133 [109, 110]. These CSC-targeting aptamers internalize into target cells through receptor-mediated endocytosis, which is capable of circumventing ATP-binding cassette transporters that function multiple drug resistance in CSCs [26]. In addition, this newly developed EpCAM RNA aptamer is more sensitive than counterpart antibodies for detecting the surface EpCAM proteins in formalin-fixed paraffin-embedded primary breast cancers, with no nonspecific staining or cross-reactivity with non-EpCAM-expression tissues [111]. This shows the potential of aptamers for specific targeting of cancers but with minimized side effects observation. To optimize promising approaches by targeting cell surface markers might be one of the answers for tracing CSCs and eventually eradiating CSCs, thereby preventing patients from suffering from cancer attacking.

5.2. Targeting ATP-driven Efflux Transporters

The failure of cancer chemotherapy mainly results from increased efflux of anticancer drugs from cancer cells, resulting in the impairment of drug cellular entrance and consequent reduction of chemotherapeutic sensitivity [112]. A considerable root of multidrug resistance (MDR) involves the augmented expression of the ABC transporter superfamily, many of these transmembrane proteins are responsible for effluxion of various xenobiotics (including anticancer agents) from cancer intracellular membranes [112, 113]. The well-characterized MDR transporters consist with ABCB1 (MDR1 or P-glycoprotein), ABCC1 (MRP1), and ABCG2 (BCRP or MXR) [112, 114–116]. Although projects focusing on understanding the mechanisms of these ABC transporters behind chemotherapy failure have been broadly developed, clinical outcomes in these fields have been generally unsatisfactory [113, 117]. The recurrence of primary and metastatic cites can occur following the escaped chemotherapy, in which CSCs, possessing enhanced efflux of therapeutic agents through ABC transporters, have been proven to provide major contributions [114, 118, 119].

Given the association of ABC transporters with cancer stem cell (CSC) characteristics, one strategy to overcome CSC-mediated chemoresistance is the application of targeted chemical inhibitors that disrupt particular functions of individual multidrug resistance (MDR) transporters [114]. Verapamil, a compound aimed at generic ABC transporters, has progressed to clinical trials; however, further investigation was halted due to dose-limiting toxicity [120]. Therefore, there is a necessity for more selective compounds that target individual MDR transporters [121]. A substantial amount of evidence indicates favorable results in surmounting CSC drug resistance by the development of physical conjugation or chemically nanoparticle-functionalized drug delivery systems for anticancer medicines. Chou et al. demonstrated that the conjugation of doxorubicin (DOX) to nanodiamonds decreased DOX efflux in MDR1-overexpressing cancer cells and enhanced anticancer activity in DOX-resistant cancer models [122]. CSC-related chemoresistance and tumor recurrence mostly result from elevated ABC transporter expression; thus, therapeutic methods designed to precisely disrupt the functions of ABC transporter proteins present a promising avenue for targeting and eliminating CSCs.

6. CONCISE SUMMARY

The CSC concept remains an evolving model progressing ahead. The recent lineage tracing approach has demonstrated the existence and roles of cancer stem cells in the growth of solid tumors. Cancer stem cells exhibiting inherent chemoresistance are responsible for tumor recurrence and the primary cause of therapy failures. Challenges persist in the efficient identification and targeting of cancer stem cells (CSCs) in vivo, as well as in monitoring CSCs following treatment. Cancer biology has demonstrated that classical clonal evolution and cancer stem cell models are not mutually exclusive but coexist in carcinogenesis. Consequently, future clarification of the molecular principles governing CSC biology should provide opportunities for effective novel therapeutic techniques that eradicate both CSCs and non-CSCs.

REFERENCES

1. Jemal A, Siegel R, Ward E, et al. Cancer statistics, 2008. CA Cancer J Clin 2008; 58: 71–96. DOI: 10.3322/CA.2007.0010
2. Herter-Sprie GS, Greulich H, Wong K-K. Activating mutations in ERBB2 and their impact on diagnostics and treatment. Front Oncol 2013; 3: 86. DOI: 10.3389/fonc.2013.00086.
3. Hanahan D, Weinberg RA. Hallmarks of cancer: the next generation. Cell 2011; 144: 646–674. DOI: 10.1016/j.cell.2011.02.013
4. Krogan NJ, Lippman S, Agard DA, Ashworth A, Ideker T. The cancer cell map initiative: defining the hallmark networks of cancer. Mol Cell 2015; 58: 690–698. DOI: 10.1016/j.molcel.2015.05.008

5. Stratton MR. Exploring the genomes of cancer cells: progress and promise. Science 2011; 331: 1553–1558. DOI: 10.1126/science.1204040
6. O'Connor ML, Xiang D, Shigdar S, et al. Cancer stem cells: a contentious hypothesis now moving forward. Cancer Lett 2014; 344: 180–187. DOI: doi: 10.1016/j.canlet.2013.11.012
7. Nowell PC. The clonal evolution of tumor cell populations. Science 1976; 194: 23–28.
8. Tsai AG, Lu H, Raghavan SC, Muschen M, Hsieh C-L, Lieber MR. Human chromosomal translocations at CpG sites and a theoretical basis for their lineage and stage specificity. Cell 2008; 135: 1130–1142. DOI: 10.1016/j.cell.2008.10.035
9. Bardelli A, Cahill DP, Lederer G, et al. Carcinogen-specific induction of genetic instability. Proc Natl Acad Sci U S A 2001; 98: 5770–5775. DOI: 10.1073/pnas.081082898
10. Gatenby RA, Gillies RJ. A microenvironmental model of carcinogenesis. Nat Rev Cancer 2008; 8: 56–61. DOI: 10.1038/nrc2255
11. Lathia JD, Heddleston JM, Venere M, Rich JN. Deadly teamwork: neural cancer stem cells and the tumor microenvironment. Cell Stem Cell 2011; 8: 482–485. DOI: 10.1016/j.stem.2011.04.013
12. Chen J, Sprouffske K, Huang Q, Maley CC. Solving the puzzle of metastasis: the evolution of cell migration in neoplasms. PloS One 2011; 6: e17933. DOI: 10.1371/journal.pone.0017933
13. Mazzone M, Dettori D, Leite de Oliveira R, et al. Heterozygous deficiency of PHD2 restores tumor oxygenation and inhibits metastasis via endothelial normalization. Cell 2009; 136: 839–851. DOI: 10.1016/j.cell.2009.01.020
14. Greaves M, Maley CC. Clonal evolution in cancer. Nature 2012; 481: 306–313. DOI: 10.1038/nature10762
15. Gilbert LA, Hemann MT. DNA damage-mediated induction of a chemoresistant niche. Cell 2010; 143: 355–366. DOI: 10.1016/j.cell.2010.09.043
16. Cabioglu N, Ozmen V, Kaya H, et al. Increased lymph node positivity in multifocal and multicentric breast cancer. J Am Coll Surg 2009; 208: 67–74. DOI: 10.1016/j.jamcollsurg.2008.09.001
17. Nguyen-Khac F, Lesty C, Eclache V, et al. Chromosomal abnormalities in transformed Ph-negative myeloproliferative neoplasms are associated to the transformation subtype and independent of JAK2 and the TET2 mutations. Genes Chromosomes Cancer 2010; 49: 919–927. DOI: 10.1002/gcc.20802
18. Visvader JE, Lindeman GJ. Cancer stem cells in solid tumours: accumulating evidence and unresolved questions. Nat Rev Cancer 2008; 8: 755–768. DOI: 10.1038/nrc2499
19. Nguyen-Khac F, Lesty C, Eclache V, et al. Chromosomal abnormalities in transformed Ph-negative myeloproliferative neoplasms are associated to the transformation subtype and independent of JAK2 and the TET2 mutations. Genes Chromosomes Cancer 2010; 49: 919–927. DOI: 10.1002/gcc.20802
20. Shackleton M, Quintana E, Fearon ER, Morrison SJ. Heterogeneity in cancer: cancer stem cells versus clonal evolution. Cell 2009; 138: 822–829. DOI: 10.1016/j.cell.2009.08.017
21. Lee HE, Kim JH, Kim YJ, et al. An increase in cancer stem cell population after primary systemic therapy is a poor prognostic factor in breast cancer. Br J Cancer 2011; 104: 1730–1738. DOI: 10.1038/bjc.2011.159
22. Beck B, Driessens G, Goossens S, et al. A vascular niche and a VEGF-Nrp1 loop regulate the initiation and stemness of skin tumours. Nature 2011; 478: 399–403. DOI: 10.1038/nature10525
23. Nguyen LV, Vanner R, Dirks P, Eaves CJ. Cancer stem cells: an evolving concept. Nat Rev Cancer 2012; 12: 133–143. DOI: 10.1038/nrc3184

24. Wenjing J, Jianhua P, Yue Z, Cho WCS, Kunlin J. The implications of cancer stem cells for cancer therapy. Int J Mol Sci 2012; 13: 16636–16657. DOI: 10.3390/ijms131216636
25. Vermeulen L, de Sousa e Melo F, Richel DJ, Medema JP. The developing cancer stem-cell model: clinical challenges and opportunities. Lancet Oncol 2012; 13: e83–e89. DOI: 10.1016/S1470-2045(11)70257-1
26. Xiang D, Shigdar S, Qiao G, et al. Nucleic acid aptamer-guided cancer therapeutics and diagnostics: the next generation of cancer medicine. Theranostics 2015; 5: 23–42. DOI: 10.7150/thno.10202
27. Chaffer CL, Brueckmann I, Scheel C, et al. Normal and neoplastic nonstem cells can spontaneously convert to a stem-like state. Proc Natl Acad Sci U S A 2011; 108: 7950–7955. DOI: 10.1073/pnas.1102454108
28. Scheel C, Eaton EN, Li SH-J, et al. Paracrine and autocrine signals induce and maintain mesenchymal and stem cell states in the breast. Cell 2011; 145: 926–940. DOI: 10.1016/j.cell.2011.04.029
29. O'Brien CA, Kreso A, Jamieson CHM. Cancer stem cells and self-renewal. Clin Cancer Res 2010; 16: 3113–3120. DOI: 10.1158/1078-0432.CCR-09-2824
30. Wei J, Wunderlich M, Fox C, et al. Microenvironment determines lineage fate in a human model of MLL-AF9 leukemia. Cancer Cell 2008; 13: 483–495. DOI: 10.1016/j.ccr.2008.04.020
31. Kim M, Moon HB, Spangrude GJ. Major age-related changes of mouse hematopoietic stem/progenitor cells. Ann N Y Acad Sci 2003; 996: 195–208. DOI: 10.1111/j.1749-6632.2003.tb03247.x
32. Quintana E, Shackleton M, Sabel MS, Fullen DR, Johnson TM, Morrison SJ. Efficient tumour formation by single human melanoma cells. Nature 2008; 456: 593–598. DOI: 10.1038/nature07567
33. Tan E, Ding XQ, Saadi A, Agarwal N, Naash MI, Al-Ubaidi MR. Expression of cone-photoreceptor-specific antigens in a cell line derived from retinal tumors in transgenic mice. Invest Ophthalmol Vis Sci 2004; 45: 764–768.
34. Limaye PB, Bowen WC, Orr AV, Luo J, Tseng GC, Michalopoulos GK. Mechanisms of hepatocyte growth factor-mediated and epidermal growth factor-mediated signaling in transdifferentiation of rat hepatocytes to biliary epithelium. Hepatology 2008; 47: 1702–1713. DOI: 10.1002/hep.22221
35. Michalopoulos GK, Barua L, Bowen WC. Transdifferentiation of rat hepatocytes into biliary cells after bile duct ligation and toxic biliary injury. Hepatology 2005; 41: 535–544. DOI: 10.1002/hep.20600
36. Vermeulen L, Snippert HJ. Stem cell dynamics in homeostasis and cancer of the intestine. Nat Rev Cancer 2014; 14: 468–480. DOI: 10.1038/nrc3744
37. Chiba T, Kita K, Zheng YW, et al. Side population purified from hepatocellular carcinoma cells harbors cancer stem cell-like properties. Hepatology 2006; 44: 240–251. DOI: 10.1002/hep.21227
38. Kimura O, Takahashi T, Ishii N, et al. Characterization of the epithelial cell adhesion molecule (EpCAM)+ cell population in hepatocellular carcinoma cell lines. Cancer Sci 2010; 101: 2145–2155. DOI: 10.1111/j.1349-7006.2010.01661.x
39. Cao L, Zhou Y, Zhai B, et al. Sphere-forming cell subpopulations with cancer stem cell properties in human hepatoma cell lines. BMC Gastroenterol 2011; 11: 71. DOI: 10.1186/1471-230X-11-71

40. Adams JM, Strasser A. Is tumor growth sustained by rare cancer stem cells or dominant clones? Cancer Res 2008; 68: 4018–4021. DOI: 10.1158/0008-5472
41. Resetkova E, Reis-Filho JS, Jain RK, et al. Prognostic impact of ALDH1 in breast cancer: a story of stem cells and tumor microenvironment. Breast Cancer Res Treat 2010; 123: 97–108. DOI: 10.1007/s10549-009-0619-3
42. Allikmets R, Schriml LM, Hutchinson A, Romano-Spica V, Dean M. A human placenta-specific ATP-binding cassette gene (ABCP) on chromosome 4q22 that is involved in multidrug resistance. Cancer Res 1998; 58: 5337–5339.
43. Abdullah LN, Chow EK. Mechanisms of chemoresistance in cancer stem cells. Clin Transl Med 2013; 2: 3. DOI: 10.1186/2001-1326-2-3
44. Todaro M, Francipane MG, Medema JP, Stassi G. Colon cancer stem cells: promise of targeted therapy. Gastroenterology 2010; 138: 2151–2162. DOI: 10.1053/j.gastro.2009.12.063
45. Sottoriva A, Verhoeff JJC, Borovski T, et al. Cancer stem cell tumor model reveals invasive morphology and increased phenotypical heterogeneity. Cancer Res 2010; 70: 46–56. DOI: 10.1158/0008-5472
46. Bonnet D, Dick JE. Human acute myeloid leukemia is organized as a hierarchy that originates from a primitive hematopoietic cell. Nat Med 1997; 3: 730–737.
47. Yang YM, Chang JW. Current status and issues in cancer stem cell study. Cancer Invest 2008; 26: 741–755. DOI: 10.1080/07357900801901856
48. Al-Hajj M, Wicha MS, Benito-Hernandez A, Morrison SJ, Clarke MF. Prospective identification of tumorigenic breast cancer cells. Proc Natl Acad Sci U S A 2003; 100: 3983–3988. DOI: 10.1073/pnas.0530291100
49. O'Brien CA, Pollett A, Gallinger S, Dick JE. A human colon cancer cell capable of initiating tumour growth in immunodeficient mice. Nature 2007; 445: 106–110. DOI: 10.1038/nature05372
50. Li C, Heidt DG, Dalerba P, et al. Identification of pancreatic cancer stem cells. Cancer Res 2007; 67: 1030–1037. DOI: 10.1158/0008-5472.CAN-06-2030
51. Shen J, Zhu Z. Catumaxomab, a rat/murine hybrid trifunctional bispecific monoclonal antibody for the treatment of cancer. Curr Opin Mol Ther 2008; 10: 273–284.
52. Medema JP, Vermeulen L. Microenvironmental regulation of stem cells in intestinal homeostasis and cancer. Nature 2011; 474: 318–326. DOI: 10.1038/nature10212
53. de Sousa EM, Vermeulen L, Richel D, Medema JP. Targeting Wnt signaling in colon cancer stem cells. Clin Cancer Res 2011; 17: 647–653. DOI: 10.1158/1078-0432.CCR-10-1204
54. Hu Y, Smyth GK. ELDA: extreme limiting dilution analysis for comparing depleted and enriched populations in stem cell and other assays. J Immunol Methods 2009; 347: 70–78. DOI: 10.1016/j.jim.2009.06.008
55. Parrish RS, Hazlett LJ. Design and estimation in the limiting dilution assay when concentrations vary widely among samples. J Biopharm Stat 2000; 10: 197–215. DOI: 10.1081/BIP-1001101022
56. Macken C. Design and analysis of serial limiting dilution assays with small sample sizes. J Immunol Methods 1999; 222: 13–29. DOI: 10.1016/S0022-1759(98)00133-1
57. Sieburg HB, Cho RH, Muller-Sieburg CE. Limiting dilution analysis for estimating the frequency of hematopoietic stem cells: uncertainty and significance. Exp Hematol 2002; 30: 1436–1443. DOI: 10.1016/S0301-472X(02)00963-3

58. Cheli Y, Giuliano S, Guiliano S, et al. Mitf is the key molecular switch between mouse or human melanoma initiating cells and their differentiated progeny. Oncogene 2011; 30: 2307–2318. DOI: 10.1038/onc.2010.598
59. Shultz LD, Sidman CL. Genetically determined murine models of immunodeficiency. Ann Rev Immunol 1987; 5: 367–403. DOI: 10.1146/annurev.iy.05.040187.002055
60. Ricci-Vitiani L, Lombardi DG, Pilozzi E, et al. Identification and expansion of human colon-cancer-initiating cells. Nature 2007; 445: 111–115. DOI: 10.1038/nature05384
61. Maitland NJ, Frame FM, Polson ES, Lewis JL, Collins AT. Prostate cancer stem cells: do they have a basal or luminal phenotype? Horm Cancer 2011; 2: 47–61. DOI: 10.1007/s12672-010-0058-y
62. Barabe F, Kennedy JA, Hope KJ, Dick JE. Modeling the initiation and progression of human acute leukemia in mice. Science 2007; 316: 600–604. DOI: 10.1126/science.1139851
63. Howarth KD, Blood KA, Ng BL, et al. Array painting reveals a high frequency of balanced translocations in breast cancer cell lines that break in cancer-relevant genes. Oncogene 2008; 27: 3345–3359. DOI: 10.1038/sj.onc.1210993
64. Summer R, Kotton DN, Sun X, Ma B, Fitzsimmons K, Fine A. Side population cells and Bcrp1 expression in lung. Am J Physiol Lung Cell Mol Physiol 2003; 285: L97–L104. DOI: 10.1152/ajplung.00009.2003
65. Kim M, Moon H-B, Spangrude GJ. Major age-related changes of mouse hematopoietic stem/progenitor cells. Ann N Y Acad Sci 2003; 996: 195–208. DOI: 10.1111/j.1749-6632.2003.tb03247.x
66. Triel C, Vestergaard ME, Bolund L, Jensen TG, Jensen UB. Side population cells in human and mouse epidermis lack stem cell characteristics. Exp Cell Res 2004; 295: 79–90. DOI: 10.1016/j.yexcr.2003.11.032
67. Choo CR, Danjoux C, Morton GC. Should pathological T3 and/or margin positive prostate cancer receive adjuvant therapy? A radiation oncologist's view. Can J Urol 2000; 7: 1043–1050.
68. Fromm MF, Kauffmann HM, Fritz P, et al. The effect of rifampin treatment on intestinal expression of human MRP transporters. Am J Pathol 2000; 157: 1575–1580. DOI: 10.1016/S0002-9440(10)64794-3
69. Pece S, Tosoni D, Confalonieri S, et al. Biological and molecular heterogeneity of breast cancers correlates with their cancer stem cell content. Cell 2010; 140: 62–73. DOI: 10.1016/j.cell.2009.12.007
70. Kim S, Alexander CM. Tumorsphere assay provides more accurate prediction of in vivo responses to chemotherapeutics. Biotechnol Lett 2014; 36: 481–488. DOI: 10.1007/s10529-013-1393-1
71. Willan PM, Farnie G. Application of stem cell assays for the characterization of cancer stem cells. In: Cancer Stem Cells in Solid Tumors. Springer; 2011. p. 259–282. DOI: 10.1007/978-1-61779-246-5_15
72. Charrier C, Coronas V, Fombonne J, et al. Characterization of neural stem cells in the dorsal vagal complex of adult rat by in vivo proliferation labeling and in vitro neurosphere assay. Neuroscience 2006; 138: 5–16. DOI: 10.1016/j.neuroscience.2005.10.046
73. Ayyanan A, Civenni G, Ciarloni L, et al. Increased Wnt signaling triggers oncogenic conversion of human breast epithelial cells by a Notch-dependent mechanism. Proc Natl Acad Sci U S A 2006; 103: 3799–3804. DOI: 10.1073/pnas.0600065103

74. Singh SK, Hawkins C, Clarke ID, et al. Identification of human brain tumour initiating cells. Nature 2004; 432: 396–401. DOI: 10.1038/nature03128

75. Toma JG, McKenzie IA, Bagli D, Miller FD. Isolation and characterization of multipotent skin-derived precursors from human skin. Stem Cells 2005; 23: 727–737. DOI: 10.1634/stemcells.2004-0134

76. Fang D, Nguyen TK, Leishear K, et al. A tumorigenic subpopulation with stem cell properties in melanomas. Cancer Res 2005; 65: 9328–9337. DOI: 10.1158/0008-5472.CAN-05-1343

77. Croker AK, Goodale D, Chu J, et al. High aldehyde dehydrogenase and expression of cancer stem cell markers selects for breast cancer cells with enhanced malignant and metastatic ability. J Cell Mol Med 2009; 13: 2236–2252. DOI: 10.1111/j.1582-4934.2008.00455.x

78. Cariati M, Naderi A, Brown JP, et al. Alpha-6 integrin is necessary for the tumourigenicity of a stem cell-like subpopulation within the MCF7 breast cancer cell line. Int J Cancer 2008; 122: 298–304. DOI: 10.1002/ijc.23103

79. Chute JP, Muramoto GG, Whitesides J, et al. Inhibition of aldehyde dehydrogenase and retinoid signaling induces the expansion of human hematopoietic stem cells. Proc Natl Acad Sci U S A 2006; 103: 11707–11712. DOI: 10.1073/pnas.0603806103

80. Ginestier C, Hur MH, Charafe-Jauffret E, et al. ALDH1 is a marker of normal and malignant human mammary stem cells and a predictor of poor clinical outcome. Cell Stem Cell 2007; 1: 555–567. DOI: 10.1016/j.stem.2007.08.014

81. Braun KM, Watt FM. Epidermal label-retaining cells: background and recent applications. J Investig Dermatol Symp Proc 2004; 9: 196–201. DOI: 10.1111/j.1087-0024.2004.09313.x

82. Kase S, Yoshida K, Ohgami K, Shiratori K, Ohno S, Nakayama KI. Phosphorylation of p27(KIP1) in the mitotic cells of the corneal epithelium. Curr Eye Res 2006; 31: 307–312. DOI: 10.1080/02713680600584687

83. Oliver JA, Maarouf O, Cheema FH, Martens TP, Al-Awqati Q. The renal papilla is a niche for adult kidney stem cells. J Clin Invest 2004; 114: 795–804. DOI: 10.1172/JCI200420921

84. Bossing T, Technau GM. The fate of the CNS midline progenitors in Drosophila as revealed by a new method for single cell labelling. Development 1994; 120: 1895–1906.

85. Jensen UB, Lowell S, Watt FM. The spatial relationship between stem cells and their progeny in the basal layer of human epidermis: a new view based on whole-mount labelling and lineage analysis. Development 1999; 126: 2409–2418.

86. Tao L, van Bragt MPA, Laudadio E, Li Z. Lineage tracing of mammary epithelial cells using cell-type-specific cre-expressing adenoviruses. Stem Cell Reports 2014; 2: 770–779. DOI: 10.1016/j.stemcr.2014.04.004

87. Chen J, Li Y, Yu T-S, et al. A restricted cell population propagates glioblastoma growth after chemotherapy. Nature 2012; 488: 522–526. DOI: 10.1038/nature11287

88. Driessens G, Beck B, Caauwe A, Simons BD, Blanpain C. Defining the mode of tumour growth by clonal analysis. Nature 2012; 488: 527–530. DOI: 10.1038/nature11344

89. Schepers AG, Snippert HJ, Stange DE, et al. Lineage tracing reveals Lgr5+ stem cell activity in mouse intestinal adenomas. Science 2012; 337: 730–735. DOI: 10.1126/science.1224676

90. Shigdar S, Lin J, Li Y, et al. Cancer stem cell targeting: the next generation of cancer therapy and molecular imaging. Ther Deliv 2012; 3: 227–244.

91. Nater A, Burri R, Kawakami T, Smeds L, Ellegren H. Resolving evolutionary relationships in closely related species with whole-genome sequencing data. Syst Biol 2015; DOI: 10.1093/sysbio/syv045

92. Hehir-Kwa JY, Pfundt R, Veltman JA. Exome sequencing and whole genome sequencing for the detection of copy number variation. Expert Rev Mol Diagn 2015; 15: 1023–1032. DOI: 10.1586/14737159.2015.1053467
93. Li J, Wang T, Zhang X, Yang X. The contribution of next generation sequencing technologies to epigenome research of stem cell and tumorigenesis. Hum Genet Embryol 2011; 01: 1–10. DOI: 10.4172/2161-0436.s2-001
94. Nanney DL. Epigenetic control systems. Proc Natl Acad Sci U S A 1958; 44: 712–717.
95. Morales La Madrid A, Hashizume R, Kieran MW. Future clinical trials in DIPG: bringing epigenetics to the clinic. Front Oncol 2015; 5: 148. DOI: 10.3389/fonc.2015.00148
96. Busch C, Burkard M, Leischner C, Lauer UM, Frank J, Venturelli S. Epigenetic activities of flavonoids in the prevention and treatment of cancer. Clin Epigenetics 2015; 7: 64. DOI: 10.1186/s13148-015-0095-z
97. Munoz P, Iliou MS, Esteller M. Epigenetic alterations involved in cancer stem cell reprogramming. Mol Oncol 2012; 6: 620–636. DOI: 10.1016/j.molonc.2012.10.006
98. Esteller M. Epigenetics in cancer. N Engl J Med 2008; 358: 1148–1159. DOI: 10.1056/NEJMra072067
99. Volkel P, Dupret B, Le Bourhis X, Angrand P-O. Diverse involvement of EZH2 in cancer epigenetics. Am J Transl Res 2015; 7: 175–193.
100. Jeter CR, Yang T, Wang J, Chao HP, Tang DG. Concise review: NANOG in cancer stem cells and tumor development: an update and outstanding questions. Stem Cells 2015; 33: 2381–2390. DOI: 10.1002/stem.2007
101. Shukla S, Meeran SM. Epigenetics of cancer stem cells: pathways and therapeutics. Biochim Biophys Acta 2014; 1840: 3494–3502. DOI: 10.1016/j.bbagen.2014.09.017
102. Mardis ER. The impact of next-generation sequencing technology on genetics. Trends Genet 2008; 24: 133–141. DOI: 10.1016/j.tig.2007.12.007
103. Morozova O, Marra MA. Applications of next-generation sequencing technologies in functional genomics. Genomics 2008; 92: 255–264. DOI: 10.1016/j.ygeno.2008.07.001
104. Visvader JE, Lindeman GJ. Cancer stem cells in solid tumours: accumulating evidence and unresolved questions. Nat Rev Cancer 2008; 8: 755–768. DOI: 10.1038/nrc2499
105. Chen K, Huang Y-h, Chen J-l. Understanding and targeting cancer stem cells: therapeutic implications and challenges. Acta Pharmacol Sin 2013; 34: 732–740. DOI: 10.1038/aps.2013.27
106. Pollyea DA, Gutman JA, Gore L, Smith CA, Jordan CT. Targeting acute myeloid leukemia stem cells: a review and principles for the development of clinical trials. Haematologica 2014; 99: 1277–1284. DOI: 10.3324/haematol.2013.085209
107. Hoang VT, Buss EC, Wang W, et al. The rarity of ALDH(+) cells is the key to separation of normal versus leukemia stem cells by ALDH activity in AML patients. Int J Cancer 2015; 137: 525–536. DOI: 10.1002/ijc.29410
108. Fan D, Li Z, Zhang X, et al. AntiCD3Fv fused to human interleukin-3 deletion variant redirected T cells against human acute myeloid leukemic stem cells. J Hematol Oncol 2015; 8: 18. DOI: 10.1186/s13045-015-0109-5
109. Shigdar S, Qiao L, Zhou S-F, et al. RNA aptamers targeting cancer stem cell marker CD133. Cancer Lett 2013; 330: 84–95. DOI: 10.1016/j.canlet.2012
110. Shigdar S, Lin J, Yu Y, Pastuovic M, Wei M, Duan W. RNA aptamer against a cancer stem cell marker epithelial cell adhesion molecule. Cancer Sci 2011; 102: 991–998. DOI: 10.1111/j.1349-7006.2011.01897.x

111. Shigdar S, Qian C, Lv L, et al. The use of sensitive chemical antibodies for diagnosis: detection of low levels of EpCAM in breast cancer. PLoS One 2013; 8: e57613. DOI: 10.1371/journal.pone.0057613

112. Fletcher JI, Haber M, Henderson MJ, Norris MD. ABC transporters in cancer: more than just drug efflux pumps. Nat Rev Cancer 2010; 10: 147–156. DOI: 10.1038/nrc2789

113. Gottesman MM, Fojo T, Bates SE. Multidrug resistance in cancer: role of ATP-dependent transporters. Nat Rev Cancer 2002; 2: 48–58. DOI: 10.1038/nrc706

114. Abdullah LN, Chow EK-H. Mechanisms of chemoresistance in cancer stem cells. Clin Transl Med 2013; 2: 3. DOI: 10.1186/2001-1326-2-3

115. Jonker JW, Merino G, Musters S, et al. The breast cancer resistance protein BCRP (ABCG2) concentrates drugs and carcinogenic xenotoxins into milk. Nat Med 2005; 11: 127–129. DOI: 10.1038/nm1186

116. Zhou S, Schuetz JD, Bunting KD, et al. The ABC transporter Bcrp1/ABCG2 is expressed in a wide variety of stem cells and is a molecular determinant of the side-population phenotype. Nat Med 2001; 7: 1028–1034. DOI: 10.1038/nm0901-1028

117. Szakacs G, Paterson JK, Ludwig JA, Booth-Genthe C, Gottesman MM. Targeting multidrug resistance in cancer. Nat Rev Drug Discov 2006; 5: 219–234. DOI: 10.1038/nrd1984

118. Scharenberg CW, Harkey MA, Torok-Storb B. The ABCG2 transporter is an efficient Hoechst 33342 efflux pump and is preferentially expressed by immature human hematopoietic progenitors. Blood 2002; 99: 507–512. DOI: 10.1182/blood.V99.2.507

119. Chow EK-H, Fan L-l, Chen X, Bishop JM. Oncogene-specific formation of chemoresistant murine hepatic cancer stem cells. Hepatology 2012; 56: 1331–1341. DOI: 10.1002/hep.25776

120. Dalton WS, Crowley JJ, Salmon SS, et al. A phase III randomized study of oral verapamil as a chemosensitizer to reverse drug resistance in patients with refractory myeloma. A Southwest Oncology Group study. Cancer 1995; 75: 815–820.

121. Lancet JE, Baer MR, Duran GE, et al. A phase I trial of continuous infusion of the multidrug resistance inhibitor zosuquidar with daunorubicin and cytarabine in acute myeloid leukemia. Leuk Res 2009; 33: 1055–1061. DOI: 10.1016/j.leukres.2008.09.015

122. Chow EK, Zhang XQ, Chen M, et al. Nanodiamond therapeutic delivery agents mediate enhanced chemoresistant tumor treatment. Sci Transl Med 2011; 3: 73ra21. DOI: 10.1126/scitranslmed.3001713

6 Chapter

IMMUNOCARRIERS TARGETED BY ANTIBODIES FOR CANCER THERAPY

1. INTRODUCTION: AN OVERVIEW

Cancer can be induced by various factors, including bacterial infections, radiation, and genetic anomalies, and it is the predominant cause of mortality globally. Currently, cancer accounts for around one in eight deaths globally. Conventional cancer treatments, including chemotherapy, surgery, and radiation therapy, have significantly advanced in the management of cancer. Nonetheless, they may still induce severe side effects or mortality due to the impairment of normal cells or organs, such hepatotoxicity, cardiotoxicity, or nephrotoxicity. Nanomedicine, as defined by the National Institutes of Health in the USA, refers to the utilization of nanotechnology in the treatment, monitoring, and management of cancer. The therapeutic index for cancer was markedly enhanced by the nanomedicines.

In contrast to conventional therapeutic techniques, novel cancer therapies utilizing nanoparticles have garnered significant interest owing to their distinct advantages. Nevertheless, certain limitations persist, including suboptimal in vivo efficacy for nanomedicine and the adverse phenomenon of tumor escape in immunotherapy. The in vivo performance is significantly influenced by the structural features of micelles; therefore, the substantial disparity between in vitro and in vivo outcomes can be mitigated through the chemical design and microstructural optimization of micelles. Furthermore, the engineering of these fine micelles can offer practical solutions to address the challenges in conventional cancer immunotherapy. This chapter examines recent advancements in antibody engineering, nanomedicine, cancer treatment, and nanoimmunotherapy. We provide an explanation of how the engineering of fine micelles, with particular emphasis on the distinctive pathophysiology of tumor microenvironments and the characteristics of immune cells, can significantly enhance in vivo performance and augment the therapeutic index of nanoimmunotherapy. This chapter will delineate four sections detailing the role of antibody-targeted immunomicelles in cancer therapy.

2. ANTIBODY MODIFICATION

Cancer-targeted therapy, designed to target malignant cells while safeguarding normal tissue, is advancing swiftly and yielding substantial enhancements. Nanomedicine represents a pivotal advancement in tumor-targeted therapy, characterized as the utilization and enhancement of nanotechnology to address medical challenges, particularly in the diagnosis, treatment, and prevention of diseases. [1, 2] Nanomedicines are engineered to modify the pharmacological characteristics of encapsulated medications, including pharmacokinetics (PK) and biodistribution (BD), or to serve as drug reservoirs, such as sustained release systems, or both. Nanomedicines can significantly mitigate the deleterious effects of traditional chemotherapeutics. [4, 5] The pharmacological qualities of traditional medications can be enhanced through the application of nanomedicines. [6, 7] Conversely, nanomedicines can safeguard the medication against premature degradation and adverse interactions with the biological milieu, promote targeting to tumors through the "enhanced permeability and retention (EPR) effect," and augment intracellular penetration. [8, 9] Recently, numerous nanomedicines have received approval or are undergoing clinical trials, including Myocet (non-PEGylated doxorubicin liposomes), DaunoXome (daunorubicin liposomes), Onco TCS (vincristine liposomes), Doxil/Caelys (PEGylated doxorubicin liposomes), and Abraxane (albumin-bound paclitaxel nanoparticles).

A notable advancement in cancer-targeted therapy is the development of monoclonal antibodies (mAbs) for cancer treatment. [10, 11] Monoclonal antibodies (MAbs) have been extensively utilized either independently or in conjunction with other chemotherapeutic drugs in oncological treatment. [10-12] The utilization of monoclonal antibodies in cancer treatment is increasing swiftly owing to their precise targeting of neoplastic cells and robust antitumor efficacy. [13] To date, over 10 monoclonal antibodies have received approval for cancer treatment. [14]

2.1. Monoclonal Antibodies

MAbs are monospecific antibodies which are made by identical immune cells cloning from the unique parent cell. MAbs are typically made by fusing myeloma cells with spleen cells of mice immunized with antigens. The first generation of mAbs of murine origins is limited in clinic use owing to their strong immunogenicity and weak activity to elicit antitumor immune response. These defects are considerably overcome by the chimeric and humanized mAbs, which contain human Fc domains and retain targeting specificity by incorporating portions of the murine variable regions. Chimeric mAbs are generated by grafting the entire murine regions into the human IgG framework, whereas humanized mAbs are developed by grafting complementary-determining regions (CDRs) into the human IgG framework. [15-17] Recently, the fully human mAbs with little immunogenicity in humans are being developed rapidly using either phage display technology or transgenic mice. [18]

MAbs have achieved significant progress in cancer therapy. The most significant advances in the application of mAbs to oncology have been the approval of bevacizumab (Avastin, anti-VEGF antibody), cetuximab (Erbitux, anti-EGFR antibody), and trastuzumab (Herceptin, anti-HER2 antibody). Bevacizumab significantly prolongs the survival of patients with metastatic cancers of the colorectum, breast, and lungs, combined with standard chemotherapy regimens. [19] Cetuximab achieved potent antitumor responses in patients with chemotherapy-refractory colorectum cancer. [20] Herceptin has been shown to prolong the disease-free and overall survival of patients with breast cancer. [21]

2.2. Immunoglobulin-like Antibodies

Immunoglobulin is a protein manufactured by plasma cells and lymphocytes and characteristic of these types of cells. Immunoglobulins play a key role in the body's immune system. Antibody, also known as an immunoglobulin, is a large Y-shaped protein used by the immune system to detect and neutralize foreign objects such as bacteria and viruses. The antibody recognizes a unique part of the foreign target, termed an antigen. Recent gene engineering could redesign the antibody by structure modification. After gene engineering, several antibodies still maintain their immunoglobulin-like structure but significantly enhanced the binding affinity or cytotoxic effects. Li et al. developed two genetically engineered tetravalent antibodies (TetraMcAb), respectively, derived from the anti-CD20 mAbs C2B8 and 2F2. [22] TetraMcAbs were not only effective in inducing complement-dependent cytotoxicity (CDC) and antibody-dependent cellular cytotoxicity (ADCC) against B-lymphoma cells as native divalent antibodies (DiMcAbs) but also had antiproliferative and apoptosis-inducing activity markedly superior to that of DiMcAbs. Wu et al. developed dual-specific and tetravalent immunoglobulin G (IgG)-like molecule-termed dual-variable-domain immunoglobulin (DVD-Ig)-that can be engineered from any two mAbs while preserving activities of the parental antibodies. [23] This molecule can be efficiently produced from mammalian cells and exhibits good physicochemical and pharmacokinetic properties. In an animal disease model, preclinical studies of a DVD-Ig protein demonstrate its potential for therapeutic application in human diseases.

2.3. Antibody Fragments

In addition to mAbs and immunoglobulin-like antibodies, antibodies could also be reduced in size, dissected into minimal binding fragments, and rebuilt into multivalent high-avidity reagents. There are many kinds of antibody fragments. (i) The scFv is a fusion protein of the variable regions of the heavy (VH) and light chains (VL) of immunoglobulins, connected with a short peptide linker consisting of 10~25 amino acids. To provide flexibility and enhance the hydrophilicity of the peptide backbone, the most commonly used linker contains a combination of glycine and serine residues. The linker is usually rich in glycine for flexibility, as well as serine or threonine for solubility, and can either connect the N-terminus of the VH with the C-terminus of the VL. Despite of the removal of the constant regions and the introduction of the linker, this engineered antibody retains the specificity of the original immunoglobulin. (ii) Multivalent antibodies are constructed by multiple Fab or scFv. [24] (iii) Domain antibodies (dAbs), derived from the "heavy chain" of the immunoglobulins from camels, are the smallest known antigen-binding fragments of antibodies, ranging from 11 kDa to 15 kDa. They are the robust variable regions of the heavy and light chains of immunoglobulins (VH and VL, respectively). Due to the small size and inherent stability, dAbs are bioactive as monomers and can be formatted into larger molecules, which could be created with prolonged serum half-lives or other pharmacological activities. [25] (iv) Qiu et al. reported that the mimetics fused by two CDRs, VHCDR1 and VLCDR3, through a cognate framework region (VHFR2) retained the antigen recognition of their parent molecules and had a superior penetration capacity. [26] The antigen-recognition abilities of these B3 kDa mimetics surpass those of comparable fragments lacking the framework region. To our knowledge, these small antibody mimetics are the smallest antibodies among all the present antibodies.

3. CAREFULLY CONSTRUCTED MICELLES TO ENHANCE ANTICANCER TREATMENT

Nearly 40% of newly identified pharmaceuticals encounter delivery issues because to their inadequate solubility, permeability, and stability. Compared to conventional small molecule therapeutic agents, nanomedicine presents significant advancements in cancer therapy by enhancing the solubility of poorly water-soluble drugs, extending the half-life of systemic drug circulation, facilitating controlled drug release, enabling targeted drug delivery with minimal side effects, mitigating drug resistance, and decreasing immunogenicity. [30] Nanomedicine was typically prohibited from being utilized for the creation of nanoscale or nanostructured materials to address medical issues through its distinctive therapeutic effects. Recent advancements in nanotechnology have led to the development of numerous cancer therapeutic agent delivery methods utilizing nanoparticles, including polymeric micelles, polymer-drug conjugates, dendrimers, liposomes, nanopolymer compositions, and inorganic particulates, all within a size range of 1-1,000 nm. Certain of these products have been launched in the pharmaceutical market. Doxil was the inaugural liposomal medication formulation for the treatment of AIDS-related Kaposi's sarcoma in 1995. [31] Abraxane, a polymer-drug combination consisting of an albumin-bound paclitaxel formulation, received approval from the Food and Drug Administration (FDA) in 2005 as a second-line treatment for breast cancer. [32-34].

However, some major challenges are raised as the clinical test of numerous ensuing nanomedicine products. The obvious drawbacks are the in vivo instability[35] and the fast clearance from the blood by the reticuloendothelial system (RES). [36] The most widely used strategy overcoming the instability is covering the carrier's with some hydrophilic polymers such as poly(ethylene glycol) (PEG) or poly(vinylalcohol) (PVA). Nanocarriers linked with highly hydrated flexible PEG successfully escaped from the RES. [37] The PVA coating also improved the particle's stability. However, it should be a commonsense that introducing too much adjuvant into the body resulted in the undesirable toxicity. Moreover, the size, structure, and surface electronic properties of the formulations were changed resulting in unfavorable therapy index. On the contrary, the micellar system mainly including the polymeric micelle and phospholipid micelle has successfully overcome the above drawbacks because these spherical nanoparticles have simple structure and no adjuvant. The lipid based micelles show high potential in the doxorubicin entrapping. [38] However, its intrinsic phospholipid structure resulted in the untunable micellar structure with D > 100 nm, which considerably limited the intratumor accumulation. Additionally, drug release from conventional liposome formulations is quite limited once these particles reach the tumor. [39]

Fortunately, the nanosized polymeric micelles (10-100 nm in diameter) self-assembled from amphiphilic block copolymers can significantly improve the hydrophobic drug solubility in the core via the similar-to-similar interaction. The micelle possesses well-defined hydrophobic core and hydrophilic corona structure in aqueous media. [40] On the other hand, the densely packed corona forming hydrophilic polymer chain can protect micellar system from the RES by reducing the interaction with serum proteins and renal filtration. [41] In comparison with lipid-based micelles, block copolymeric micelles provide a unique and powerful nanoplatform for anticancer drug delivery. The size of polymeric micelles can be easily tuned by varying the block lengths of the amphiphilic copolymer. It is also easy to modify micellar surface via the functional shell forming polymer. Both the tunable size range and the tailorable structure successfully reduce the renal filtration and obviously enhance tumor penetration. Some nanosized micelles such as PEG-PLA/PCL or PEG-PPO-PEG have significantly improved the in vitro /vivo application. Several polymeric micellar formulations are currently undergoing phase I/II clinical trials, which have shown significant antitumor efficacy and reduced systemic toxicity. [40, 41]

It is known that the endothelial cells of the tumor blood vessels proliferate at a 30- to 40-fold higher rate than those in normal tissues, which results in the larger endothelial cells gaps (200-700 nm, or sometimes even larger, up to 1. 2 μm) than 7 nm in the normal tissue. [42] Additionally, the high metabolism of tumor cells requires much more oxygen, nutrients, gas exchange, and waste removal. However, the heterogeneity structure and distribution of the tumor blood vessels as well as the blood capillaries slow down the energy exchange between intra- and extratumor. All these result in unique characteristics of tumor, that is, the unnormal tumor blood vessels with gap in 200-700 nm, [43] the relative high temperature of tumor (T > 37°C), [44] and the relative low pH (5~6). In order to further improve micellar delivering profile, including the lesion's accumulating, cellular uptake, and intracellular release, many new stimulate-responsive micelles were extensively investigated with special focus on the tumor microenvironment. Utilizing the lower pH value in solid tumors and endosomes (5. 5), Kataoka's group explored the novel multifunctional pH-sensitive doxorubicin-conjugated PEG-p(Asp-Hyd-DOX) copolymer micelles. The pH linker broke as pH <6. 0 ensued a sustain release. [46] An enhanced accumulation in lung and colon tumors of the micelle-forming PEO-PAsp (ADR) conjugates after 24 h (ca. 10% dose per g tumor) was much higher than the free ADR (ca. 0. 90% dose per g tumor). Later, they further investigated the pH triggered intracellular release profile of poly(ethyleneglycol)-

poly(aspartate hydrazone adriamycin) micelles and observed that the micelles can stably circulated in physiological conditions (pH 7. 4) and selectively release drug by sensing the intracellular low pH (pH 5-6). In vitro and in vivo studies show that the micelles had a good pH-triggered drug release capability, tumor-infiltrating permeability, and effective antitumor activity with extremely low toxicity. [45, 46] Okano's group used the temperature-sensitive poly(*N*-isopropylacrylamide) (PNIPAM) to investigate the cellular uptake of bovine carotid endothelial cells. As T>LCST, the cell uptake was significantly enhanced. In addition, the LCST of such PNIAPM can be tuned to ~39°C by introducing some hydrophilic monomer into the chain backbone. Thus, the system can shabbily circulate at 37°C but be disassociated as T approaching to 39°C. This PNIPAM was designed to enhance the intracellular release because the cargo structure was disrupted as phase transition. [47, 48] The oxidative condition in the extracellular medium and reductive conditions in the tumor was used to enhance intracellular release. For example, the bioreducible PEG-SS-P[Asp(DET)] micelles bearing the disulfide bridge showed both 1-3 orders of magnitude higher gene transfection efficiency and a more rapid onset of plasmid DNA release than micelles without disulide linkages. [49] Feng's group recently developed a micellar system containing a functional polymer of D-α-tocopheryl polyethylene polyethylene glycol succinate (Vitamin E TPGS or TPGS), which stabilized the micelle and further promotes synergistic effects with the encapsulated drug. [50] This is a novel micellar system. The formulation formed by folic acid-conjugated D-α-tocopheryl polyethylene glycol succinate 2000 (Vitamin E TPGS2k) micelles successfully suppress the tumor cell growth. [51] For improving the therapeutic effect, some other intelligent micellar systems such as light responsive poly(methacrylate) and poly(acrylic acid) (PAzoMA-PAA) micelle were developed. This trans-cis photoisomerization of the azobenzene group improved drug release. [52] In addition, the polymeric micelles conjugated tumor targeting V3lig-and cyclic-(arginine-glycine-aspartic acid-D-phenylalanine-lysine) (cRGDfK) to DOXO-loaded polyethylene glycol-polycaprolactone (PEG-PCL) micelles greatly enhanced internalization of the micelles through receptor-mediated endocytosis. [53]

These substantial advancements in intelligent block copolymer micelles have ushered in a new age for nanomedicine. Nonetheless, a significant gap remains in transferring an optimum micelle to clinical practice due to insufficient understanding of the relationship between the particular characteristics of tumors (needs) and the physical chemistry qualities of micelles (seeds) in vitro versus in vivo. The in vitro/vivo performance of micelles is significantly influenced by their physicochemical features, including composition, size, microstructure, and intelligence characteristics. The primary impetus for self-assembly is the substantial solubility disparity between the hydrophobic and hydrophilic blocks, as delineated by the Flory-Huggins parameter.

4. IMMUNOLIPOSOME

Although liposomes have already achieved significant advance, antitumor activity could be further ehanced for liposomes through ligand-mediated targeting. For liposomes, the ligands would promote the selective binding and facilitate the intracellular delivery. The most commonly used ligands include mAbs or antibody fragments, folic acid, or receptor ligands. [54-59] MAbs or their derivatives (e. g. , Fab fragments, single-chain variable fragments (scFv)) are often adopted as the targeted ligands in LTLs. LTLs decorated with mAbs or their derivatives are termed as immunoliposomes. Immunoliposomes can be used to deliver various drugs, like chemotherapeutics, gene, or protein drugs, and significantly improve the therapeutic efficacy of conventional strategies in cancer. [60-64] When conjugated with antibodies as targeting ligands, immunoliposomes can target tumor cells with high specificity and affinity, resulting in significantly improved antitumor activity over untargeted liposomes. [65] The development of immunoliposomes, which perfectly combine antibody engineering and liposomes, is becoming a possible state-of-the-art in liposome research. This review discusses the recent development and therapeutic effect of immunoliposomes in cancer therapy. This review includes the following sections: antibody engineering, antibody conjugation strategies, therapeutic potential of immunoliposomes in cancer, challenges, and future perspectives of immunoliposomes.

4.1. Conjugation of Thiolated Antibody with Liposomes

The most common conjugation strategy employs the reaction between thiol functions and maleimide groups, which form thioether bonds. This strategy consists of two steps. First, after reaction with traut's reagent (2-imiothiolane), the antibodies modified with free sulfhydryl are obtained. [66] Alternately, antibodies reacts with the heterobifunctional crosslinking agents such as *N*-succinimidyl 3-(2-pyridyldithio) propionate (SPDP) or succinimidyloxycarbonyl-α-methyl-α-(2-pyridyldithio) toluene (SMPT). Once modified with SPDP or SMPT, antibodies are treated with dithiothreitol (DTT) and form the free sulfhydryl. [67, 68] Also, antibodies react with the heterobifunctional crosslinking agents such as *N*-succinimidyl S-acetylthioacetate (SATA), S-acetylmercaptosuccinic anhydride (SAMSA), or succinimidyl acetylthiopropionate (SATP). [69-71] Once modified with SATA, SAMSA, or SATP, antibodies are treated with hydroxylamine and form free sulfhydryl. Second, thiolated antibody bearing the free sulfhydryl reacted with maleimide groups on the liposomes, and the resultant liposomes conjugated with antibodies were obtained. Attachment of antibodies to liposomes via a disulfide linkage A disulfide bond formed by two thiols is easily obtained. However, the disulfide bond is relatively unstable under reductive conditions. Thiolated antibodies could react with the pyridyldithio moiety of the anchor (PE-PDP) to form a disulfide linkage. This coupling strategy achieved efficient conjugation of antibodies to liposomes without denaturation of antibodies. [72-74]

4.2. Crosslinking between Carboxylic Acid on Liposomes and the Ligand

Antibodies could be conjugated to the liposomes by an amide bond using the membrane-anchored lipid functionalized with carboxylic acid end groups. This conjugation commonly used distearoyl-*N*-(3-carboxypropionoyl poly(ethylene glycol) succinyl) phosphatidylethanolamine (DSPE-PEG-COOH) offering carboxylic acid groups at the distant end of surface-grafted PEG chains as the membrane-anchored lipid. [75, 76] In the coupling reaction, 1-ethyl-3-(3-dimethylaminopropyl) carbodiimide (EDAC) and *N*-hydroxysulfosuccinimide (NHS) are usually used to form an acyl amino ester, which subsequently react with the primary amine of the ligand, yielding an amide bond. Suzuki et al. prepared liposomes conjugated with transferrin specific for transferrin receptor overexpressing solid colon 26 tumor cells, and the results indicated that the immunoliposomes recognized and bound specifically to target cells in vivo.

4.3. Antibody Conjugation with Liposomes via a Hydrazone Bond

Antibodies can be covalently bound to hydrazide groups of the liposomes through their carbohydrate moieties to form a hydrazide bond. In the conjugation strategy, the carbohydrates groups on the constant region of the heavy chain of the antibody are oxidized by sodium periodate to produce reactive aldehydes, which form hydrazone linkages with the hydrazide groups on the PEG-terminus. [77, 78] It is has to be noted that the oxidation reaction should be performed in mild conditions to avoid the loss of antibody activity. The antibodies are correctly orientated on the surface of the liposomes because only the Fc region is involved in the conjugation reaction and the antigen binding site are protected. Furthermore, this conjugation strategy avoids the recognition of the immunoliposomes by the macrophages, resulting in longer circulation time of immunoliposomes.

4.4. Crosslinking between Primary Amines on Liposomes with the Antibody

Direct amine-amine crosslinking has also been investigated in antibody conjugation. [79] In the conjugation, two homobifunctional crosslinkers including glutaraldehyde and suberimidate are used, and no prior modification is required to add functional groups to the antibody. Briefly, the primary amine of phosphatidylethanolamine of the liposomes is firstly activated using the crosslinkers and subsequently conjugated to the antibody. It is reported that almost 60% of the antibodies were coupled to the liposomes, and these conjugated antibodies still retained their binding affinity. However, this conjugation strategy was rarely applied because the uncontrollable homopolymerization of antibodies or liposomes would happen during the crosslinking reaction.

4.5. Noncovalent Methods for Antibodies Conjugated with Liposomes

A noncovalent technique is an alternative means to for antibody conjugation to liposomes. The unique advantage of a noncovalent technique is easy and rapid performance without the need of aggressive reagents. For example, simply mixing antibodies and phospholipids during the preparation of the liposomes would achieve the binding of antibodies to the liposomes. [80] However, the disadvantages of the noncovalent technique are obvious. The conjugation efficiency of antibodies is relatively low and liposome aggregation would happen. Furthermore, the amount of antibody conjugated to the liposome is not easily controllable, and the correct orientation of the antibodies is not guaranteed. Finally, conjugated antibodies are not stable and may detach easily. Thus, due to the weak interaction between the liposome and the antibodies, the noncovalent technique has not been widely used. However, it is noteworthy that one noncovalent technique, which uses the binding between streptavidin and biotin for attachment of antibodies to liposomes, is an exception. The binding of streptavidin to biotin is simple, highly stable, and reproducible; thus, the attachment of antibodies to liposomes using such a strategy is rather favorable and promising. [81] Generally, two strategies of antibody conjugation use the streptavidin-biotin interaction.

First, the streptavidin-modified antibodies were conjugated to the anchor lipid DSPE-PEG-biotin. The immunoliposomes redirected the biodistribution of entrapped drugs and showed specific targeting to the targeted organ overexpressing specific antigens, leading to significant accumulation in the targeted organ. [82] Second, the biotinylated antibodies were incubated with the targeted cells overexpressing specific antigens. Then streptavidin was added, followed by biotinylated liposomes. The results showed that the liposomes specifically bound to the targeted cells coated with antibodies but not to the control cells, which do not express the specific antigen. [83]

5. Precisely Engineered Nanocarriers for Immunotherapy

Various immune cells, including B cells, T-lymphocytes, and dendritic cells, are recruited to the tumor. Immunotherapy refers to the alteration of the host immune system and/or the application of immune system components for cancer treatment, primarily encompassing active and passive forms. Passive immunotherapy involves administering substantial quantities of effector molecules, such as tumor-specific monoclonal antibodies (mAbs), to enhance the immune system. Active immunotherapy involves the deployment of humoral and/or cytotoxic T-cell effector mechanisms of the immune system subsequent to vaccination, specifically cancer vaccines. This approach can concurrently activate antigen presentation cells (APCs), CD4+ T cells, CD8+ T cells, B cells, and innate immune cells, such as granulocytes and NK cells. Dendritic cells are the most specialized and crucial antigen-presenting cells, essential for eliciting an adaptive immune response. Vaccines utilizing lipid-based nanocarriers can enhance accumulation in dendritic cells within tumor-bearing animals and significantly impact dendritic cell functionality. Poly(D, L-lactic acid-co-glycolic acid) (PLGA) nanoparticles containing the cancer-associated antigen MUC1 mucin peptide (BLP25) and mouse-specific peripheral lymphocyte antigen (MPLA) significantly enhanced native T-cell activation in both normal and MUC1-transgenic mice. [86] The efficacy of immunization is significantly influenced by tumor-specific antigens (TSAs) and the vaccine delivery mechanism. Polymeric nanoparticles garner significant interest owing to their easily adjustable composition, customizable structure, distinctive intelligence features, and considerable potential in cancer immunotherapy, namely nanoimmunotherapy.

Immunotherapy cannot only kill tumor cells in a specific manner but also alert the immune system to eradicate the disseminated tumor cells in blood circulation and micrometastases in distant organs. [87, 88] However, tumor cells can survive when they either maintain chronically or immunologically sculpt by immune "editors." This well-known "immunoediting" refers to the elimination, equilibrium, and escape. [88] The new populations of tumor variants may eventually evade the immune system and escape from host immune surveillance by a variety of mechanisms including loss of MHC-I, adhesion molecules, tumor-associated antigens (TAAs), generation of regulatory T-(Treg-) lymphocyte, expansion of myeloid-derived suppressor cells ($CD11b^+$ $Gr\text{-}1^+$ cells, MDSCs), immunosuppression, blocking of NKG2D-mediated activation, and apoptosis induction of antitumor effector cells. [89, 90] Tumor-specific immune activation and nonspecific immune activation have been applied for overcoming such tumor escape. The tumor-specific immune responses are teaching the immune cells to recognize tumor cells specifically. B cells secrete antigen-specific antibodies that recognize, bind, and help to destroy the targets with the help of the $CD4^+$T cells. $CD4^+$ T cells recognize the antigens presented by MHC-II molecules and then stimulate B cells to produce antibodies to that specific antigen. Such antibody-coated cancer cells recognized and killed by NK cells, macrophage, and activated monocytes are called antibody-dependent cell-mediated cytotoxicity (ADCC). The nonspecific immune activation strategy mainly utilizes the cytokines (IL2 and IL8), the interferons (IFN-α, β, and IFN-γ), and the Toll-like receptors (TLRs) for trigging DC maturation, stimulating proliferation of $CD4^+$ and $CD8^+$ T cells and modulating the suppressive function of regulatory T cells (Treg cells). [91] Treg cells suppress TAA-specific immunity by inhibiting TAA-specific priming in tumor draining lymph nodes and further recruiting into the tumor microenvironment. [92] Thus, depletion, blocking, and tracking Treg cells in tumors or reducing their differentiation and suppressive mechanisms represent new strategies for cancer treatment. It was known that the knockdown of transcription factor Foxp3 gene in mature Treg cells resulted in the loss of their suppressive function. [93] However, the transfection efficiency is very low. The newly developed novel carbon nanotubes (CNTs) can enhance the transfection of Treg cells. [92] The PLGA nanoparticle (PLGA-NP) carrying murine melanoma antigenic peptides $hgp100_{25\text{-}33}$ and $TRP2_{180\text{-}188}$ can also induce cytotoxic T lymphocyte responses against tumor-associated self-antigens in C57BL/6 mouse. [94]

Thus, finely engineering nanocarriers from homopolymers, copolymers, and lipids with high loading and transferring efficiency, site-specific targeting to immune cells, high in vitro/vivo stability, and intelligent responsive to tumor microenvironment show high potential in nanoimmunotherapy. [95, 96] Tumor microenvironment is the main battlefield for tumor escape and immune system activation. As shown in Figure, the high proliferation and metabolism of tumor endothelial cells resulted in the unique properties of tumor microenvironment, including large endothelial cells gaps (200-1000 nm), the relative high temperature (T>37°C), low pH (5~6), lacking lymphatic nodes, and lymph vessels. [97] This unique pathological condition of microenvironment offers challenges for novel nanocarrier's engineering. Based on the self-assembly mechanism, well-defined micelle and vesicle with surface targeting decorating were finely engineered. [98] We found that the temperature-regulated passive and mAb-tuned active dual targeting immunomicelles significantly enhanced intratumor accumulation and cellular uptake. The nanostructure and the dimension were also tailored to match the large endothelial cells gaps in tumors with enhanced permeability and retention (EPR). [86] The extracellular pH is ~7. 4, but the pH in the endosome and microenvironment is ~6. 0. This value is still lowered to ~5. 0 in the lysosome. The hydrolysis rates of polyester such as polylactic acid, polyglycolic acid, and their copolymers can thus be tuned for endosomal and/or lysosomal delivery. [99] Additionally, the endosome is reductive, but the lysosomal is oxidative. This difference is very important for spatial delivery antigens for MHC presentation. The antigens for MHC class I pathways must be available in cytosol, whereas those for MHC class II molecules must be present in endolysosome. The finely engineered lipids with protein antigens in nanovesicle core and lipid-based immunostimulatory molecules in the walls successfully elicits endogenous T cell and antibody responses, which showed rapid release adjuvants in the presence of endolysosomal lipases. [100] Some danger signals (adjuvants) for APC activation are present on the plasma membrane. So nanocarriers engineered from polycations such as polyethyleneimine (PEI) or its graft copolymers (Figure) hold favorable effect on membrane destabilization by the "proton-sponge" effect, which can also control the endosomal release. [101] Both structural defects and fibrosis of the interstitial matrix result in poor/dysfunctional T-cell priming in tumor microenvironment. However, the forced expression of the tumor necrosis factor (TNF) can induce naive T-cell priming. Thus, delivery stimulator such asCD80, interleukin-4 (IL-4), and cytokines by intelligent nanocarriers to tumor microenvironment can produce T-cell priming with the microenvironment reversion. [102]

DCs appear in most peripheral tissues where antigens typically first encounter the immune system. Immature DCs phagocytose the encountered antigens followed by the activation, maturation, and migration to draining lymph nodes. They present antigens to their cognate naive T-cell partners and instruct the anergy, tolerance, or immunity. Then the antigen-specific T-cell immunity is initiated. Noted here is the timing at which antigen and adjuvant reach DCs is crucial. If the maturation stimulus is too late, tolerance will be induced. If the antigens reach mature DCs, they will not be efficiently presented. The intelligent responsive polymer carriers can be finely designed to regulate the antigen's communication with DCs. Some lipids had successfully been used to promote the lymphatic trafficking and endue the DCs mutation. [103] The DCs preferentially take up smaller particles with size similar to viral (~20 nm), whereas macrophages ingest the large particles with size around bacterial. It is also worth mentioning that PLGA-NPs (500 nm) are more effective than microparticles (~2 nm) in stimulating CTL responses. The DC's phagocytosis is also affected by nanoparticle's surface charge. [104] Cationic particles are particularly effective for uptake by DCs and macrophages due to that the ionic attraction increases the particle binding and internalization. Above-mentioned nanocarrier's size, microstructure, charge, and intelligent properties can be facilely engineered by tuning polymer composition and particle formation process. In addition, specific DC-specific antibodies such as anti-CD11c and anti-DEC205 can enhance nanocarrier's accumulation in DCs. The PLA nanoparticles loaded dacarbazine (DTIC) decorated with TRAIL-receptor2 (DR5) mAb (DTIC-NPs-DR5) showed high internalization by DR5-overexpressing metastatic melanoma and chemo-immunocooperative therapeutic effects. [105] Informed by our comprehension of the molecular mechanisms of immune evasion and the physiological conditions of tumors, nanocarriers in nanoimmunotherapy require meticulous engineering with well-defined dimensions, intelligent characteristics, precise targeting, advanced lymphatic imaging, and exact intracellular release to optimize the therapeutic index.

REFERENCES

1. Archakov A. I. 2010. Nanobiotechnologies in medicine: nanodiagnostics and nanodrugs. Biochemistry (Moscow) 4:2-14.
2. Feng S. S. 2006. New-concept chemotherapy by nanoparticles of biodegradable polymers: where are we now? Nanomedicine (Lond) 1:297-309.
3. Allen T. M. , Cullis P. R. 2004. Drug delivery systems: entering the mainstream. Science 303:1818-22.
4. Moghimi S. M. , Hunter A. C. , Murray J. C. 2005. Nanomedicine: current status and future prospects. FASEB Journal 19:311-30.
5. Bawarski W. E. , Chidlowsky E. , Bharali D. J. , Mousa S. A. 2008. Emerging nanopharmaceuticals. Nanomedicine 4:273-82.
6. Duncan R. Polymer conjugates as anticancer nanomedicines. 2006. Nature. Review Cancer 6:688-701.
7. Gao J. , Feng S. S. , Guo Y. 2012. Nanomedicine against multidrug resistance in cancer treatment. Nanomedicine (Lond.) 7:465-8.
8. Matsumura Y. , Maeda H. 1986. A new concept of macromolecular therapies in cancer chemotherapy: mechanism of tumortropic accumulation of proteins and the titumor agent. SMANCS. Cancer Research 6:6387-92.
9. Davis M. E. , Chen Z. G. , Shin D. M. 2008. Nanoparticle therapeutics: an emerging treatment modality for cancer. Nature Reviews. Drug Discovery2:771-82.
10. Torchilin V. P. 2005. Recent advances with liposomes as pharmaceutical carriers. Nature Reviews. Drug Discovery 2:145-60.
11. Schrama D. , Reisfeld R. A. , Becker J. C. 2006. Antibody targeted drugs as cancer therapeutics. Nature. Reviews. Drug Discovery 5(2):147-59.
12. Adams G. P. , Weiner L. M. 2005. Monoclonal antibody therapy of cancer. Nature. Biotechnol 23:1147-57.
13. Zhang T. , Herlyn D. 2009. Combination of active specific immunotherapy or adoptive antibody or lymphocyte immunotherapy with chemotherapy in the treatment of cancer. Cancer Immunol. Immunother 58 : 475-92.
14. Beckman R. A. , Weiner L. M. , Davis H. M. 2007. Antibody constructs in cancer therapy: protein engineering strategies to improve exposure in solid tumors. Cancer 109:170-79.
15. Kolkman J. A. , Law D. A. 2010. Nanobodies—from llamas to therapeutic proteins. Drug Discovery Today: Technologies 2:139-46.

16. Dai J., Jin J., Li B., Wang H., Hou S., Qian W., Kou G., Zhang D., Li J., Tan M., Ma J., Guo Y. 2007. A chimeric SM5-1 antibody inhibits hepatocellular carcinoma cell growth and induces caspase-dependent apoptosis. Cancer Letters 258 : 208-14.
17. Wu L., Wang C., Zhang D., Zhang X., Qian W., Zhao L., Wang H., Li B., Guo Y. 2010. Characterization of a humanized anti-CD20 antibody with potent antitumor activity against B-cell lymphoma. Cancer Letters 292 :208-14.
18. Li B., Wang H., Zhang D., Qian W., Hou S., Shi S., Zhao L., Kou G., Cao Z., Dai J., Guo Y. 2007. Construction and characterization of a high-affinity humanized SM5-1 monoclonal antibody. Biochemical Biophysical Research Communications 357:951-56.
19. Lonberg, N. 2005. Human antibodies from transgenic animals. Nature Biotechnol 23:111725.
20. Jain R. K., Duda D. G., Clark J. W., Loeffler J. S. 2006. Lessons from phase III clinical trials on anti-VEGF therapy for cancer. Nature Clinical Practice Oncology 3:24-40.
21. Cunningham D., Humblet Y., Siena S., Khayat D., Bleiberg H., Santoro A., Bets D., Mueser M., Harstrick A., Verslype C., Chau I., Van Cutsem E. 2004. Cetuximab monotherapy and cetuximab plus irinotecan in irinotecan-refractory metastatic colorectal cancer. New England Journal of Medicine 351:337-45.
22. Hortobagyi G. N. 1998. Treatment of breast cancer. New England Journal of Medicine 339:974-84.
23. Li B., Shi S., Qian W., Zhao L., Zhang D., Hou S., Zheng L., Dai J., Zhao J., Wang. H., Guo Y., 2008. Development of novel tetravalent anti-CD20 antibodies with potent antitumor activity. Cancer Research 68 :2400-08.
24. Wu C., Ying H., Grinnell C., Bryant S., Miller R., Clabbers A., Bose S., McCarthy D., Zhu R. R., Santora L., Davis-Taber R., Kunes Y., Fung E., Schwartz A., Sakorafas P., Gu J., Tarcsa E., Murtaza A., Ghayur T. 2007. Simultaneous targeting of multiple disease mediators by a dual-variable domain immunoglobulin. Nature Biotechnol 25:1290-97.
25. Hudson P. J., Kortt A. A. 1999. High avidity scFv multimers; diabodies and triabodies. Journal of Immunological Methods 231:177-189.
26. Holt L. J., Herring C., Jespers L. S., Woolven B. P., Tomlinson I. M. 2003. Tomlinson domain antibodies: proteins for therapy. Trends Biotechnol 21:484-90.
27. Lin J. H., Lu A. Y. H. 1997. Role of pharmacokinetics and metabolism in drug discovery and development. Pharmacological Reviews 49:403-449
28. Lukyanov A. N., Torchilin V. P. 2004. Micelles from lipid derivatives of water-soluble polymers as delivery systems for poorly soluble drugs. Advanced Drug Delivery Reviews 56:1273-1289
29. Kwon G. S., Kataoka K. 1995. Block copolymer micelles as long-circulating drug vehicles. Advanced Drug Delivery Reviews 16:295-309,
30. Jeong B., Bae Y. H., Kim S. W. 2000. Drug release from biodegradable injectable thermosensitive hydrogel of PEG-PLGA-PEG triblock copolymers. Journal of Controlled Release 63:155-163
31. Barenholz Y. 2012. Doxil®—the irst FDA-approved nano-drug: lessons learned. Journal of Controlled Release 160:117-134.
32. Wagner V., Dullaart A., Bock A-K., Zweck A. 2006. The emerging nanomedicine landscape. Nature Biotechnology 24:1211-1217
33. Ferrari, M. 2005. Cancer nanotechnology: opportunities and challenges. Nature Reviews Cancer 5:161-171.

34. He L. , Wang G. L. , Zhang Q. 2003. An alternative paclitaxel microemulsion formulation: hypersensitivity evaluation and pharmacokinetic profile. International Journal of Pharmaceutics 250:45 50.

35. Feng Z. , Zhao G. , Yu L. , Gough D. , Howell S. B. 2010. Preclinical efficacy studies of a novel nanoparticle-based formulation of paclitaxel that out-performs Abraxane. Cancer Chemotherapy and Pharmacology 65:923-930.

36. Alexis F. , Pridgen E. , Molnar L. K. , Farokhzad O. C. 2008. Factors affecting the clearance and biodistribution of polymeric nanoparticles. Molecular Pharmaceutics 5:505-515.

37. Matsumura Y. , Maeda H. 1986. A new concept for macro-molecular therapeutics in cancer chemotherapy: mechanism of tumoritropic accumulation of proteins and the antitumor agent smancs. Cancer Research 46:6387-6392.

38. Talelli M. , Iman M. , Varkouhi A. K. 2010. Core-crosslinked polym-eric micelles with controlled release of covalently entrapped, doxorubicin. Biomaterials 31:7797-7804,

39. Lukyanov A. N. , Torchilin V. P. 2004. Micelles from lipid derivatives of water-soluble polymers as delivery systems for poorly soluble drugs. Advanced Drug Delivery Reviews 56:1273-1289.

40. Kakizawa Y. , Kataoka K. 2002. Block copolymer micelles for delivery of gene and related compounds. Advanced Drug Delivery Reviews 4:203-222.

41. Kabanov A. V. , Nazarova I. R. , Astaieva I. V. 1995. Micelle formation and solubilization of luorescent probes in poly (oxyethylene-b-oxypropylene-b-oxyethylene) solutions. Macromolecules 28:2303-2314.

42. Brown J. M. , Giaccia A. J. 1998. The unique physiology of solid tumors: opportunities (and problems) for cancer therapy. Cancer Research 58:1408-1416.

43. Yahara T. , Koga T. , Yoshida S. , Nakagawa S. , Deguchi H. , Shirouzo K. 2003. Relationship between microvessel density and thermographic hot areas in breast cancer. Surgery Today 33:243-248,

44. Bae Y. , Nishiyama N. , Fukushima S. , Koyama H. , Yasuhiro M. , Kataoka K. 2005. Preparation and biological characterization of polymeric micelle drug carriers with intracellular pH-triggereddrug release property: tumor permeability, controlled subcellular drug distribution, and enhanced in vivo antitumor eicacy. Bioconjugate Chemistry 16:122-130,

45. Kwon G. , Suwa, S. , Yokoyama M. , Okano T. , Sakurai Y. , Kataoka K. , 1994. Enhanced tumor accumulation and prolonged circulation times of micelle-forming poly(ethylene oxide-aspartate)block copolymer-adriamycin conjugates. Journal of Controlled Release 29:17-23,

46. Nakayama, M. Okano, T. Miyazaki, T. Kohori, F. Sakai, K. Yokoyama, M. 2006. Molecular design of biodegradable polymeric micelles for temperature-responsive drug release. Journal of Controlled Release 115:46-56,

47. Akimoto J. , Nakayama M. , Sakai K. , Okano T. , 2009. Temperature-induced intracellular uptake of thermorespon-sive polymeric micelles. Biomacromolecules 10:1331-1336.

48. Takae S. , Miyata K. , Oba M. 2008. PEG-detachable poly-plex micelles based on disulide-linked block catiomers as bioresponsive nonviral gene vectors. Journal of the American Chemical Society 130:6001-6009.

49. Zhang Z. Z. , Tan S. W. , Feng, S. S. 2012. Vitamin E TPGS as a molecular biomaterial for drug delivery. Biomaterials 33: 4889-4906.

50. Mi Y. , Liu Y. , Feng S. S. 2011. Formulation of Docetaxel by folic acid-conjugated D-tocopheryl polyethylene glycol succinate 2000 (Vitamin E TPGS2k) micelles for targeted and synergisticchemotherapy. Biomaterials 32:. 4058-4066,

51. Lee H. I. , Wu W. , Oh J. K. 2007. Light-induced reversible formation of polymeric micelles. Angewandte Chemie 46:2453-2457.

52. Nasongkla N. , Bey E. , Ren J. 2006. Multifunctional polymeric micelles as cancer-targeted, MRI-ultrasensitive drug delivery systems. Nano Letters 6:. 2427-2430.

53. Li W. , Li J. 2011. The ine-tuning of thermosensitive and degradable polymer micelles for enhancing intracellular uptake and drug release in tumors. Biomaterials 32:3832-3844,

54. Lee R. J. , Low P. S. 1994. Delivery of liposomes to cultured KB cells via folate receptor-mediated endocytosis. Journal of Biological Chemistry 269:3198-3204.

55. Lopes de Menezes D. E. , Pilarski L. M. , Allen T. M. 1998. In vitro and in vivo targeting of immunoliposomal doxorubicin to human B-cell lymphoma. Cancer Research 58:3320-30.

56. Lopes de Menezes D. E. , Kirchmeier M. J. , Gagne J. F. , Pilarski L. M. , Allen T. M. 1999. Cellular trafficking and cytotoxicity of anti-CD19-targeted liposomal doxorubicin in B lymphoma cells. Journal of Liposome Research 9:199-228.

57. Singh M. 1999. Transferrin As A targeting ligand for liposomes and anticancer drugs. Current Pharmaceutical Design 5:443-51.

58. Sugano M. , Egilmez N. K. , Yokota, S. J. , et al. 2000. Antibody targeting of doxorubicin-loaded liposomes suppresses the growth and metastatic spread of established human lung tumor xenografts in severe combined immunodeficient mice. Cancer Research 60:6942-49.

59. Abra R. M. , Bankert R. B. , Chen F. , et al 2002. The next generation of liposome delivery systems: recent experience with tumor-targeted, sterically-stabilized immunoliposomes and active-loading gradients. Journal of Liposome Research 12:1-3.

60. Gao J. , Kou G. , Wang H. , et al. 2009. PE38KDELloaded anti-HER2 nanoparticles inhibit breast tumor progression with reduced toxicity and immunogenicity. Breast Cancer Research and Treatment 115:29-41.

61. Gao J. , Kou G. , Chen H. W. , et al. 2008. Treatment of hepatocellular carcinoma in mice with PE38KDEL type I mutant-loaded poly(lactic-co-glycolic acid) nanoparticles conjugated with humanized SM5-1 F(ab') fragments. Molecular Cancer Therapeutics 7:3399-407.

62. Gao J. , Sun J. , Guo Y. , et al. 2010. Lyophilized HER2-specific PEGylated immunoliposomes for active siRNA gene silencing. Biomaterials 31:2655-64.

63. Gao J. , Feng S. S. , Guo Y. 2010. Antibody engineering promotes nanomedicine for cancer treatment. Nanomedicine (Lond) 5:1141-5.

64. Kou G. , Gao J. , Wang H. , et al. 2007. Preparation and characterization of paclitaxel-loaded PLGA nanoparticles coated with cationic SM5-1 single-chain antibody. Journal of Biochemistry Molecular Biology 40:731-39.

65. Sapra P. , Tyagi P. , Allen T. M. 2005. Ligand-targeted liposomes for cancer treatment. Current Drug Delivery 2 :369-381

66. Traut R. R. , Bollen A. , Sun R. R. , et al. 1973. Methyl 4-mercaptobutyrimidate as a cleavable cross-linking reagent and its application to the Escherichia coli 30s ribosome. Biochemistry 12:3266-73.

67. Carlsson J. , Drevin H. , Axen R. 1978. Protein thiolation and reversible protein-protein conjugation. N-succinimidyl 3(2-pyridyldithio) propionate, a new heterobifunctional reagent. Biochemical Journal 173:723-37.

68. Thorpe P. E. , Wallace P. M. , Knowles P. P. , et al. 1987. New coupling agents for the synthesis of immunotoxins containing a hindered disulfide bond with improved stability in vivo. Cancer Research 47:5924-31.

69. Duncan R. J. , Weston P. D. , Wrigglesworth, R. 1983. A new reagent which may be used to introduce sulfhydryl groups into proteins, and its use in the preparation of conjugates for immunoassay. Analytical Biochemistry 132:68-73.

70. Klotz I. M. , Heiney R. E. 1962. Introduction of sulfhydryl groups into proteins using acetylmercaptosuccinic anhydride. Archives Biochemistry Biophysics 96:605-12.

71. Wegner G. J. , Lee H. J. , Marriott G. , et al. 2005. Fabrication of histidine-tagged fusion protein arrays for surface plasmon resonance imaging studies of protein-protein and protein-DNA interactions. Analytical Chemistry 75:4740-6.

72. Martin F. J. , Hubbell W. L. , Papahadjopoulos D. 1981. Immunospecific targeting of liposomes to cells: a novel and efficient method forcovalent attachment of Fab fragments via disulfide bonds. Biochemistry 20:4229-38.

73. Ivanov V. O. , Preobrazhensky S. N. , Tsibulsky V. P. , et al. 1985. Liposome uptake by cultured macrophages mediated by modified low-density lipoproteins. Biochimica Biophysica. Acta 846:76-84.

74. Leserman L. D. , Barbet J. , Kourilsky F. , et al. 1980. Targeting to cells of fluorescent liposomes covalently coupled with monoclonal antibody or protein A. Nature 288:6024.

75. Suzuki R. , Takizawa T. , Kuwata Y. , et al. 2008. Effective anti-tumor activity of oxaliplatin encapsulated in transferrin-PEG-liposome. International Journal of Pharmaceutics 346:43-50.

76. Ying X. , Wen H. , Lu W. L. , et al. 2010. Dual-targeting daunorubicin liposomes improve the therapeutic efficacy of brain glioma in animals. Journal of Control Release 141:183-92.

77. Koning G. A. , Kamps J. A. , Scherphof G. L. 2002. Efficient intracellular delivery of 5-fluorodeoxyuridine into colon cancer cells by targeted immunoliposomes. Cancer Detection Prevention 26:299-307.

78. Harding J. A. , Engbers C. M. , Newman M. S. , et al. 1997. Immunogenicity and pharmacokinetic attributes of poly(ethylene glycol)-grafted immunoliposomes. Biochimica Biophysica. Acta 1327:181-92.

79. Torchilin V. P. , Khaw B. A. , Smirnov V. N. , et al. 1979. Preservation of antimyosin antibody activity after covalent coupling to liposomes. Biochemical and Biophysical. Research Communications 89:1114-9.

80. Torchilin V. P. , Goldmacher V. S. , Smirnov V. N. 1978. Comparative studies on covalent and noncovalent immobilization of protein molecules on the surface of liposomes. Biochemical and Biophysical. Research Communications 85:983-90.

81. Huang L. , Kennel S. J. 1979. Binding of immunoglobulin G to phospholipid vesicles by sonication. Biochemistry 18:1702-7.

82. Ko Y. T. , Bhattacharya R. , Bickel U. 2009. Liposome encapsulated polyethylenimine/ODN polyplexes for brain targeting. Journal of Control Release 133:230-7.

83. Xiao Z. , McQuarrie S. A. , Suresh M. R. , et al. 2002. A three-step strategy for targeting drug carriers to human ovarian carcinoma cells in vitro. Journal of Biotechnology 94:171-84.

84. Feldmann M. , Steinman L. 2005. Design of effective immunotherapy for human autoimmunity. Nature 435:612-619

85. Herber D. L. , Cao W. , Nefedova Y. , et al. 2010. Lipid accumulation and dendritic cell dysfunction in cancer. Nature Medicine 16:880-886

86. Elamanchili P. , Diwan M. , Cao M. , et al. 2004. Characterization of poly(D, L-lactic-co-glycolic acid) based nanoparticulate system for enhanced delivery of antigens to dendritic cells. Vaccine 22:2406-2412.

87. Schietinger A. , Philip M. , Liu R. B. , et al. 2010. By stander killing of cancer requires the cooperation of CD4+ and CD8+ T cells during the effect or phase. Journal of Experimental Medicine 207:2469-2477.

88. Schuster M. , Nechansky A. , Kircheis R. 2006. Cancer immunotherapy. Biotechnology Journal 1:138-147.

89. Ganss R. , Hanahan D. 1998. Tumor microenvironment can restrict the effectiveness of activated antitumor lymphocytes. Cancer Research 58: 4673-4681.

90. Kim R. , Emi M. , Tanabe K. 2007. Cancer immunoediting from immune surveillance to immune escape. Immunology 121:1365-2567.

91. Dunn G. P., Old L. J., Schreiber R. D. 2004. The immunobiology of cancer immunosurveillance and immunoediting. Immunity 21:137-148

92. Liu Z. , Winters M. , Holodniy M. M. , et al. 2007. siRNA delivery into human T cells and primary cells with carbon-nanotube transporters. Angewandte Chemie 46:2023-2027

93. Williams L. M. , Rudensky A. Y. 2007. Maintenance of the Foxp3-dependent developmental program in mature regulatory T cells requires continued expression of Foxp3. Nature Immunology 8:277-284.

94. Zhang Z. , Tongchusak S. , Mizukami Y. , et al. 2011. Induction of anti-tumor cytotoxic Tcell responses through PLGA-nanoparticle mediated antigen delivery. Biomaterials 32:3666-3678.

95. Li W. , Zhang L. , Zhang G. , etal. 2013. The finely regulating well-defined functional polymer nanocarriers for anti-tumor immunotherapy. Mini-Reviews in Medicinal Chemistry 13:643-652.

96. Li W. , Guo Q. , Zhao H. , et al. 2012. Noveldual-controlpoly (Nisopropylacryla mide-c-chlorophyllin) nanogels for improving drug release. Nanomedicine 7:383-392,

97. Li W. , Feng S. S. , Guo Y. 2013. Nanocarrier's engineering for immunotherapy. Nanomedicine 8: 643-52.

98. Li W. , Li J. , Li H. , et al. 2012. Self-assembled supramolecular nano vesicles for safe and highly efficient gene delivery to solid tumors. International Journal of Nanomedicine 7:4661-4677.

99. Ayano E., Karaki M., Ishihara T., Kanazawa H., Okano T. 2012. Poly (N-isopropylacrylamide)-PLA and PLA blend nanoparticles for temperature-controllable drug release and intracellular uptake. Colloids and Surfaces B 99:4661-4677

100. Moon J. J. , Suh H. , Bershteyn A. et al. 2011. Interbilayer-crosslinked multilamellar vesicles as synthetic vaccines for potent humoral and cellular immune responses. Nature Materials 10:243-251.

101. Fischer D. , Li Y. , Ahlemeyer B. J. , et al. 2003. In vitro cytotoxicity testing of polycations: inluence of polymer structure on cell viability and hemolysis. Biomaterials 24:1121-1131

102. Zou W. 2005. Immunosuppressive networks in the tumour environment and their therapeutic relevance. Nature Reviews Cancer 5:263-274

103. Zhuang Y. , Ma Y. , Wang C. , et al. 2012. PEGylated cationic liposomes robustly augment vaccine-induced immune responses: role of lymphatic tracking and biodistribution. Journal of Controlled Release 159:135-142.

104. Champion J. A., Mitragotri S. 2006. Role of target geometry in phagocytosis. Proceedings of the National Academy of Sciences of the United States of America 103:4930-4934,

105. Ding B, Wu X., Fan W., et al. 2011. Anti-DR5 monoclonal antibody-mediated DTIC-loaded nanoparticles combining chemotherapy and immunotherapy for malignant melanoma: target formulation development and in vitro anticancer activity. International Journal of Nanomedicine 6:1991-2005.

7 Chapter

GRAPHENE QUANTUM DOTS - FROM INCEPTION TO NANOTHERANOSTIC APPLICATIONS

1. INTRODUCTION: AN OVERVIEW

Nanotechnology is unequivocally the most promising research domain that has profoundly impacted biology and medicine, and it can be regarded as the foremost technology of the 21st century. In addition to biological pursuits, nanotechnology enables novel approaches and applications in electronics, computer science, and aerospace technology. In the current socioeconomic context, nanotechnology can significantly contribute to addressing several health and environmental challenges. "Nano" is derived from Latin, signifying "dwarf," and an object with one dimension at the nanoscale is classified as a nanomaterial. At the nanoscale, the physicochemical properties of a substance undergo significant alterations, including increased surface area, modifications in thermal and optical characteristics, and the predominance of quantum effects associated with the transition to nanoscale dimensions. The notion of nanotechnology was initially articulated by physicist Richard P. Feynman in 1959, while the term 'nanotechnology' was introduced by Norio Taniguchi in 1974.

Since its inception, nanotechnology has established a notable presence in various fields, including medical, biology, electronics, space exploration, and agriculture.

Nanotechnology intervention has established a novel domain known as "nanomedicine" inside the medical research and healthcare sector. The primary domains of nanotechnology application in the pharmaceutical business encompass medication delivery, biosensors, and diagnostic imaging. This chapter will primarily concentrate on the use of graphene quantum dots (GQDs) in drug delivery and bioimaging, despite the known uses of various nanoparticles (metal, polymeric, liposomes, and dendrimers) in drug delivery and disease diagnostics.

1.1. History of Graphene Quantum Dots

A quantum dot (QD) is a semiconductor crystal measuring between 1 and 10 nanometers. Due to their particular size range, quantum dots show quantum processes that provide substantial advantages in optical qualities. It is a well-established principle that upon excitation, the smaller the size of the quantum dot, the greater the energy and intensity of the produced light. Quantum dots (QDs) can be obtained from metals (such as gold), semiconductors (e.g., selenium, cadmium), or carbon-based materials (including carbon dots and graphene). Quantum dots (QDs), owing to their unique features, serve as photodiodes and have diverse applications in analytical chemistry; nevertheless, the possible toxicity linked to semiconductor quantum dots hinders their usage in biology and medicine. The limitations of quantum dots prompted the search for new alternatives, leading to the development of graphene-based quantum dots, which have emerged as a more biocompatible option for biomedical applications due to advancements in nanotechnology. Graphene is a carbon allotrope, a zero-band-gap, two-dimensional (2D) sheet composed of a single layer of sp2-hybridized carbon, exhibiting exceptional thermoelectric properties [1, 2]. Initially, R. Wallace examined its characteristics in 1947 [3], then in 1963, Hoffman et al. extracted pure graphene from graphene oxide using hydrazine reduction [4]. The term "graphene" was coined by Mouras et al. in 1987 [5]. Although early findings on graphene received little attention, significant interest in study into its properties was sparked following the pioneering efforts of Geim and Novoselov in separating graphene from highly oriented pyrolytic graphite (HOPG). GQDs, first reported by Peng et al., are zero-dimensional graphene segments that are small enough to exhibit quantum confinement and size effect. Unlike graphene sheets, they exhibit band gap that is responsible for their unique electrical and optoelectronic properties. Moreover, GQDs also possess size-dependent strong photoluminescence properties [6–9]. These are relatively new nano-dimension entities with a size range between 1 and 10 nm, having a "molecule-like structure," nontoxic, and can be easily handled compared with colloidal QDs. GQDs are gradually attaining significance due to their potential applications in sensors, electronics, and biology from the standpoint of less health concerns than their traditional semiconductor counterparts due to their less toxicity, ease of functionalization, and favorable electro-optic properties [10–12].

2. METHODS FOR SYNTHESIZING GRAPHENE QUANTUM DOTS

Significant advancements have been achieved in the development of novel synthesis methodologies for graphene quantum dots. GQDs can be synthesized using two primary approaches: top-down and bottom-up procedures. The initial method involves the cleavage and exfoliation of bulk graphene-derived material (graphite) under extreme circumstances. The bottom-up strategy primarily involves the synthesis of GQDs from polycyclic aromatic compounds or aromatic molecular structures.

Despite the cost-effectiveness of the top-down approach with many synthesis steps, its principal drawbacks are severe reaction conditions and inadequate morphological control. The primary advantage of this strategy is that the GQDs produced possess oxygen-containing functional groups that affect their solubility and functionalization. Bottom-up methodologies provide exact control over morphology, size, and form; nevertheless, they are hindered by drawbacks such as the requirement for costly precursors and intricate synthesis procedures. The GQDs produced by this method have a pronounced propensity for aggregation, which constrains the usefulness of this technique. This segment will provide a concise summary of modern methodologies for GQD synthesis.

2.1. Top-down approaches

The basic route of implementing top-down methods is either chemical reactions or physical methods. Based on their mechanism, these approaches can be described as "defect-mediated fragmentation processes." Mostly, chemical approaches are applied due to some distinguished benefits. Generally, graphene oxide (GO) is cleaved to generate GQDs, and chemical methods generate defects due to the presence of oxygen-containing reactive epoxy and hydroxyl groups. The reactive groups generate a cleavage site, thus allowing GO sheets to be cut into smaller sheets [13]. During the oxidation procedure of graphene, epoxy groups appear linearly on the carbon lattice and this alignment causes the cleavage of C–C bond. The emergence of epoxy groups on GO makes it energetically favorable to convert these groups into stable carbonyl pairs at room temperature. Graphene sheets become fragile due to these chemical transformation and defects and can be readily attacked by chemicals to generate GQDs. The presence of aromatic sp^2 domains having epoxy groups on graphene, GO, carbon black, and carbon nanotubes makes them excellent starting candidates for GQD synthesis.

2.1.1. Hydrothermal and solvothermal synthesis

Particle size of GQDs and formation mechanisms are deeply influenced by hydrothermal synthesis. Water, as a green solvent used in this procedure, is a key player in atom-economical reactions [14]. These methods generally require a high amount of strong alkali (NaOH and ammonia) for cutting carbon precursors into GQDs. First, Pan et al. reported this method to synthesize water-soluble blue luminescent quantum dots. The diameter of QDs was 5–13 nm and they exhibited strong fluorescence in alkali conditions, while in acidic conditions the fluorescence got quenched. The basic synthesis step involved was the oxidation of graphite to GO that produces epoxy groups, which cause the rupture of C–C bonds. Further, these epoxy groups are oxidized into stable carbonyl groups responsible for the water dispersiblity of GQDs as shown in Figure 1. Later, Pan et al. put forth a modified high-temperature synthesis procedure to synthesize fine crystalline GQDs with green fluorescence [14, 15].

In recent years, graphene-based materials have seen extensive applications in the field of electronics, pollution treatment, solar cells, Li-ion batteries, and sensing. The modification of graphene by nitrogen or boron doping significantly amends its optical and electronic properties. Similarly, a change in photoluminescence and electric properties can be attained by tuning the band gap of GQDs [16].

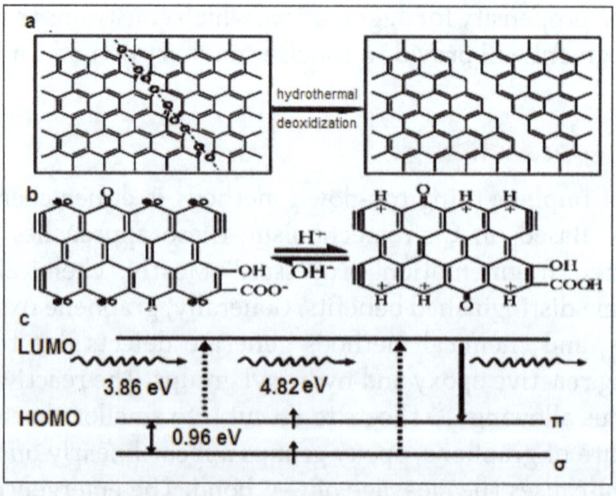

Figure 1. Synthesis mechanism of GQDs via cutting of graphite sheets. This was a multistep process and GQDs were prepared by the reduction of epoxy groups generated in oxidation and cutting step. (Ref [14]: Pan et al.)

Hydrothermal approach deeply influences the size and morphology of GQDs. In one report, Tetsuka et al. [17] synthesized amine-functionalized graphene quantum dots (NH_2-GQDs) using oxidized graphene sheets and ammonia using this method by bond-scission reaction. Concentration variation of ammonia played a key role in controlling the luminescence of GQDs from violet to yellow. The nucleophilic substitution upon ammonia addition to graphene triggered the reaction of ring-opening epoxide, and sp^2 domains were cut out to generate amino-functionalized GQDs of 2.5 nm size and 1.1 nm thickness (Figure 2). In this series, few researchers have reported altered optical properties of GQDs after functionalization with polymers or small molecules. Feng et al. have put forth their idea of fluorinated GQDs (F-GQDs) prepared by hydrothermal procedure. Xenon difluoride was utilized for fluorinated graphene synthesis at high temperatures and then F-GQDs were obtained by hydrothermal procedure [18].

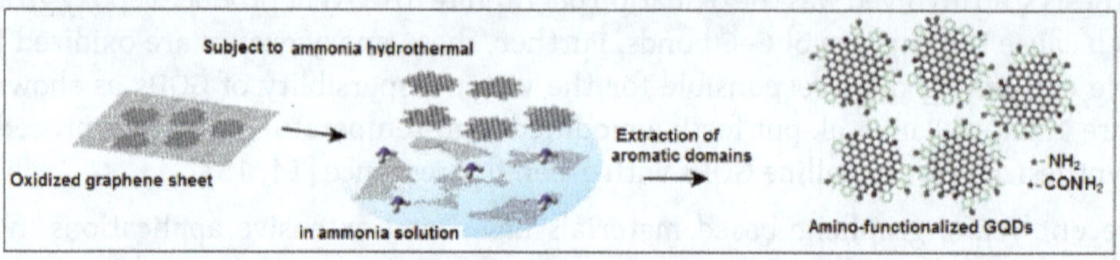

Figure 2. Illustration of hydrothermal synthesis of amino-functionalized GQDs. (Ref [17]: Tetsuka et al.)

Hu et al. [19] came up with a new methodology by synthesizing nitrogen-doped GQDs (N-GQDs) from oxidized debris (ODs) on graphene oxide by the hydrothermal treatment of GO at 180°C in the presence of ammonia without any strong acid treatment. The as-prepared N-GQDs were highly blue luminescent, 2–6 nm in size, with a quantum yield (QY) of 24.6. Aqueous route and novel application of ODs for the synthesis of

N-GQDs were the major highlights of their work. The prime advantage associated with this approach was its cost effectiveness due to aqueous reaction conditions in the absence of any surface-passivation agent or strong acids. Liu et al. and Zhang and coworkers also reported similar procedures for the synthesis of functionalized GQDs [20, 21]. Recently, Nigam et al. have reported a novel reducing agent Lawsone for hydrothermal synthesis of GQDs of 3-6 nm size and green fluorescence from graphene oxide reduction. The GQDs were stable and showed good biocompatibility at higher concentrations [22]. In another approach, Shen et al. prepared surface-passivated GQDs from hydrazine hydrate reduction of GO that were further passivated by poly(ethylene glycol) diamine (PEG_{1500N}) as depicted in Figure 3. By this method, they obtained GQDs of broad diameter in the range of 5–19 nm with blue fluorescence; hence, they further modified the procedure, and the GQDs were synthesized via one-pot hydrothermal synthesis route using GO and PEG as starting materials. The basic advantage of PEG-surface passivation was high photoluminescence (PL) quantum yield, better photon-to-electron conversion, and improved unconverted PL properties than native GQDs [23].

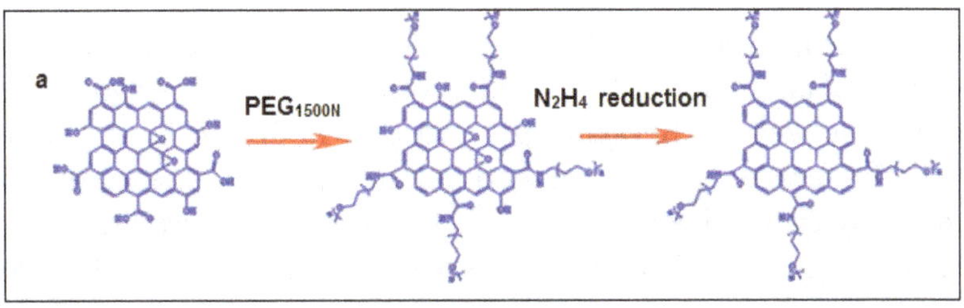

Figure 3. Synthesis of surface-passivated GQDs with hydrazine hydrate reduction and surface passivation by PEG_{1500N}. (Ref. [23]: Shen et al.)

In solvothermal reaction, organic solvents (dimethyl sulfoxide (DMSO), dimethylformamide (DMF), and benzene) are utilized instead of water to obtain GQDs. The size and morphology of the GQDs are greatly influenced by the physicochemical properties of solvents. In a recent approach reported by Zhu et al. [24], DMF was used as a solvent to split graphene oxide into green fluorescent GQDs under ultrasonication followed by heating at 200°C in a Teflon autoclave. Column chromatography on silica gel was performed to obtain GQDs instead of dialysis treatment with water as eluent. As an improvisation, they later increased the reaction time to 8 h using methanol/methylene chloride and water as mobile phase for GQD synthesis [25]. Shin et al. put forth a new solvothermal approach based on novel acid-free and oxone-oxidant-assisted synthesis of GQDs using various natural carbon resources, including graphite, multiwall carbon nanotubes (MWCNTs), carbon fibers (CFs), and charcoal (C) [26].

2.1.2. Microwave-assisted cutting and ultrasonic approach

Hydrothermal/solvothermal techniques are the most applied processes for GQD synthesis, but due to their tedious synthesis protocols, researchers have reported a few procedures based on microwave-assisted synthesis as this technique has the advantage of both hydrothermal and microwave processes. In a recent work by Luk et al., nitrogen-doped GQDs (N-GQDs) were prepared by mixing 3 wt% of glucose dissolved in aqueous ammonia (25%) at room temperature. The homogeneous solution was heated in a microwave reactor (300 W power) for 5 min at 180°C. Using this method, GQDs with 6 nm size and excitation-dependent luminescence spectra were obtained. Upconversion emission spectrum was another important feature of their work. According to their findings, nitrogen doping played the key role in two-photon luminescence [27]. Recently, a one-step-microwave-assisted solvothermal method for fabricating sulfur- and nitrogen-doped GQDs (S-, N-GQDs) has been reported based on the reaction of GO and reduced glutathione in N,N-dimethylformamide (DMF) at 200° C under microwave irradiation [28].

Tang et al. have reported glucose-derived GQDs through a microwave-assisted hydrothermal (MAH) approach. The basic advantage of this method was uniform heating that produced particles of small sizes. The authors have synthesized GQDs of average size of 4 nm. Based on the microwave heating time, GQDs of varying sizes were obtained [29].

In another approach, Li et al. [30] have developed a method for facile microwave-assisted synthesis of two-color GQDs in acidic conditions. Figure 4 shows the schematic of basic steps involved in the synthesis procedure. Greenish yellow luminescent GQDs (gGQDs) of average size 4–5 nm were obtained. The as-synthesized GQDs were further moderately reduced with $NaBH_4$, and blue GQDs were produced with the same dimensions. The quantum yield of blue and green GQDs was 23% and 12%, respectively.

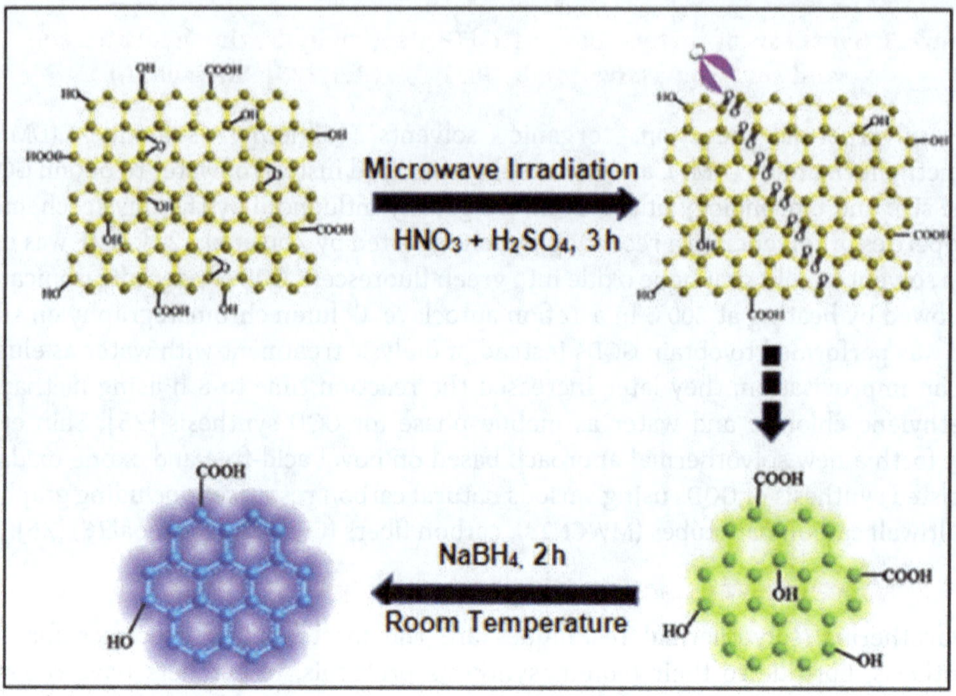

Figure 4. Schematic of synthesis of green and blue GQDs. (Ref [30]: Li et al.)

Ultrasonication is a simpler procedure to prepare GQDs, because of the fact that ultrasound can generate alternating low-pressure and high-pressure waves in liquid that can be useful for shearing the carbon layer materials into GQDs. Zhu et al. [31] have reported one-step synthesis using ultrasonication with only graphene oxide and $KMnO_4$, and luminescent graphene quantum dots of 3 nm in high quantum yield were prepared.

2.1.3. Electrochemical exfoliation approaches

Electrochemical approaches were already established for the synthesis of carbon dots at a potential of 1.5–3 V, where electrochemical exfoliation and intercalation are the basic steps to obtain the desired product by generating hydroxyl and oxygen radicals that play the role of electrochemical "scissors" in an oxidative cleavage reaction [32, 33].

Li et al. [34] extended this strategy further to synthesize GQDs of 3–5 nm size through an electrochemical method that involved the breaking up of a graphene film that has been treated with oxygen plasma to increase hydrophilicity. The as-synthesized GQDs exhibited green luminescence and enhanced stability in water dispersion. Zhang et al. [35] put forth another approach for synthesizing water-soluble GQDs by electrochemical exfoliation of graphite and further reducing the as-synthesized nanoscale GQDs with hydrazine at room temperature in contrast to earlier reported high-temperature reductions. It was the first report of strong yellow fluorescence in high yield and uniform sizes. The yellow fluorescence can be attributed to hydrazide groups on the surface of GQDs, produced during the low-temperature hydrazine reduction step. Though carbon nanotubes are not very suitable materials for GQD synthesis due to their potential toxicity, recently Pillai and Shinde have described an electrochemical procedure for GQDs based on multiwalled nanotubes. Figure 5 illustrates the mechanism of GQD synthesis. This method is a new procedure to synthesize size-tunable quantum dots by the oxidation time [36]. Due to the toxic base material, applicability of GQDS prepared by such methods is limited and it involves extra efforts to coat the GQDs with any polymer or compound to enhance their biocompatibility. However, in another report, Shinde et al. put forth a two-step electrochemical strategy of synthesizing nitrogen-doped GQDs (N-GQDs) from multiwall CNTs. The presence of nitrogen dopants in the carbon framework caused faster unzipping of N-MWCNTs, and also provided lower activation energy site that was beneficial for enhanced electrocatalytic activity for oxygen reduction reaction [37].

Recently, a facile electrochemical exfoliation of graphite in $K_2S_2O_8$ solution for the synthesis of uniform small-sized red fluorescent GQDs (RF-GQDs) was demonstrated by Tan et al. with no chemical modification. This method was relatively simple, and water-soluble GQDs of uniform size (3 nm diameter) with excellent PL properties and less cytotoxicity were obtained with *in vivo* applicability in bioimaging applications.

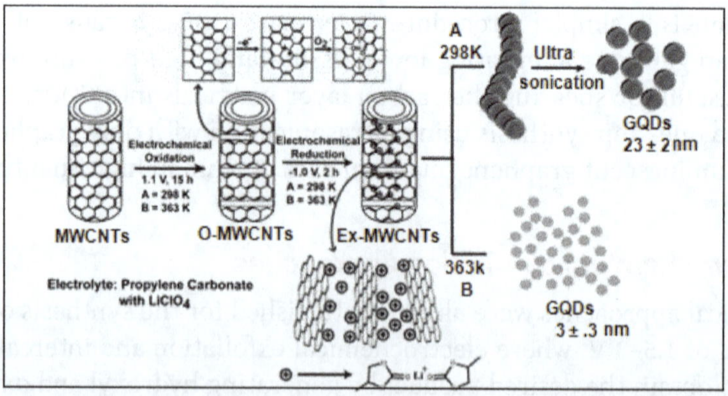

Figure 5. Synthesis stages involved in electrochemical synthesis of GQDs from MWCNTs. (Ref [36]: Shinde et al.)

2.1.4. Nanolithography

Nanolithography is a high-precision technique but gives low yield, and expensive instrumentation is required, which is the prime reason for very few reports being available on this methodology. Ponomarenko et al. [39] used ultrahigh-resolution electron beam lithography to cut graphene to desired sizes. In another work by Lee and coworkers [40], chemical vapor deposition method was used to generate GQDs of uniform size from self-assembled block copolymers (BCP) as an etch mask on graphene films. Although this was a low-yielding method, uniform particles were synthesized for probing effects of size and functionalization.

2.2. Bottom-up approaches

As compared to top-down approaches, very few bottom-up procedures have been reported.

2.2.1. Pyrolysis

Pyrolysis is one of the simplest methods of synthesizing graphene quantum dots. In this method, GQDs are formed via carbonization of small organic molecules. However, apart from its simplicity, GQDS of low quantum yield are produced in most of the cases. Few recent reports based on this method are described here. GQDs from hexa-peri-hexabenzocoronene (HBC) were reported by Liu et al. [41]. HBC is a polycyclic aromatic hydrocarbon that resembles nanoscaled fragments of graphene that stack via π–π interactions. This method produced monodisperse disk-like GQDs of ≈60 nm and 2–3 nm thickness. Pyrolysis, unfunctionalization, and oxidation processes are shown in Figure 6. Further, GQDs from citric acid (CA) and glutathione (GSH) as starting materials were also prepared. Glutathione is a tripeptide containing glutamate, cysteine, and glycine. The core advantage of glutathione is enhanced biocompatibility and high quantum yield. In this method, a 33.6% QY was obtained that can be attributed to the amination reaction between the amine group of GSH and the epoxy and carboxylic groups of GQDs [42]. It has been reported earlier that carboxylic and epoxy groups act like non-radiative electron-hole combination centers [18], and during amination reaction, reduction in number of these centers leads to better emission properties.

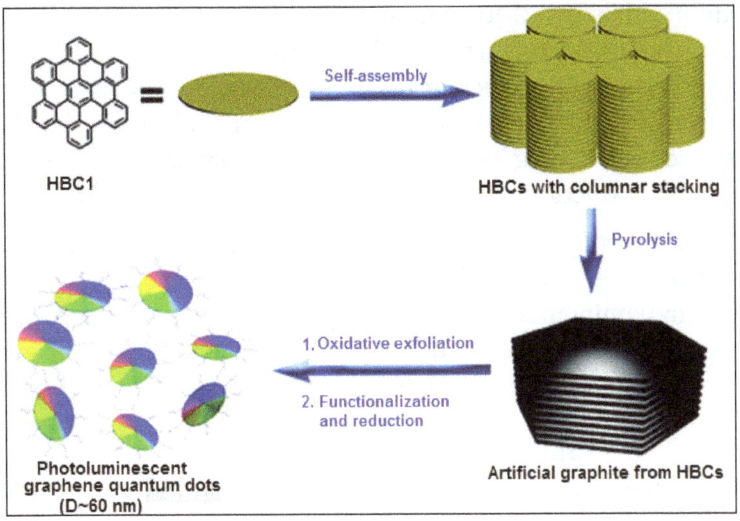

Figure 6. Illustration of pyrolysis procedure of HBC for synthesis of GQDs. Monodisperse disk like GQDs with 2-3 nm thickness and 60 nm diameters were obtained. (Ref [41]: Liu et al.)

In another approach, Wu and coworkers synthesized GQDs via a simple one-step pyrolysis of L-glutamic acid in a heating mantle. With this method, GQDs with a broad emission range (from visible to near infrared (NIR)) with excellent quantum yield of 55% were obtained. Figure 7a illustrates the basic steps of pyrolysis procedure, while Figure 7 b, c depicts the characteristic features of GQDs. These quantum dots exhibited tremendous bioimaging potential, and as shown in Figure 7d they can be successfully utilized for in vitro and *in vivo* cell imaging [43].

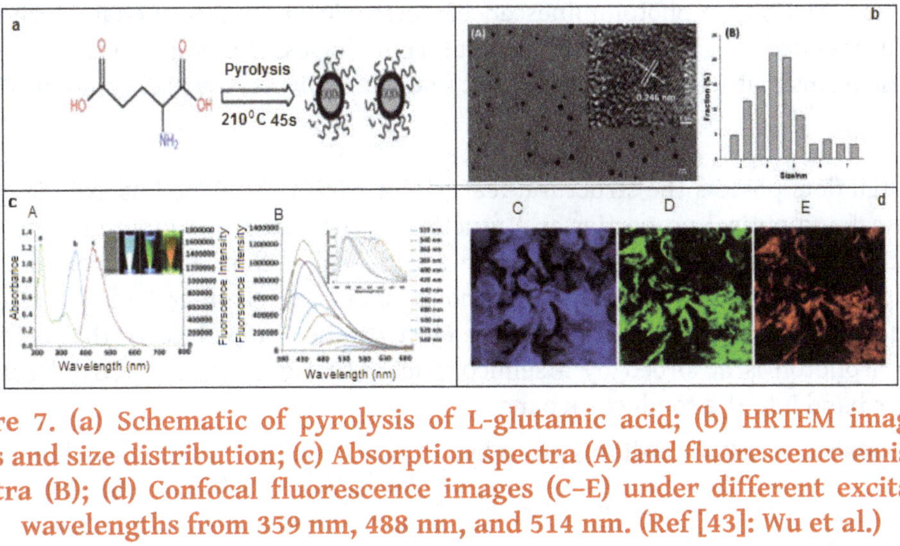

Figure 7. (a) Schematic of pyrolysis of L-glutamic acid; (b) HRTEM image of GQDs and size distribution; (c) Absorption spectra (A) and fluorescence emission spectra (B); (d) Confocal fluorescence images (C-E) under different excitation wavelengths from 359 nm, 488 nm, and 514 nm. (Ref [43]: Wu et al.)

Citric acid was also explored as the staring material to synthesize blue luminescent GQDs by tuning its carbonization degree. The as-synthesized GQDs were 15 nm in width and 0.5–2.0 nm in thickness. GQDs obtained by this method were self-passivated due to incomplete carbonization of citric acid [13]. Gram-scale synthesis of functionalized GQDs from pyrene via facile molecular fusion route was described by Wang et al. [44]. The single-crystalline GQDs were having excellent optical properties such as bright excitonic fluorescence, strong excitonic absorption bands extending to the visible region, large molar extinction coefficients, and long-term photostability.

Recently, a facile bottom-up method producing fluorescent nitrogen-doped graphene quantum dots (N-GQDs) based on one-step pyrolysis of citric acid and tris(hydroxymethyl)aminomethane was reported. These nitrogen-doped GQDs emitted strong blue fluorescence under 365 nm ultraviolet (UV) light excitation with the highest reported quantum yield of 59.2% [45].

2.2.2. From fullerene

Lu et al. [46] reported a mechanistic approach for the synthesis of geometrically well-defined GQDs on a ruthenium surface using C_{60} molecules as a precursor. Ruthenium (Ru) catalyzed the cage opening reaction of C_{60}. The strong C60–Ru interaction initiated the formation of surface vacancies in the Ru single crystal and a subsequent embedding of C60 molecules in the surface. At high temperatures, embedded molecules get fragmented and form carbon clusters that undergo diffusion and aggregation to form GQDs.

3. PHYSICOCHEMICAL PROPERTIES OF GRAPHENE QUANTUM DOTS

GQDs are nanosized graphene sheets. In this chapter, we will deal with Bohr radius and quantum confinement effect to explain the optical properties of GQDs. It is believed that the variations in photoluminescence, electronic, and physical characteristics of GQDs are related with these two important terminologies. Therefore, let us briefly look at these terms that will enhance our basic understanding on the properties of GQDs.

Bohr radius

Quantum dots possess the structural features of parent molecule but exhibit unique electrical and optical properties as a function of their size. The quantum size effect occurs when these nanostructures attain a size smaller than a fundamental unit of exciton Bohr radius. An exciton is a bound state of an electron and an electron hole, which are attracted to each other by the electrostatic Coulomb force that is formed when a photon is absorbed by a semiconductor that excites an electron from the valence band into the conduction band.

In Gaussian unit, a Bohr radius is given by:

$$a_0 = \hbar^2 / m_e e^2 \quad (1)$$

where a_0 is the Bohr radius, ħ is the reduced Plank's constant, and m_e is the electron rest mass. Bohr radius has an approximate value of 0.53 Å [47].

Quantum confinement effect

When the size of quantum dot becomes smaller and approaches toward the Bohr radius of bulk exciton, the quantum confinement effect becomes apparent. Depending on the dimension of the confinement, three kinds of structures can be defined: quantum well (QW), quantum wire (QWR), and quantum dot (QD) based on the reduced dimension. Material size is reduced in one direction in a QW and the exciton is free to move in other two directions, while in a QWR the material size is reduced in both the directions leaving only a single direction for the movement of exciton. In a QD, all directions are reduced restricting the free movement of exciton in any direction [48].

Due to this confinement effect exciton nature gets modified, which leads to distinguished optical and electrical properties of quantum dots.

3.1. Electrochemical properties

The 2010 Nobel Prize was awarded to Geim and Novoselov for their remarkable work in graphene. This not only validated the importance of graphene but also paved the way for their applications in different research areas of electronics and optics as well as commercial applications. GQDs are so closely related to graphene that a discussion on GQD would be incomplete without describing the basics of graphene. With technological advancements in different fields, demand for carbon and carbon-related materials like graphene, carbon nanotubes is increasing rapidly for electrical, mechanical, and biomedical applications due to their tremendous thermal, electrical, mechanical, optical, and other unique properties [49–51]. Although graphene has an upper hand in comparison to CNTs due to low toxicity, it has the disadvantages of aggregation and low dispersity. The nanoparticles of GQDs are more advantageous due to their better physicochemical properties.

Graphene is known as a zero-band-gap material having infinite exciton Bohr radius, because of the linear energy dispersion of the charge carriers [52, 53]. Quantum confinement is a phenomenon that evolves in a finite-size graphene sheet and GQDs are best examples of this prominent effect. GQDs exhibit non-zero, tunable band gap than graphene and luminescence on excitation. Moreover, GQDs provide the flexibility of tuning the band gap by size and surface chemistry amendments. Eda et al. have reported that electrical properties of GQDs are size tunable. According to their findings of density functional theory (DTF), the band gap of GQDs consisting of 20 aromatic rings is approximately 2 eV, while for a benzene ring the value is 7 eV [54]. GQDs are a very new addition to the family of quantum dots and a great deal is left to explore their electronic and electrochemical properties. Graphene has been widely explored in field-effect transistors but GQDs are applied in single electron transistor (SET)-based charge sensors [55–57]. SETs are newer switching devices that use controlled electron tunneling to amplify a current [58]. Apart from charge variation detection, GQDs are applied for electronic sensors for humidity detection based on the modulation of electron tunneling distances caused by humidity and pressure.

3.2. Absorption and photoluminescence properties

GQDs are widely explored for their photoluminescence properties. They generally show a strong absorbance in UV region. The basic absorption spectra of GQDs show a prominent peak at about 230 nm, which is assigned to the $\pi \rightarrow \pi^*$ excitation of the π bonds of aromatic C=C, and a shoulder peak at 300 nm is assigned to the n–π^* transition of C=O bonds [59]. GQDs also exhibit size-dependent UV–Vis absorption spectrum due to quantum confinement effect. Peng et al. [60] analyzed that the absorbance peak red shifted from 270 nm to 330 nm, with increase in the size from 1–4 nm to 7–11 nm (Figure 8a). It was also observed that varying the average size of GQDs from 5 nm to 35 nm, the peak energy of the absorption spectra monotonously decreases from 6.2 ev to 4.6 ev (Figure 8b) [61]. According to the findings of Fuyuno et al., the absorption spectra of GQDs showed increases in absorbance with decreasing wavelength for each sample. GQD samples were collected via high-performance liquid chromatography (HPLC) at different intervals.

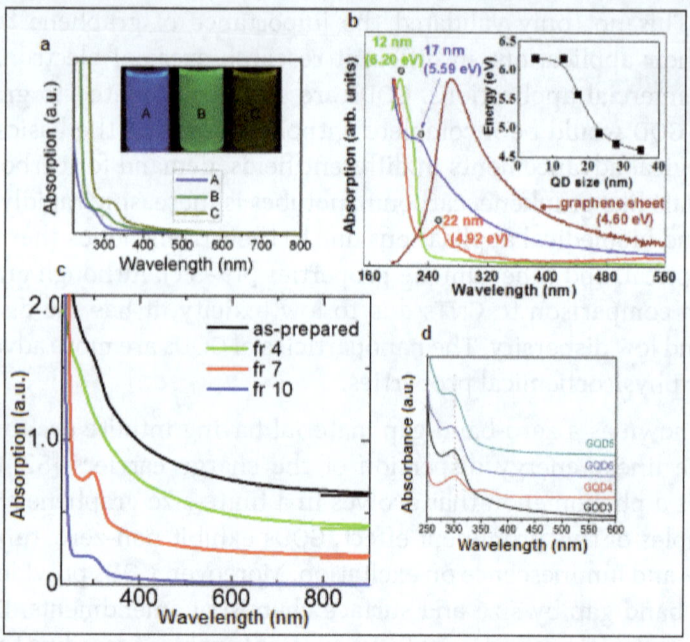

Figure 8. Variation in absorption spectra of GQDs with synthesis parameters (a) UV–Vis spectra of GQDs A, B, and C correspond to synthesized reaction temperature at 120, 100, and 80°C, respectively (Ref [60]: Peng et al.); (b) Absorption spectra for three typical GQDs of 12, 17, and 22 nm average sizes dispersed in DI water and a graphene sheet. Inset: absorption peak energy as a function of average GQD size (Ref [61]: Kim et al.); (c) Spectra of different sizes of GQDs at different collection times (4, 7, 10 h) (Ref [62]: Fuyuno et al.); (d) Presence of oxygen functional groups variation and its effect on UV spectra (Ref [65]: Yang et al.)

A gradual change in the absorption spectra of HPLC-GQDs was observed depending on the retention time (i.e., with the size of the GQDs). For the GQD samples collected at 4 h, no distinct energy gap and peak structure were obtained, while for the GQDs of 7 h and 10 h, peak structures were observed at ~300 nm, which corresponds to n–π^* transitions of nonbonding electrons in the C=O bonds (Figure 8c). However, the size dependency was not visible and the absorbance peaks were independent of size variation from 1.7 nm to 21 nm with GQDs prepared via glucose carbonization [62]. Moreover, absorption spectra also vary with difference in the method of synthesis [63, 64]. The presence of oxygen-containing groups also plays a governing role in the absorption peak position of GQDs, as illustrated in Figure 8d. The two electronic transitions at 300 nm (3.81 eV) in the absorption spectra of the GQDs can be attributed to electronic transitions from s and p orbitals or from highest occupied molecular orbital (HOMO) to lowest unoccupied molecular orbital (LUMO) [65].

Another attractive feature of GQDs is their photoluminescence profile. Though the exact mechanism of PL is still not completely validated, researchers have revealed that the possible causes can be quantum confinement effect, aromatic structures, presence of functional groups and oxygen-containing groups, free zigzag sites, and edge defects, due to which GQDs show new absorption features that affect the photoluminescence profile of GQDs [66–69]. It is a well-known fact that GQDs exhibit quantum confinement and edge effects, the key players of PL properties. Researchers have identified that the band gap is a function of size of QDs and decreases with an increase in size. Eda et al. [55] in their hypothesis proposed that the radiative recombination of e–h pairs generated within localized states can be the possible cause of blue PL spectra. The energy gap between the π and π^* states generally depends on the size of sp^2 clusters [27] or conjugation length [18]. According to their findings, it is the interaction between the nanometer-sized sp^2 clusters and the finite-sized molecular sp^2 domains which is the key in optimizing the blue emission. Moreover, the synthesis procedure of GQDs in top-down approaches and cutting of large graphene fragments in different crystallographic directions generates edges (zigzag and arm chair). These edges are prima facie responsible for diverse emission properties, as suggested by Kim et al. [61]. Zigzag sites are either carbine like with a triplet ground state or carbyne-like with a singlet ground state, and the irradiation decay of activated electrons from LUMO to HOMO is the most probable cause of blue emission [14].

In this segment, we will discuss some aspects of GQDs and their effect on PL spectra. Size dependency of PL of GQDs was reported by Alam et al. [70]. In their analysis, emission wavelengths of pristine zigzag-edged GQDs of different diameters were calculated. On varying the size from 0.46 nm to 2.31 nm, GQDs exhibited PL spectra from deep UV to near infrared as shown in Figure 9a. The smallest GQD (benzene) showed an emission peak at 235.2 nm while a peak at 999.5 nm was exhibited by GQDs of size 2.31 nm. They reported a linear and steep size dependence and concluded that emission covers the entire visible-light spectrum (400–770 nm) on varying the diameter of GQD from 0.89 nm to 1.80 nm [70].

Depending on the method of synthesis, GQDs possess oxygen-containing groups, that is, hydroxyl, carboxy, carbonyl, and epoxy ether groups; the difference in energy levels of surface groups and emission traps on GQDs governs the difference in emission spectra and PL with different colors including red, green, blue, and yellow [52, 71].

As reported by Zhu et al., surface defects on GQDs that arise from oxidation of surface groups also result in red-shifted PL spectra [72].In addition, not only the surface defects and functional groups but also the synthesis parameters (pH and solvent), size, and excitation wavelength have marked their impact on the PL spectra of GQDs. As described above, quantum confinement effect is a major phenomenon of QDs that arises when the size of QDs is less than the Bohr exciton radius. This size dependency of band gap of GQDs is responsible for their unique optical and spectroscopic characteristics. It is reported that by decreasing the size of QDs, emission spectra show blue or high energy shift [73–76]. Figure 9 illustrates various effects of physiological parameters on emission spectrum of GQDs.

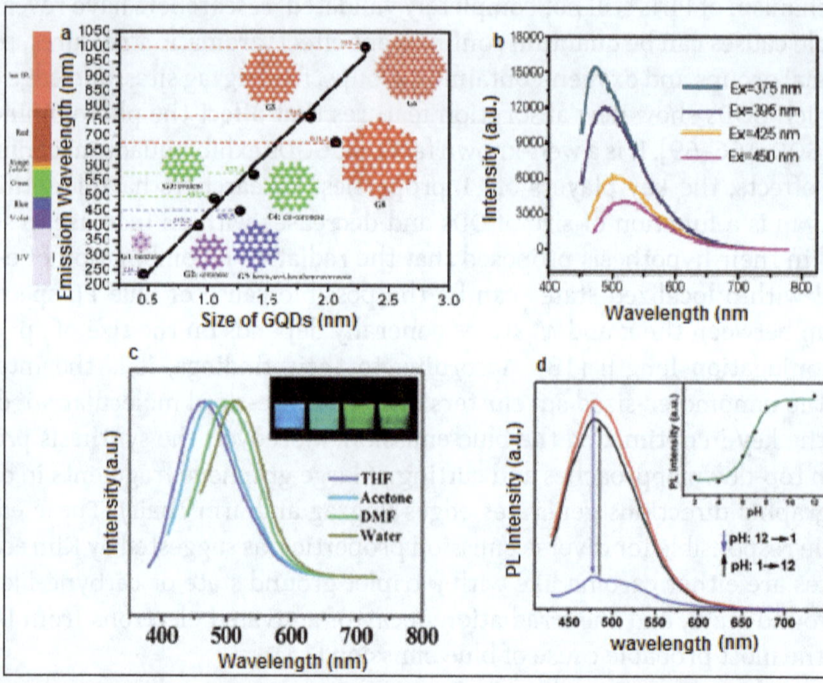

Figure 9. Illustrating the change in emission spectra of GQDs based on (a) size (Ref [70]: Alam et al.); (b) Excitation dependent (Ref [71]: Tang et al.); (c) in different solvents (Ref [75], Zhu et al.); (d) with pH of the GQD solution (Ref [15]: Pan et al.)

In an interesting finding, few reports deal with the upconversion luminescence properties exhibited by GQDs. As reported by Shen et al., surface-passivated GQDs showed strong upconversion PL when illuminated with 980 nm. An unconverted PL spectrum at 525 nm was obtained (Figure 10a). The upconversion emissions also showed peak shifts from 390 nm to 460 nm when excited with wavelengths of 600–800 nm. They further demonstrated that the PL spectrum was a transition from the lowest unoccupied molecular orbital to the highest occupied molecular orbital [23]. Similar phenomena were also observed by Zhu et al., and when their GQDs were illuminated with 600–900 nm wavelengths, a significant red shift was obtained. The possible cause for this can be explained by the multi-photon active process as reported for carbon dots earlier [77, 78]. The possible cause of upconversion effect was depicted by anti-Stokes transition, as shown in Figure 10c. In comparison to excitation-dependent upconversion effect, Zhou et al. observed an excitation-independent upconversion effect with GQDs synthesized via ultrasonication as illustrated in Figure 10d [79].

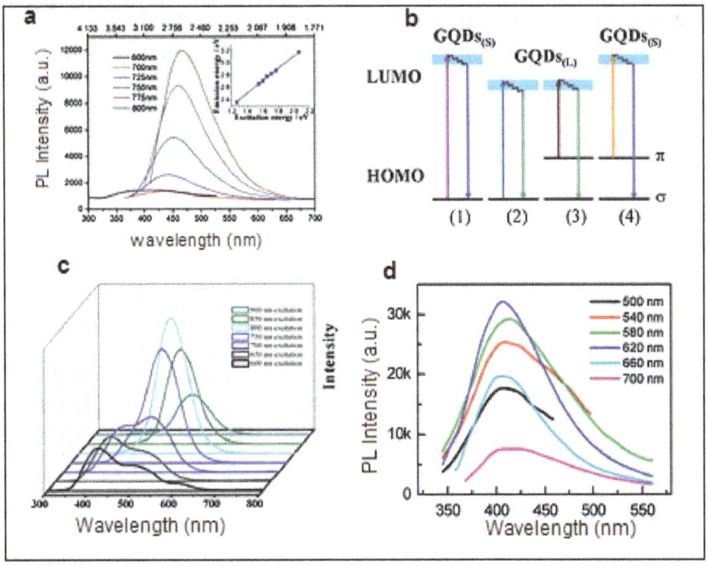

Figure 10. (a) Upconversion luminescence properties exhibited by GQDs; (b) A schematic illustration of various typical electronic transitions processes of GQDs (Ref [23]: Shen et al.) (c) PL spectra of GQDs upconversion GQDs on illumination of 600–900 nm (Ref [78]: Zhu et al.); (d) Upconverted excitation-independent PL spectra of the ultrasonically synthesized GQDs at different excitation (Ref [79]: Zhou et al.)

3.3. Quantum Yield

Quantum yield is another important aspect associated with the PL of GQDs. The highest value reported was 28%. However, Wu et al. have reported a high QY of ~55% by the pyrolysis method of GQD synthesis [43]. In general, the QY depends on the fabrication methods and surface chemistry. It was reported by Liu et al. and Loh and coworkers that the removal of oxygen-containing groups and surface passivation can drastically enhance the QY of GQDs [80–82]. The possible reasons for this can be the non-radiative electron-hole recombination tendency of oxygen-containing groups. Though GQDs have optical properties similar to semiconductor QDs, few basic differences in PL spectra in terms of bandwidth (GQDs have broad bandwidth) and spectral shift toward red that decreases with increasing excitation clearly distinguish them from the semiconductor QDs [82].

3.4. Electrochemiluminescence

Another unique characteristic of GQDs is electrochemiluminescence (ECL), a phenomenon of showing luminescence during electrochemical reactions. GQDs are electro-active species and few reports deal with their ECL properties [83, 84]. Figure 11 is an illustration of ECL and PL spectra of GQDs synthesized by hydrothermal method. GQDs exhibited bright blue emission under ultraviolet irradiation (~365 nm) in a water solution of neutral pH, an excitation-independent photoluminescence feature, and interestingly, it also exhibited a novel anodic ECL by using H_2O_2 as a co-reactant [83]. The possible mechanism can be the formation of excited-state GQDs* through electron transfer (ET) annihilation of negatively and positively radical species.

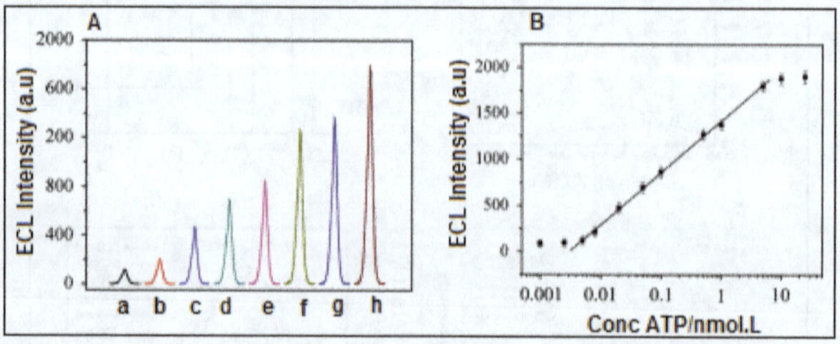

Figure 11. ECL intensity curves at different ECL intensities and ATP concentration. (Ref [83]: Lu et al.)

3.5. Biocompatibility of GQDs

GQDs are basically carbon materials and show low toxicity. As graphene and related materials have shown great potential in disease diagnosis and bioimaging, the potential toxicity of GQDs in biological systems has become a cause of concern. It is previously reported that graphene or graphene oxide can cause pulmonary inflammation upon inhalation [55], and graphene family materials were found to be toxic to bacteria [85–87]. In vitro studies on animal cell lines were also conducted and it was reported that the cytotoxicity of graphene and GQDs is also dependent on the method of synthesis and starting material. GQDs synthesized from carbon nanotubes are more toxic than those synthesized from graphene oxide and amino acids. Few reports have shown that GQDs can be well tolerated at low concentrations (50 μg/ml) but at higher concentrations (1 mg/ml), they show acute toxicity. In this regard, it is imperative to find out new strategies for less-toxic graphene materials for their practical biological applications with enhanced bioavailability. Surface functionalization of GQDs and graphene material can play an important role in mitigating the cytotoxicity of GQDs. These are the materials of future with potential biomedical applications, and surface modification of GQDs is an important criterion for their wide applicability. Many researchers have reported the emergence of unique properties with variations in surface properties. Production of reactive oxygen species (ROS) from GQDs by blue laser ablation and surface passivation by polyethylene glycol was reported by Christensen et al. in cell-free conditions [88] In another study by Yuan and coworkers, on functionalized GQDs, very encouraging results of cytotoxicity were observed; even at higher concentrations (200 μg/ml), quantum dots showed good biocompatibility as depicted in Figure 12 a, b. Their analysis proved that surface functionalization can be a better alternative to reduce the cytotoxity of GQDs [89]. Jastrz□bska et al. have summarized the toxicological analysis of graphene-related materials in a recent review [90]. As an interesting fact, many researchers have reported that GQDs are less toxic than GO and the possible cause may be less damage to cell membrane owing to their smaller size and their fast clearance [91].

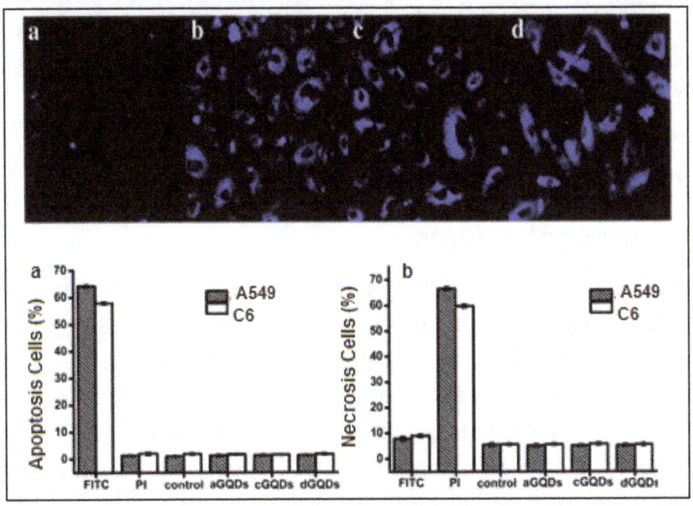

Figure 12. Biocompatibility analysis of GQDs *in vitro*. (Ref [89]: Yuan et al.)

Furthermore, the rising biological uses of GQDs and graphene materials necessitate consideration of their in vivo hazardous effects. Wang et al. observed that elevated dosages (0.4 mg) of graphene oxide induced persistent toxicity in mice [91, 92]. In a separate investigation, PEGylated GQDs exhibited no toxicity in mice, however PEG–GO demonstrated toxicity due to its buildup in the liver and spleen. They saw micrometer-sized black patches, significantly larger than the dimensions of GO in animal organs. This clearly indicated the aggregation of PEG–GO in organs, which is responsible for organ damage and potential fatalities [93].Based on the data available, it can be concluded that GQDs are less toxic than other graphene family materials and that is the prime reason for newer applications of GQDs in the field of biology and medicine.

4. NANOTHERANOSTIC APPLICATIONS OF GQDS

Due to the excellent optical and physical properties of GQDs, they have wide biological applications as a sensitive probe for disease marker screening in fluids, precise marker for tissue biopsy classification, and high-resolution contrast agent for biomedical cell/tissue imaging that can be applied for detecting tiny tumors. Moreover, the most distinctive feature of GQDs is their precise detection from macroscale visualization, down to atomic resolution using electron microscopy. Though many reports are there dealing with the wide applications of GQDs in energy-related [94, 95] biosensing [96,

97] and light-emitting diodes [98, 99], in this section we will only emphasize the role of GQDs in drug delivery and bioimaging or specifically nanotheranostic application of GQDs in medical biology. "Theranostics" is a new term coined by Funkhouser in 2002 that describes any "material that combines the modalities of therapy and diagnostic imaging" into a single package [100].

With the advancement in the field of nanotechnology, the field of nanotheranostics has emerged that not only provides a platform for simultaneous drug distribution and release monitoring but also enables us to evaluate the therapeutic efficacy of a noninvasive treatment in real time that will guide toward personalized therapy based on patients' individual responses and needs, minimizing the chances of the adverse side effects due to over- or under-dosing [101, 102].

In this segment, recent advances in the application of graphene quantum dots in drug delivery and bioimaging will be discussed.

4.1. Drug Delivery Applications

GQDs are emerging as an effective drug carrier for nanotheranostics application due to their unique properties as quantum dots as well as goodness of graphene. To date, many reports deal with GQDs as drug carrier and bioimaging. Recently, Wang et al. [103] synthesized PEGylated green fluorescent GQDs for carrying doxorubicin (Dox) for cancer treatment. Surface passivation by PEG enhanced the fluorescence and improved the solubility of GQDs. Moreover, GQDs were synthesized via reduction of GO by L-ascorbic acid so they adopted the green route for better biocompatibility. Figure 13a represents the schematic of Dox-loaded GQDs. GQD–PEG showed distinctly different loading capacities toward Dox at different pH values. The maximum loading capacity of Dox on GQD–PEG is 0.9 mg/mg at pH 5.5; 2.5 mg/mg at pH 7.4; and 1.1 mg/mg at pH 9 (Figure 13b, c).

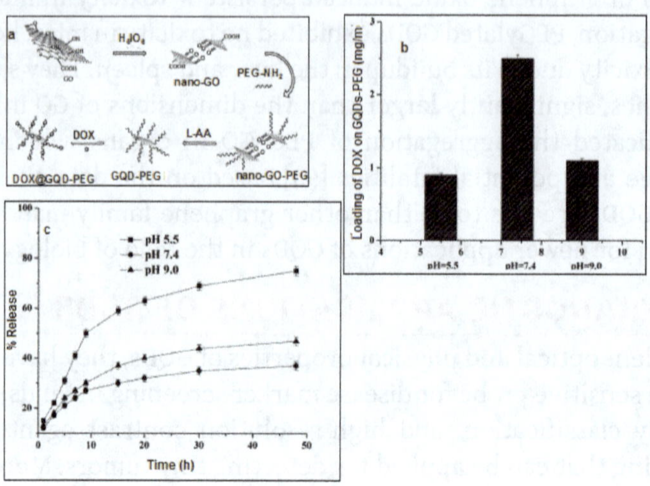

Figure 13. (a) Illustration of drug loading on GQDS; (b) Drug loading capacity of GQDs; (c) Percentage release profile of drugs at different pH. (Ref [103]: Wang et al.).

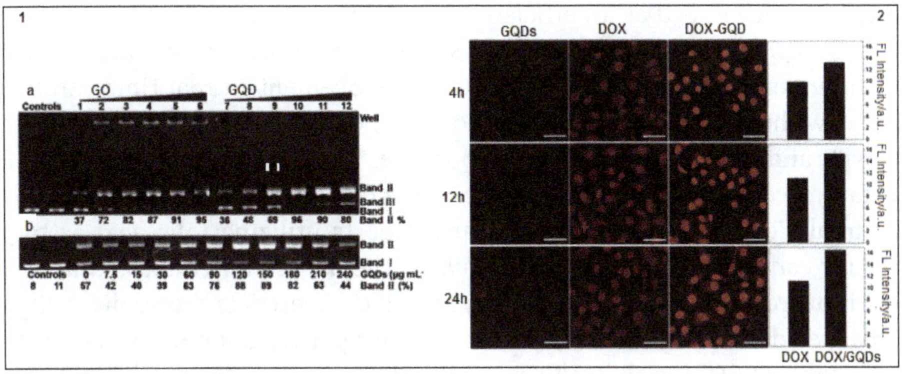

Figure 14. (a) Illustrating DNA (38 μM) cleavage with Cu $(Phen)_2$ (di-1,10-phenanthroline-copper) with GO and GQDs; 1(b) Cleavage with different concentrations of GQDS and DOX. 2: CLSM images of MCF-7 cells incubated with GQDs, DOX and GQD-DOX. (Ref [105]: Wang et al.)

In another similar application, Zhu et al. [104] fabricated paclitaxel-loaded multifunctional core–shell structure capsules composed of olive oil, dual-layer porous TiO2 shell, Fe_3O_4, and GQDs. The olive oil core for hydrobhic drug loading was the novel aspect of this formulation. The TiO_2 shell suppressed the initial burst release, while Fe_3O_4 and GQDs were utilized for magnetic targeting and fluorescence imaging, respectively. In two different interesting applications, DNA cleavage activity with drug delivery of GQDs was reported. Wang et al. [105] prepared GQD–Dox complex for enhanced nucleus accumulation and DNA cleavage efficiency. They achieved efficient delivery of doxorubicin to the nucleus through Dox/GQD conjugates, as the conjugates assumed different cellular and nuclear internalization pathways compared to free Dox. Furthermore, with drug-resistant cancer cells, the Dox/GQD conjugates increased the nuclear uptake and cytotoxicity of Dox, capable of increasing the chemotherapy efficacy of anticancer drugs that are suboptimal due to the drug resistance. Figure 14 shows the DNA cleavage activity and cellular internalization of GQD–Dox complex via diffusion and the release of drug in nucleus after interaction with DNA. In another approach, Zhou et al. [106] have reported GQDs in DNA cleavage system. According to their findings, by using GQDs and Cu^{2+}, about 90% supercoiled DNA was converted into nicked DNA, while only about 59% supercoiled DNA was cleaved with the same amount of large-sized GO and Cu^{2+}. According to their hypothesis, the as-prepared GQD sheets with smaller lateral size performed as a better intercalator to DNA molecules than micron GO sheets and therefore, under the same conditions, GQDs exhibited better efficiency than GO for DNA cleavage.

A nanocomposite based on conglomeration of Au–Fe_3O_4 core–shell with GQDs is reported by Oza et al. [107]. This modular design enabled Au-Fe_3O_4-GQD-based magnetic combined therapeutic nanoplatform to perform multiple functions simultaneously, such as in multimodal imaging, drug delivery, and real-time monitoring. Dox was loaded by cystamine linker and the drug release was a temperature-dependent phenomenon. With folic acid (FA) as the targeted moiety, this formulation showed potential to be developed as an efficient drug delivery system. Another FA-mediated Dox-loaded GQD-based targeted delivery system was reported by Wang et al. [108]. Due to the inherent fluorescence of GQDs, cell movement in real time can be easily monitored without employing external dyes, and simultaneous localization of the drug carrier and the loaded drug can be possible. The nanoassembly was internalized by the target cells via receptor-mediated endocytosis with prolonged Dox release and accumulation. Though there are many reports utilizing folic acid as targeting moieties for cancer-cell-specific drug delivery, the major constraint is that folic acid receptor is overexpressed on healthy cells as well that restricts the applicability of FA-functionalized delivery system. Nahain et al. [109] put forth a new targeting strategy by functionalizing GQDs with hyaluronic acid (HA). HA is a natural polysaccharide and a targeting receptor for CD44 cells. CD44 are cancer stem cells responsible for drug resistance and reoccurrence of pancreatic cancer. Hence, by targeting CD44 by HA, an effective targeting strategy was developed. Figure 15 illustrates Dox-loaded green fluorescent GQD nanoformulation. The authors also evaluated the in vivo efficacy of GQDs in bioimaging and therapy. Figure 15b shows the in vivo imaging of mice model studies performed. HA-functionalized GQDs showed enhanced stability and stable fluorescence in vivo that could pave the way for future applications of GQDs in targeted drug delivery for cancer, the most fatal disease of human history (Figure 16b).

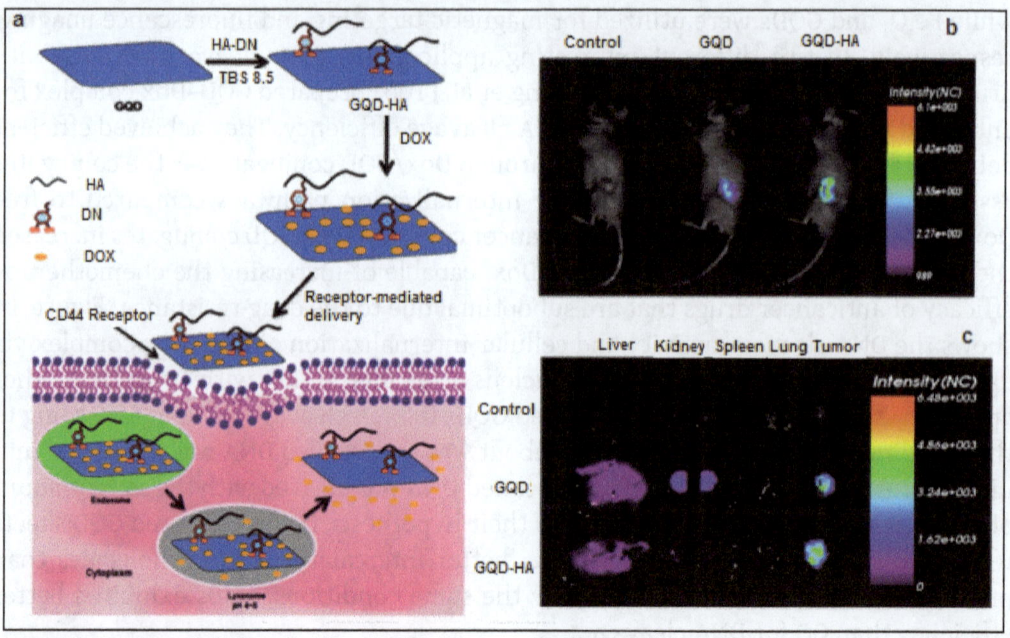

Figure 15. (a) Schematic of target delivery of GQDs using hyaluronic acid and subsequent release of the drug from the surfaces of GQD in a tumor-cell environment; (b) In vivo fluorescence images of GQD-HA in mice after tail vein injection; (c) Ex vivo images of liver, kidney, spleen, heart, and tumor after dissection. (Ref [109]: Nahain et al.)

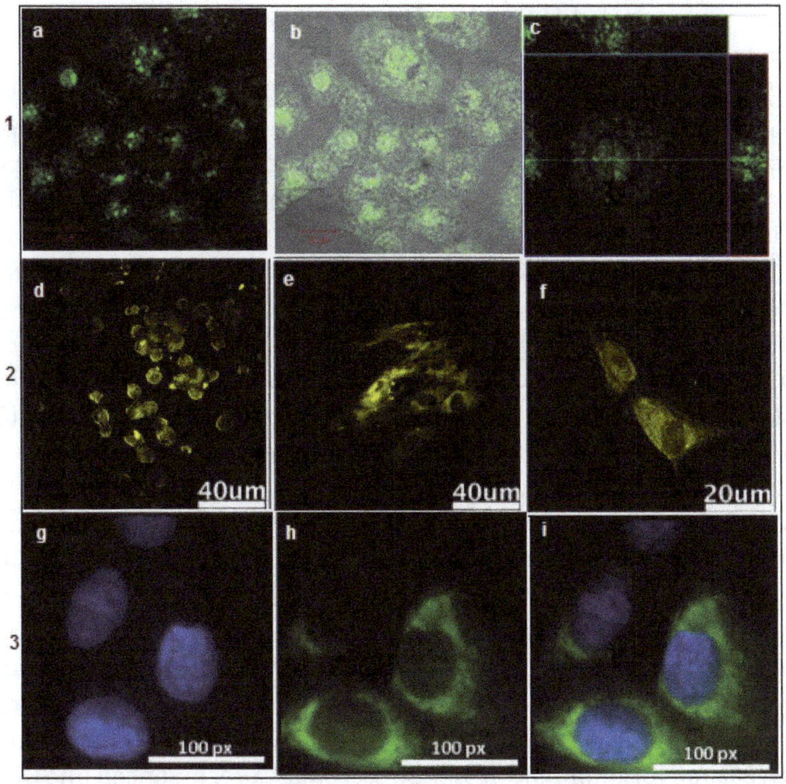

Figure 16. Confocal Images of MCF-7 cells labeled with GQDs 1 (a) Fluorescent image; (b) Bright field; (c) Merged fluorescent and bright field; (d) Section analysis (Ref [114]: Dong et al.); 2. Stem cells images of (d) Neurospheres cells (NSCs); (e) Pancreas progenitor cells (PPCs); (c) Cardiac progenitor cells (CPCs) (Ref [35] Zhang et al.); 3. High-contrast bioimaging via GQDs for breast cancer cell line (T47D). (Ref [9]: Peng et al.)

4.2. Applications of Bioimaging

Traditional semiconductor quantum dots like CdSe or CdS and their core-shell nanoparticles have been exploited for applications in in vitro and in vivo cell imaging [110, 111], but the toxicity and potential health and environmental hazards associated with them restrict their applicability in live systems. In this regard, GQDs with their tunable PL, ecofriendly nature, and emergence of GQDs to date have shown remarkable potential for their successful application in the field of biotechnology and medicine owing to their excellent optical properties and low cytotoxicity up to very high concentrations of 400 μg/ml [112]. The authors also noted good uptake of GQDs by cells, as shown by the bright PL observed. Another example of bioimaging potential of GQDs, made from CX-72 carbon black, was reported by Dong et al. [113] in human breast cancer MCF-7 cells. They obtained effective luminescence inside the cell nucleus along with the cell membrane and cytoplasm. It was the first example that illustrated that GQDs have the ability to penetrate the cell nucleus and is another promising feature of GQDs to prove their strong candidature in nanotheranostic applications

(Figure 16a). Sun et al. [114] compared the cytotoxicity and bioimaging capabilities of chemically reduced and photoreduced brightly blue luminescent GQDs in A549 cells using the MTT (3-(4,5-dimethylthiazol-2-yl)-2,5-diphenyltetrazolium bromide) assay. According to their findings, the cytotoxicity of the chemically reduced GQDs (cGQDs) was significantly greater than that of the photoreduced GQDs (pGQDs). The possible reason for this was the use of toxic reagents ($NaBH_4$ and $N_2H_4 \times H_2O$) during the chemical reduction. Photoreduced GQDs also exhibited stronger fluorescence indicating better cellular uptake due to the presence of less negative charge on the GQD surface. A very interesting approach was presented by Zhang et al. [35] by utilizing GQDs to label stem cells. The ability of GQDs to penetrate stem cell without reducing cell viability was exploited. Three different types of stem cells (neurosphere cells (NSCs), pancreas progenitor cells (PPCs), and cardiac progenitor cells (CPCs)) with GQDs at a final concentration of 25 μg/ml were labeled and strong fluorescence was observed in the cytoplasm of the stem cells, but not in the nuclei. They obtained good penetration into cytoplasmic areas but not inside the cell nucleus. The authors also found that the GQDs were able to easily penetrate tumor cells (human lung cancer (A549) and human breast cells (MCF-7) and showed little cytotoxicity (Figure 16b). In most of the cases, downconversion PL imaging is reported, but Zhu et al. came up with upconversion GQDs. In downconversion, mainly UV or blue excitations are involved that are considered unsafe for living systems. In this scenario, Zhu et al. could attain more biocompatibility with their upconversion GQDs excited at near-infrared light of wavelength 808 nm for illuminating mouse osteoblast precursor cell line (MT3T3) cells. A blue or bright green fluorescence was observed inside the cells even after 20 min of continuous excitation. This indicated the successful internalization of GQDs inside the cells and photostability of GQDs as well [115].

Recently, Nigam et al. [20] have also reported the excellent bioimaging potential in a human serum-albumin-based multifunctional drug delivery system for pancreatic cancer. A strong and stable green fluorescence with good biocompatibility was observed in their analysis. In another report, Peng et al. [9] incubated breast cancer cell line T47D. The cell nucleus was stained with DAPI (blue color). Figure 16c illustrates the images of T47D cells treated with green GQDs with a 4-h incubation time, which clearly visualized the phase contrast image of T47D cells with nucleus stained with blue DAPI and green fluorescence from the cytoplasm. This bioimaging data proved that GQDs can be utilized in high-contrast bioimaging applications. Recently, GQDs synthesized by polycyclic aromatic compound via bottom-up approach by Zhou et al. were applied for illuminating MCF-7 (breast cancer cell lines). A stable green fluorescence inside the cytoplasm was obtained [116].

Zheng et al. have demonstrated a novel application of GQDs for insulin receptor dynamics, using total internal reflection fluorescence microscopy (TIRFM), by functionalizing insulin with GQDs [117]. According to their observation, small discrete clusters of GQDs after pre-incubating adipocytes with insulin GQDs were detected. The steady lateral movement of GQD-enlightened clusters to the cell membrane and vertical movement between the inner cytosol and the plasmalemmal region were also tracked by following the GQD fluorescence (Figure 17). This application is a good example of the potential of the edge-functionalized GQDs for investigating dynamic cellular processes.

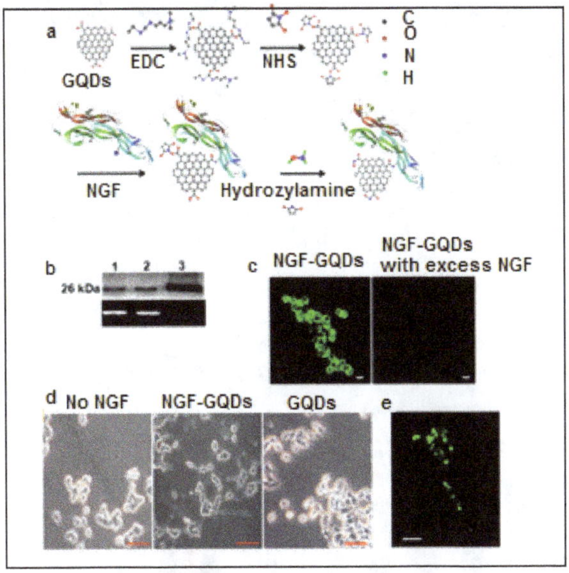

Figure 17. (a) Schematic illustration of conjugating a GQD with NGF; (b) Gel electrophoresis of NGF-GQD (lane 1), FITC-NGF (lane 2), and NGF (lane 3); (c) Fluorescence images of living PC12 cells incubated with 200 ng/mL NGF-GQDs (left) or NGF-GQDs together with 20 μg/mL free NGF (right) for 15 min; (d) Representative phase-contrast images of PC12 cells after 2-day incubation; (e) Distribution of NGF-GQDs in PC12 cells differentiated by 200 ng/mL NGF-GQDs for 24 h. (Ref [117]: Zheng et al.)

GQDs are gradually attaining popularity for their in vivo applications also. The basic flaw related with in vivo imaging is background signal associated with autofluorescence of animal tissues. Moreover, the Rayleigh scattering of short wavelength light absorbed by water is another undesirable effect that is to be considered. It was reported by Nurunnabi et al. that carboxylated GQDs can be efficiently explored for superficial tissue imaging but short-wavelength excitation limits their use for deep tissue bioimaging [118]. However, With GQDs of near-infrared photoluminescence, after 8 h of GQD injection, fluorescent signals were obtained near heart, spleen, and kidney [119]. In another approach, Ge and coworkers synthesized GQDs with polythiophene derivatives via hydrothermal approach and they observed an emission wavelength of 680 nm that enables these GQDs for in vivo applications. Another important finding of their work was the application of as-synthesized GQD in photodynamic therapy as it was observed that GQDs could produce $^1O_2$ via multistate sensitization process (Figure 18) with a quantum yield of about 1.3, the highest yield reported for photodynamic therapy (PDT) agents to date [120].

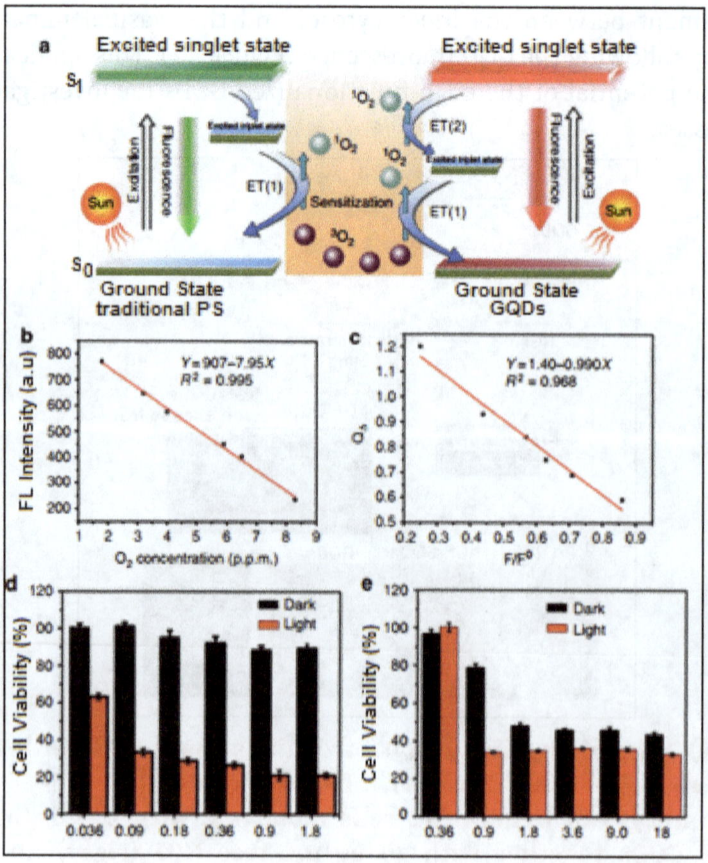

Figure 18. (a) Schematic illustration of the $^1O_2$ generation mechanisms by conventional PDT agents (left) and GQDs (right); (b) Fluorescence intensity of GQDs at 680 nm versus the O_2 concentration in solution; (c) The dependence of the $^1O_2$ quantum yield (Q_Δ) on the fluorescence intensity ratio at 680 nm (F/F^0); (d) GQDs in the concentration range 0.036–1.8 μM; (e) Protoporphyrin (PpIX) in the concentration range 0.36–18 μM. (Ref [120]: Ge et al.)

Although the cytotoxicity of GQDs in cells has been reported to be relatively low, contradictory findings were reported by Markovic et al. [121]. According to their observation, GQDs could be cytotoxic to U251 human glioma cells. They postulate that the GQDs can induce oxidative stress and activate apoptosis and autophagy-type cell deaths by generating reactive oxygen species (ROS).

5. CONCISE SUMMARY AND FUTURE PROSPECTS

Graphene quantum dots (GQDs) have attracted considerable interest in several fields, such as biology, electronics, and medicine, due to their exceptional optical and physical properties, biocompatibility, and chemical durability. Nevertheless, the study of GQDs is nascent, offering significant prospects for additional investigation into their utility. The principal problems related to GQDs encompass low quantum yield, low productivity, surface chemistry, size tunability, and inadequate control over photoluminescence and optical properties. Nevertheless, despite these constraints, GQDs provide a potential future for carbon materials. We expect that forthcoming research on GQDs will concentrate on the subsequent issues.

Advancement in Synthesis Approaches

Low production yield is the major problem associated with GQDs. Hence, the development of better synthesis strategies by solvent selection, reaction conditions, and appropriate cutting methodology in top-down approaches and better size and solubility control in bottom-up methods should be explored.

Multifunctionality of GQDs

To extend the applicability of GQDs in bioimaging and drug delivery, novel approaches are to be developed. Still there are very few reports dealing with in vivo imaging and drug delivery mediated with multifunctional GQDs. Based on their application potential, it is imperative to explore the newer techniques for generating functionalized GQDs for their application in MRI and CT scan.

Quantum Yield Enhancement

To date, the GQDs with QY ranging from 10% to 55% have been reported. To increase the QY and PL efficiency of GQDs, new surface-passivation strategies are needed so that GQDs with better bioimaging and stable fluorescence can be obtained.

Applicability in Newer Areas

There is no report to date on application of GQDs in brain. A great deal can be done by tuning the excitation and emission properties of GQDs and they can be potentially exploited for blood–brain barrier penetration and brain gene therapy for neurodegenerative diseases.

Toxicological Evaluation

The toxicity of nanoparticles is an expanding field of inquiry. Graphene quantum dots (GQDs) represent a novel category within nanoparticles, raising apprehensions over potential adverse effects linked to their use. The biodistribution, organ accumulation, and genotoxicity of GQDs produced using various processes, forms, sizes, and surface functional groups must be assessed.

Graphene quantum dots have demonstrated significant potential in a brief period. Current research in this domain will unveil new opportunities that will transform the future of medicinal and biotechnological applications.

REFERENCES

1. Novoselov KS, Geim AK, Morozov SV, Jiang D, Zhang Y, Dubonos SV, Grigorieva V, Firsov A. Electric field effect in atomically thin carbon films. Science. 2004; 306: 666–669. DOI:10.1126/science.1102896.
2. Novoselov KS, Geim AK, Morozov SV, Jiang D, Katsnelson MI, Grigorieva IV, Dubonos SV,

Firsov AA. Two-dimensional gas of massless Dirac fermions in graphene. Nature. 2005; 438: 197–200. DOI:10.1038/nature04233.

3. Wallace PR. The band theory of graphite. Phu. Rev. 1947; 71: 622. DOI:http://dx.DOI.org/10.1103/PhysRev.71.622.
4. Boehm HP, Clauss A, Fischer GO, Hofmann U, Anorg Z. Das Adsorptionsverhalten sehr dünner Kohlenstoff-Folien. Allg. Chem. 1962; 316: 119–127. DOI:10.1002/zaac.19623160303.
5. Mouras S, Hamwi A, Djurado D, Cousseins JC. Synthesis of first stage graphite intercalation compounds from fluoride. Rev. Chim. Miner. 1987; 24: 572–582.
6. Li LS, Yan X. Collioidal quantum dots. J. Phys. Chem. Lett. 2010; 1: 2572–2576. DOI:10.1021/jz100862f.
7. Ye R, Peng Z, Metzger A, Lin J, Mann JA, Huang K, Xiang C, Fan X, Samuel ELG, Alemany LB, Marti AA, Tour JM. Bandgap engineering of coal-derived graphene quantum dots. ACS Appl. Mater. Interface. 2015; 7: 7041–7048. DOI:10.1021/acsami.5b01419.
8. Mueller, X Yan, JA McGuire, L Li. Triplet states and electronic relaxation in photoexcited graphene quantum dots. Nano Lett. 2010; 10: 2679–2682. DOI:10.1021/nl101474d.
9. Peng J, Gao W, Gupta BK, Liu K, Romero-Aburto R, Ge L, Song L, Alemany LB, Zhan X, Gao G, Vithayathil SA, Kaipparettu B, Marti AA, Hayashi T, Zhu TT, Ajayan PM. Graphene quantum dots derived from carbon fibers. Nano Lett. 2012; 12: 844–849. DOI:10.1021/nl2038979.
10. Yan X, Cui X, Li B, Li L. Large, solution-processable graphene quantum dots as light absorbers for photovoltaics. Nano Lett. 2010; 10: 1869–1873. DOI:10.1021/nl101060h.
11. Dutta M, Sarkar S, Ghosh T, Basak D. ZnO/Graphene quantum dot solid-state solar C\cell. J. Phys. Chem. C. 2012; 116: 20127–20131. DOI:10.1021/jp302992k.
12. Gupta V, Chaudhary N, Srivastava R, Sharma GD, Bhardwaj R, Chand S. Luminescent graphene quantum dots for organic photovoltaic devices. J. Am. Chem. Soc. 2011; 133: 9960–9963. DOI:10.1021/ja2036749.
13. Dong Y, Shao J, Chen C, Li H, Wang R, Chi Y, Lin X, Chen G. Blue luminescent graphene quantum dots and graphene oxide prepared by tuning the carbonization degree of citric acid. Carbon. 2012; 50: 4738–4743. DOI:10.1016/j.carbon.2012.06.002.
14. Pan DY, Zhang JC, Li Z, Wu MH. Hydrothermal route for cutting graphene sheets into blue-Luminescent graphene quantum dots. Adv Mater. 2010; 22: 734–738. DOI:10.1002/adma.200902825.
15. Pan D, Guo L, Zhang L, Xi C, Xue Q, Huang H, Li J, Zhang Z, Yu W, Chen Z, Zu M. Cutting sp^2 clusters in graphene sheets into colloidal graphene quantum dots with strong green fluorescence. J. Mater. Chem. 2012; 22: 3314–3318. DOI:10.1039/C2JM16005F.
16. Yan X, Li B, Cui X, Wei Q, Tajima K, LS Li. Independent tuning of the band gap and redox potential of graphene quantum dots. J. Phys. Chem. Lett. 2011 ; 2: 1119–1124. DOI:10.1021/jz200450r.
17. Tetsuka H, Asahi R, Nagoya A, Okamoto K, Tajima I, Ohta R, Okamoto A. Optically tunable amino-functionalized graphene quantum dots. Adv. Mater. 2012; 24: 5333–5338. DOI:10.1002/adma.201201930.
18. Feng Q, Cao QQ, Li M, Liu FC, Tang NJ, Du YW. Synthesis and photoluminescence of fluorinated graphene quantum dots. Appl. Phys. Lett. 2013; 102: 013111–013114. DOI:10.1063/1.4774264.

19. Hu CF, Liu YL, Yang YH, Cui JH, Huang ZR, Wang YL, Yang LF, Wang HB, Xiao Y, Rong JH. One-step preparation of nitrogen-doped graphene quantum dots from oxidized debris of graphene oxide. J. Mater. Chem. B. 2013; 1: 39–42. DOI:10.1039/C2TB00189F.
20. Zhang ZH, Wu PY. Hydrothermal aggregation induced crystallization: a facial route towards polycrystalline graphite quantum dots with blue photoluminescence. Cryst. Eng. Comm. 2012; 14: 7149–7152. DOI:10.1039/C2CE26117K.
21. Liu Y, Wu PY. Graphene quantum dot hybrids as efficient metal-free electrocatalyst for the oxygen reduction reaction. ACS Appl. Mater. Interface. 2013; 5: 3362–3369. DOI:10.1021/am400415t.
22. Nigam P, Waghmode S, Louis M, Wangnoo S, Chavan P, Sarkar D. Graphene quantum dots conjugated albumin nanoparticles for targeted drug delivery and imaging of pancreatic cancer. J. Mater. Chem. B. 2014; 2: 3190–3195. DOI:10.1039/C4TB00015C.
23. Shen J, Zhu Y, Chen C, Yang X, Li C. Facile preparation and upconversion luminescence of graphene quantum dots. Chem. Commun. 2011; 47: 2580–2582. DOI:10.1039/C0CC04812G.
24. Zhu SJ, Zhang JH, Qiao CY, Tang SJ, Li YF, Yuan WJ, Li B, Tian L, Liu F, Hu R, Gao HN, Wei HT, Zhang H, Sun HC, Yang B. Strongly green-photoluminescent graphene quantum dots for bioimaging applications. Chem. Commun. 2011; 47: 6858–6860. DOI:10.1039/C1CC11122A.
25. Zhu SJ, Zhang JH, Liu X, Li B, Wang XF, Tang SJ, Meng QN, Li YF, Shi C, Hu R, Yang B. Graphene quantum dots with controllable surface oxidation, tunable fluorescence and up- conversion emission. RSC Adv. 2012; 2: 2717–2720. DOI:10.1039/C2RA20182H.
26. Shin Y, Park J, Hyun D, Yang J, Lee J, Kim J, Lee H. Acid-free and oxone oxidant-assisted solvothermal synthesis of graphene quantum dots using various natural carbon materials as resources. Nanoscale. 2015; 7: 6533–5637. DOI:10.1039/C5NR00814J.
27. Chan CF, Lau SP, Luk CM, Tsang MK. Two-photon fluorescence in N-doped graphene quantum dots. Int. J. Chem. Nucl. Mater. Metall. Eng. 2014: 8; 1313–1316.
28. Luo Z, Yang D, Qi G, Shang J, Yang H, Wang Y, Yuwen L, Yu T, Huang W, Wang L. Microwave-assisted solvothermal preparation of nitrogen and sulfur co-doped reduced graphene oxide and graphene quantum dots hybrids for highly efficient oxygen reduction. J. Mat. Chem. A. 2014; 2: 20605–20611. DOI:10.1039/C4TA05096G.
29. Tang L, Ji R, X C, Lin L, Jiang H, Li X, Teng KS, Luk CM, Zeng S, Hao J, Lau SP. Deep ultraviolet photoluminescence of water-soluble self-passivated graphene quantum dots. ACS Nano. 2012; 6: 5102–3110. DOI:10.1021/nn300760g
30. Li LL, Ji J, Fei R, Wang CZ, Lu Q, Zhang JR, Jiang LP, Zhu JJ. A facile microwave avenue to electrochemiluminescent two-color graphene quantum dots. Adv. Funct. Mater. 2012; 22: 2971–2979. DOI:10.1002/adfm.201200166.
31. Zhu Y, Wang G, Jiang H, Chen L, Zhang X. One-step ultrasonic synthesis of graphene quantum dots with high quantum yield and their application in sensing alkaline phosphatase. Chem. Commun. (Camb). 2015; 5: 948–951. DOI:10.1039/c4cc07449a.
32. Lu J, Yang JX, Wang J, Lim A, Wang S, Loh KP. One-pot synthesis of fluorescent carbon nanoribbons, nanoparticles, and graphene by the exfoliation of graphite in ionic liquids. ACS Nano. 2009; 3: 2367–2375. DOI:10.1021/nn900546b.
33. Zheng L, Chi Y, Dong Y, Lin J, Wang B. Electrochemiluminescence of water-soluble carbon nanocrystals released electrochemically from graphite. J. Am. Chem. Soc. 2009; 131: 4564–4565. DOI:10.1021/ja809073f.

34. Li Y, Hu Y, Zhao Y, Shi G, Deng L, Hou Y, Qu L. An Electrochemical avenue to green-luminescent graphene quantum dots as potential electron-acceptors for photovoltaics. Adv. Mater. 2011; 23: 776–780. DOI:10.1002/adma.201003819.

35. Zhang M, Bai L, Shang W, Xie W, Ma H, Fu Y, Fang D, Sun H, Fan L, Han M, Liu C, Yang S. Facile synthesis of water-soluble, highly fluorescent graphene quantum dots as a robust biological label for stem cells. J. Mater. Chem. 2012; 22: 7461–7467. DOI:10.1039/C2JM16835A.

36. Shinde DB, Pillai VK. Electrochemical preparation of luminescent graphene quantum dots from multiwalled carbon nanotubes. Chem. Eur. J. 2012; 18: 12522–12528. DOI:10.1002/chem.201201043.

37. Shinde DB, Dhavle VM, Kurungot S, Pillai VM. Electrochemical preparation of nitrogen-doped graphene quantum dots and their size-dependent electrocatalytic activity for oxygen reduction. Bull. Mater. Sci. 2015; 38: 435–442. DOI:10.1007/s12034-014-0834-3.

38. Tan X, Li Y, Li X, Zhou S, Fan L, Yang S. Electrochemical synthesis of small-sized red fluorescent graphene quantum dots as a bioimaging platform. Chem. Comm. 2015; 51: 2544–2546. DOI:10.1039/C4CC09332A.

39. Ponomarenko LA, Schedin F, Katsnelson MI, Yang R, Hill EW, Novoselov KS, Geim AK. Chaotic dirac billiard in graphene quantum dots. Science. 2008; 320: 356–358. DOI:10.1126/science.1154663.

40. Lee J, Kim K, Park WI, Kim BH, Park JH, Kim TH, Bong S, Kim CH, Chae G, Jun M, Hwang Y, Jung YS, Jeon S. Uniform graphene quantum dots patterned from self-assembled silica nanodots. Nano Lett. 2012; 12: 6078–6083. DOI:10.1021/nl302520m.

41. Liu R, Wu D, Feng X, Müllen K. Bottom-up fabrication of photoluminescent graphene quantum dots with uniform morphology. J. Am. Chem. Soc. 2011; 133: 15221–15223. DOI:org/10.1021/ja204953k.

42. Liu JJ, Zhang XL, Cong ZX, Chen ZT, Yang HH, Chen GN. Glutathione-functionalized graphene quantum dots as selective fluorescent probes for phosphate-containing metabolites. Nanoscale. 2013; 5: 1810–1815. DOI:10.1039/C3NR33794D.

43. Wu X, Tian F, Wang W, Chen J, Wub M, Zha JX. Fabrication of highly fluorescent graphene quantum dots using L-glutamic acid for in vitro/in vivo imaging and sensing. J. Mat. Chem. C. 2013; 1: 4676–4684. DOI:10.1039/C3TC30820K.

44. Wang L, Wang Y, Xu T, Yao C, Liu Y, Li Z, Chen Z, Pan D, Sun L, Wu M. Gram-scale synthesis of single-crystalline graphene quantum dots with superior optical properties. Nat. Commun. 2014; 5: 1–9. DOI:10.1038/ncomms6357.

45. Lin L, Rong M, Lu S, Song X, Zhong Y, Yan J, Wang Y, Chen Xi. A facile synthesis of highly luminescent nitrogen-doped graphene quantum dots for the detection of 2,4,6-trinitrophenol in aqueous solution. Nanoscale. 2015; 7: 1872–1878. DOI:10.1039/C4NR06365A.

46. Lu J, Yeo PSE, Gan CK, Wu P, Loh KP. Transforming C_{60} molecules into graphene quantum dots. Nat. Nanotechnol. 2011; 6: 247–252. DOI:10.1038/nnano.2011.30.

47. Sinclair J, Dr. Dagotto, "An introduction to quantum dots: confinement, synthesis, artificial atoms and applications," Solid State II Lecture Notes, University of Tennessee, Knoxville, 2009.

48. Chukwuocha EO, Onyeaju MC, Harry TST. Theoretical studies on the effect of confinement on quantum dots using the Brus Equation. World J. Condens. Matter. Phys. 2012; 2: 96–100. DOI:10.4236/wjcmp.2012.22017.

49. Dinadayalane TC, Leszczynski J. Remarkable diversity of carbon–carbon bonds: structures and properties of fullerenes, carbon nanotubes, and graphene. Struct. Chem. 2010; 21: 1155–1169. DOI:10.1007/s11224-010-9670-2.

50. Geim A. Graphene: status and prospects. Science. 2009; 324: 1530–1534. DOI:10.1126/science.1158877.

51. Allen MJ, Tung VC, Kaner RB. Honeycomb carbon: a review of graphene. Chem. Rev. 2010; 110: 132–145. DOI:10.1021/cr900070d.

52. Li L, Wu G, Yang G, Peng J, Zhao J, Zhu JJ. Focusing on luminescent graphene quantum dots: current status and future perspectives. Nanoscale. 2013; 5: 4015–4039. DOI:10.1039/C3NR33849E.

53. Baker SN, Baker GA. Luminescent carbon nanodots: emergent nanolights. Angew. Chem. Int. Ed. 2010; 49: 6726–6744. DOI:10.1002/anie.200906623.

54. Eda G, Lin YY, Mattevi C, Yamaguchi H, Chen HA, Chen IS, Chen CW, Chhowalla M. Blue photoluminescence from chemically derived graphene oxide. Adv. Mater. 2010; 22: 505–509. DOI:10.1002/adma.200901996.

55. Güttinger J, Seif J, Stampfer C, Capelli A, Ensslin K, Ihn T. Time-resolved charge detection in graphene quantum dots. Phys. Rev. B. 2011; 83: 165445–165452. DOI:http://dx.doi.org/10.1103/PhysRevB.83.165445.

56. Li HO, Tu T, Cao G, Wang LJ, Guo GC, Guo GP. Quantum transport in graphene quantum dots. Nanotechnology and nanomaterials: new progress on graphene research DOI:10.5772/52873.

57. González JW, Delgado F, Fernández-Rossier J. Graphene single-electron transistor as a spin sensor for magnetic adsorbates. Phys. Rev. B. 2012; 87: 085433. DOI:http://dx.DOI.org/10.1103/PhysRevB.87.085433.

58. Ihn T, Güttinger J, Molitor F, Schnez S, Schurtenberger E, Jacobsen A, Hellmüller S, Fery T, Ensslin K. Graphene single-electron transistors. Mater. Today. 2010; 13: 44–50. DOI:10.1016/S1369-7021(10)70033-X.

59. Luo Z, Lu Y, Somers LA, Johnson ATC. High yield preparation of macroscopic graphene oxide membranes. J. Am. Chem. Soc. 2009; 131: 898–899. DOI:10.1021/ja807934n.

60. Peng J, Gao W, Gupta BK, Liu Z, Ge RRL, Song L, Alemany LB, Zhan X, Gao G, Vithayathil SA, Kaipparettu BA, Marti AA, Hayashi T, Zhu JJ, Ajayan PM. Graphene quantum dots derived from carbon fibers. Nano Lett. 2012; 12: 844–849. DOI:10.1021/nl2038979.

61. Kim S, Hwang SW, Kim MK, Shin DY, Shin DH, Kim CO, Yang SB, Park JH, Hwang E, Choi SH, Ko G, Sim S, Sone S, Choi HJ, Bae S, Hong BH. Anomalous behaviors of visible luminescence from graphene quantum dots: interplay between size and shape. ACS Nano. 2012; 6: 8203–8208. DOI:10.1021/nn302878r.

62. Fuyuno N, Kozawa D, Miyauchi Y, Mouri S, Kitaura R, Shinohara H, Yasuda T, Komatsu N, Matsuda K. Size-dependent luminescence properties of chromatographically-separated graphene quantum dots. https://scirate.com/arxiv/1311.1684.

63. Liu R, Wu D, Feng X, Muellen K. Bottom-Up Fabrication of photoluminescent graphene quantum dots with uniform morphology. J. Am. Chem. Soc. 2011; 133: 15221–15223. DOI:10.1021/ja204953k.

64. Qu D, Zheng M, Zhang L, Zhao H, Xie Z, Jing X, Haddad RE, Fan H, Sun Z. Formation mechanism and optimization of highly luminescent N-doped graphene quantum dots. Sci. Rep. 2014; 4: 1–9. DOI:10.1038/srep05294.

65. Yang F, Zhao M, Zheng B, Xiao D, Wu L, Guo Y. Influence of pH on the fluorescence properties of graphene quantum dots using ozonation pre-oxide hydrothermal synthesis. J. Mater. Chem. 2012; 22: 25471–25479. DOI:10.1039/C2JM35471C.

66. Li H, He X, Liu Y, Huang H, Lian S, Lee ST, Kang Z. One-step ultrasonic synthesis of water-soluble carbon nanoparticles with excellent photoluminescent properties. Carbon. 2011; 49: 605–609. DOI:10.1016/j.carbon.2010.10.004.

67. Li H, He X, Kang Z, Huang H, Liu Y, Liu J, Lian S, Tsang CHA, Yang X, Lee ST. Water-soluble fluorescent carbon quantum dots and photocatalyst design. Angew. Chem. Int. Ed. 2010; 49: 4430–4434. DOI:10.1002/anie.200906154.

68. Qiao ZA, Wang Y, Gao Y, Li H, Dai T, Liu Y, Huo Q. Commercially activated carbon as the source for producing multicolor photoluminescent carbon dots by chemical oxidation. Chem. Commun. 2010; 46: 8812–8814. DOI:10.1039/C0CC02724C.

69. Li H, Kang Z, Liu Y, Lee ST. Carbon nanodots: synthesis, properties and applications. J. Mater. Chem. 2012; 22: 24230–24253. DOI:10.1039/C2JM34690G.

70. Mahasin Alam SK, Ananthanarayanan A, Huang L, Lim KH, Chen P. Revealing the tunable photoluminescence properties of graphene quantum dots. J. Mater. Chem. C. 2014; 2: 6954–6960. DOI:10.1039/C4TC01191K.

71. Tang L, Ji R, Cao X, Lin J, Jiang H, Li X, Teng KS, Luk CM, Zeng S, Hao J, Lau SP. Deep ultraviolet photoluminescence of water-soluble self-passivated graphene quantum dots. ACS Nano. 2012 ; 6: 5102–5110. DOI:10.1021/nn300760g.

72. Zhu S, Zhang J, Liu X, Li B, Wang X, Tang S, Meng Q, Li Y, Shi C, Hu R, Yang B. Graphene quantum dots with controllable surface oxidation, tunable fluorescence and up-conversion emission. RSC Adv. 2012; 2: 2717–2720. DOI:10.1039/C2RA20182H.

73. Michalet X, Pinaud FF, Bentolila LA, Tsay JM, Doose S, Li JJ, Sundaresan G, Wu AM, Gambhir SS, Weiss S. Quantum dots for live cells, in vivo imaging, and diagnostics. Science. 2005; 307: 538–544. DOI:10.1126/science.1104274.

74. Smith AM, Nie S. Semiconductor nanocrystals: structure, properties, and band gap engineering. Acc. Chem. Res. 2010; 43: 190–200. DOI:10.1021/ar9001069.

75. Fan T, Zeng W, Tang W, Yuan C, Tong S, Cai K, Liu Y, Huang W, Min Y, Epstein AJ. Controllable size-selective method to prepare graphene quantum dots from graphene oxide. Nanoscale Res. Lett. 2015; 10: 55. DOI:10.1186/s11671-015-0783-9.

76. Tian L, Liu F, Hu R, Gao H, Wei H, Zhang H, Sun H, YangB. Strongly green-photoluminescent graphene quantum dots for bioimaging applications. Chem. Commun. 2011; 47: 6858–6860. DOI:10.1039/C1CC11122A.

77. Zhu S, Zhang J, Tang S, Qiao C, Wang L, Wang H, Liu X, Li B, Li Y, Yu W, Wang A, Sun H, Yang B. Surface chemistry routes to modulate the photoluminescence of graphene quantum dots: From fluorescence mechanism to up-conversion bioimaging applications. Adv. Funct. Mater. 2012; 22: 4732–4740. DOI:10.1002/adfm.201201499.

78. Shen WJ, Zhu Y, Chen C, Yang X, Li C. Facile preparation and upconversion luminescence of graphene quantum dots. Chem. Comm. 2011; 47: 2580–2582. DOI:10.1039/C0CC04812G.

79. Zhuo S, Shao M, Lee S. Upconversion and downconversion fluorescent graphene quantum dots: ultrasonic preparation and photocatalysis. ACS Nano. 2012; 6: 1059–1064. DOI:10.1021/nn2040395.

80. Liu R, Wu D, Feng X, Muellen K. Bottom-up fabrication of photoluminescent graphene quantum dots with uniform morphology. J. Am. Chem. Soc. 2011; 133: 15221–15223. DOI:10.1021/ja204953k.

81. Loh KP, Bao Q, Eda G, Chhowalla M. Graphene oxide as a chemically tunable platform for optical applications. Nat. Chem. 2010; 2: 1015–1024. DOI:10.1038/nchem.907.

82. Pan D, Zhang J, Li Z, Wu M. Hydrothermal route for cutting graphene sheets into blue-luminescent graphene quantum dots. Adv. Mater. 2010; 22: 734–738. DOI:10.1002/adma.200902825.

83. Lu J, Yan M, Ge L, Ge S, Wang S, Yan J, Yu J. Electrochemiluminescence of blue-luminescent graphene quantum dots and its application in ultrasensitive aptasensor for adenosine triphosphate detection. Biosens. Bioelect. 2013; 47: 271–277. DOI:10.1016/j.bios.2013.03.039.

84. Li LL, Ji J, Fei R, Wang CZ, Lu Q, Zhang JR, Jiang LP, Zhu JJ. A Facile microwave avenue to electrochemiluminescent two-color graphene quantum dots. Adv. Funct. Mater. 2012; 22: 2971–2979. DOI:10.1002/adfm.201200166.

85. Hu W, Peng C, Luo W, Lv M, Li X, Li D, Huang Q, Fan C. Graphene-based antibacterial paper. ACS Nano. 2010; 4: 4317-4323. DOI:10.1021/nn101097v.

86. Ruiz OR, Fernando KAS, Wang B, Brown NA, Luo PG, McNamara ND, Vangsness M, Sun Y, Bunker CE. Graphene oxide: a nonspecific enhancer of cellular growth. ACS Nano. 2011; 5: 8100–8107. DOI:10.1021/nn202699t.

87. Zhang D, Liu X, Wang X. Green synthesis of graphene oxide sheets decorated by silver nanoprisms and their anti-bacterial properties. J. Inorg. Biochem. 2011; 105: 1181–1186. DOI:10.1016/j.jinorgbio.

88. Christensen IL, Sun YP, Juzenas P. Carbon dots as antioxidants and prooxidants. J. Biomed. Nanotechnol. 2011; 7: 667–676. DOI:10.1007/s11434-013-6058.

89. Yuan X, Liu Z, Guo Z, Ji Y, Jin M, Wang X. Cellular distribution and cytotoxicity of graphene quantum dots with different functional groups. Nanoscale Res. Lett. 2014; 9: 108. DOI:10.1186/1556-276X-9-108.

90. Jastrz□bska AM, Kurtycz P, Olszyna AR. Recent advances in graphene family materials toxicity investigations. J. Nanopart. Res. 2012; 14: 1320–1327. DOI:10.1007/s11051-012-1320-8.

91. Wang A, Pu K, Dong B, Liu Y, Zhang L, Zhang Z, Duan W, Zhu Y. Role of surface charge and oxidative stress in cytotoxicity and genotoxicity of graphene oxide towards human lung fibroblast cells. J. Appl. Toxicol. 2013; 33: 1156–1164. DOI:10.1002/jat.2877.

92. Wang K, Ruan J, Song H, Zhang J, Wo Y, Guo S, Cui D. Biocompatibility of graphene oxide. Nanoscale Res. Lett. 2011; 6: 1–8. DOI:10.1007/s11671-010-9751-6.

93. Chong Y, Ma Y, Shen H, Tu X, Zhou X, Xu J, Dai J, Fan F, Zhang Z. The in vitro and in vivo toxicity of graphene quantum dots. Biomaterials. 2014; 35: 5041–5048. DOI:10.1016/j.biomaterials.2014.03.021.

94. Pan D, Xi C, Li Z, Wang L, Chen Z, Lu B, Wu M. Electrophoretic fabrication of highly robust, efficient, and benign heterojunction photoelectrocatalysts based on graphene-quantum-dot sensitized TiO_2 nanotube arrays. J. Mater. Chem. A. 2013; 1: 3551–3555. DOI:10.1039/C3TA00059A.

95. Hamilton IP, Li B, Yan X, Li L. Alignment of colloidal graphene quantum dots on polar surfaces. Nano Lett. 2011; 11: 1524–1529. DOI:10.1021/nl200298c.

96. Li X, Zhu S, Xu B, Ma K, Zhang J, Yang B, Tian W. Self-assembled graphene quantum dots induced by cytochrome c: a novel biosensor for trypsin with remarkable fluorescence enhancement. Nanoscale. 2013; 5: 7776–7779.

97. Shi J, Chan C, Pang Y, Ye W, Tian F, Lyu J, Zhang Y, Yang Mo. A fluorescence resonance energy transfer (FRET) biosensor based on graphene quantum dots (GQDs) and gold nanoparticles (AuNPs) for the detection of mecA gene sequence of Staphylococcus aureus. Biosens Bioelectron. 2015; 67: 595–600. DOI:10.1016/j.bios.2014.09.059.

98. Gupta V, Chaudhary N, Srivastava R, Sharma GD, Bhardwaj R, Chand S. Luminescent graphene quantum dots for organic photovoltaic devices. J. Am. Chem. Soc. 2011; 133: 9960–9963. DOI:10.1021/ja2036749.

99. Luk CM, Tang LB, Zhang WF, Yu SF, Teng KS, Lau SP. An efficient and stable fluorescent graphene quantum dot–agar composite as a converting material in white light emitting diodes. J. Mater. Chem. 2012; 22: 22378–22381. DOI:10.1039/C2JM35305A.

100. Funkhouser J. Reinventing pharma: the theranostic revolution. Curr. Drug Discov. 2002; 2: 17–25.

101. Luk BT, Zhang L. Current advances in polymer-based nanotheranostics for cancer treatment and diagnosis. ACS Appl. Mater. Interface. 2014; 6: 21859–21873. DOI:10.1021/am5036225.

102. Lammers T, Kiessling F, Hennink WE, Storm G. Nanotheranostics and image-guided drug delivery: current concepts and future directions. Mol. Pharm. 2010; 7: 1899–1912. DOI:10.1021/mp100228v.

103. Wang Z, Xia J, Zhou C, Via B, Xia Y, Zhanga F, Lia Y, Xia L, Tang J. Synthesis of strongly green-photoluminescent graphene quantum dots for drug carrier. Colloid Surf B Biointerface. 2013; 112: 192–196. DOI:10.1016/j.colsurfb.2013.07.025.

104. Jing Y, Zhu Y, Yang X, Shen J, Li C. Ultrasound-triggered smart drug release from multifunctional core-shell capsules one-step fabricated by coaxial electrospray method. Langmuir. 2010; 27: 1175–1180. DOI:10.1021/la1042734.

105. Wang C, Wu C, Zhou X, Han T, Xin X, Wu J, Zhang J, Guo S. Enhancing cell nucleus accumulation and DNA cleavage activity of anti-cancer drug via graphene quantum dots. Sci. Rep. 2013; 3: 2852. DOI:10.1038/srep02852.

106. Zhou X, Zhang Y, Wang, Wu X, Yang Y, Zheng B, Wu H, Guo S, Zhang J. Photo-fenton reaction of graphene oxide: a new strategy to prepare graphene quantum dots for DNA cleavage. ACS Nano. 2012; 6: 6592–6599. DOI:10.1021/nn301629v.

107. Oza G, Ravichandran OM, Velumani S, Ramirez JT, Garcia-Sierra F, Asomoza R. Designing a drug-delivery vehicle with Au-Fe3 O4 -graphene quantum dots: a tri-pronged mechanism for bioimaging, synaptic delivery and apoptosis induction in cancer cells. J. Nanomed. Nanotechnol. 2014; 5: 5. DOI.org/10.4172/2157-7439.S1.018.

108. Wang X, Sun X, Lao J, He H, Cheng T, Wang M, WangS, Huang F. Multifunctional graphene quantum dots for simultaneous targeted cellular imaging and drug delivery. Colloid Surf. B Biointerface. 2014; 122: 638–644. DOI:10.1016/j.colsurfb.2014.07.043.

109. Nahain AA, Lee JE, In I, Lee H, Lee KD, Jeong JH, Park SY. Target delivery and cell imaging using hyaluronic acid-functionalized graphene quantum dots. Mol. Pharm. 2013; 10: 3736–3744. DOI:10.1021/mp4003283.

110. Vibin M, Vinayakan R, John A, Raji V, Rejiya CS, Vinesh NS, Abraham A. Cytotoxicity and fluorescence studies of silica-coated CdSe quantum dots for bioimaging applications. J. Nanopart. Res. 2011; 13: 2587–2596. DOI:10.1007/s11051-010-0151-8.

111. Liu LW, Hu S, Pan Y, Zhang J, Feng Y, Zhang X. Optimizing the synthesis of CdS/ZnS core/shell semiconductor nanocrystals for bioimaging applications. Beilstein J. Nanotechnol. 2014; 5: 919–926. DOI:10.3762/bjnano.

112. Zhu S, Zhang J, Qiao C, Tang S, Li Y, Yuan W, Li B, Tian L, Liu F, Hu R, Gao H, Wei H, Zhang H, Sun H, Yang B. Strongly green-photoluminescent graphene quantum dots for bioimaging applications. Chem. Commun. 2011; 47: 6858–6560. DOI:10.1039/C1CC11122A.

113. Dong Y, Chen C, Zheng X, Gao L, Cui Z, Yang H, Guo C, ChI Y, Li CM. One-step and high yield simultaneous preparation of single- and multi-layer graphene quantum dots from CX-72 carbon black. J. Mater. Chem. 2012; 22: 8764–8766. DOI:10.1039/C2JM30658A.

114. Sun H, Wu L, Gao N, Ren J, Qu X. Improvement of photoluminescence of graphene quantum dots with a biocompatible photochemical reduction pathway and its bioimaging application. ACS Appl. Mater. Interface. 2013; 5: 1174–1179. DOI:10.1021/am3030849.

115. Zhu S, Zhang J, Tang S, Qiao C, Wang L, Wang H, Liu X, Li B, Li Y, Yu W, Wang X, Sun H, Yang B. Surface chemistry routes to modulate the photoluminescence of graphene quantum dots: from fluorescence mechanism to up-conversion bioimaging applications. Adv. Funct. Mater. 2012; 22: 4732–4740. DOI:10.1002/adfm.201201499.

116. Zhou L, Geng J, Liu B. Graphene quantum dots from polycyclic aromatic hydrocarbon for bioimaging and sensing of Fe^{3+} and hydrogen peroxide. Part. Part. Syst. Charact. 2013; 30: 1086–1092. DOI:10.1002/ppsc.201300170.

117. Zheng XT, Than A, Ananthanaraya A, Kim DH, Chen P. Graphene quantum dots as universal fluorophores and their use in revealing regulated trafficking of insulin receptors in adipocytes. ACS Nano. 2013; 7: 6278–6286. DOI:10.1021/nn4023137.

118. Nurunnabi M, Khatun Z, Huh KM, Park SY, Lee DY, Cho KJ, Lee Y. In vivo biodistribution and toxicology of carboxylated graphene quantum dots. ACS Nano. 2013; 7: 6858–6867. DOI 10.1021/nn402043c.

119. Nurunnabi M, Khatun J, Reeck GR, Lee DY, Lee YK. Near infra-red photoluminescent graphene nanoparticles greatly expand their use in noninvasive biomedical imaging. Chem. Commun. 2013; 49: 5079–5081. DOI:10.1039/C3CC42334D.

120. Ge J, Lan M, Zhou B, Liu W, Guo L, Wang H, Jia Q, Niu G, Huang X, Zhou, Meng X, Wang P, Lee CS, Zhang W, Han X. A graphene quantum dot photodynamic therapy agent with high singlet oxygen generation. Nat. Commun. 2014; 5 : 4596. DOI:10.1038/ncomms5596.

121. Markovic ZM, Ristic BZ, Arsikin KM, Klisic DG, Harhaji-Trajkovic LM, Todorovic-Markovic BM, Kepic DP, Kravic-Stevovic TK, Jovanovic SP, Milenkovic MM, Milivojevic DD, Bumbasirevic VZ, Dramicanin MD, Trajkovic VS. Graphene quantum dots as autophagy-inducing photodynamic agents. Biomaterials. 2012; 33: 7084–7092. DOI:10.1016/j.biomaterials.2012.06.060.

8 Chapter

NONINVASIVE APPROACHES FOR SYSTEMIC ADMINISTRATION OF THERAPEUTIC PROTEINS: OPPORTUNITIES AND OBSTACLES

1. INTRODUCTION: AT A GLANCE

Proteins and peptides are polymers composed of amino acids that vary in chain length. These substances represent a diverse category of biological macromolecules defined by an amino acid sequence and a distinctive three-dimensional structure [1]. The three-dimensional structure is essential for biochemical reactions and is also beneficial for feedback mechanisms, transport, and solubility in physiological fluids. Proteins serve numerous vital physiological functions, attributable to their capacity for precise binding to corresponding biological entities. Enzymes, hormones, antibodies, globulins, hemoglobin, myoglobin, and other lipoproteins are proteins and peptides that facilitate catalysis and the movement of substances inside the body.

In 2010, around 20 antibody products and 150 protein-based medicines were approved for usage in the US market.

In that same year, it was reported that >100 approved protein drugs were in use, and ~800 were being developed to treat numerous conditions, including cancer, Alzheimer's, Huntington's, and Parkinson's diseases [4], with worldwide sales figures estimated to be around $70 billion [5]. It is clear that the protein drug class is continuing its strong economic growth, with the global market for bioengineered protein drugs being valued at $151.9 billion in 2013 and expectations that the market could reach $222.7 billion by 2019 (http://www.bccresearch.com/pressroom/bio/global-market-for-bioengineered-protein-drugs-to-reach-$222.7-billion-in-2019). The majority of protein and peptide-based products continue to be delivered by daily or weekly injections.

In addition to the administration route, shelf life presents a significant problem to the pharmaceutical sector, as there are no universal guidelines for stabilizing protein products and ensuring their safety and efficacy beyond the intended market duration [6].

Protein drugs are biopharmaceuticals that encompass several biological medications, including nucleic acid-based therapies, monoclonal antibodies, and recombinant proteins. Despite recent developments in genomes and proteomics yielding numerous protein therapeutic candidates, the majority do not demonstrate pharmacological efficacy in vivo [5]. Proteins are inherently susceptible to denaturation and structural alterations due to heat and agitation when in aqueous environments or organic solvents.

Significant barriers that lead to diminished biological action include low stability, immunogenicity, and toxicity [7]. The interplay of these elements yields a shortened plasma half-life, spanning from minutes to several hours, necessitating repeated dosages, hence increasing expenses and reducing patient compliance [7]. To address the challenges posed by protein drugs, the formulation of strategies aimed at enhancing drug bioavailability through alternative delivery routes (parenteral, oral, nasal, pulmonary, etc.) and novel formulation techniques (spray-freeze drying, supercritical fluid methods, fluidized-bed spray coating, lyophilization, jet milling, and spray drying) are prominent subjects in the field of protein delivery. The objective of these procedures is to enhance protein stability throughout production, storage, and in vivo post-drug administration, facilitating the drug's delivery to the specified biological target. Moreover, the formulation of novel techniques to address drug delivery obstacles, like Nanomedicine and PEGylation, may ultimately enhance the pharmacokinetics of certain protein drug candidates. This chapter will analyze the principal hurdles associated with noninvasive protein drug delivery and the techniques to mitigate these issues.

2. MAJOR PROTEIN DELIVERY CHALLENGES

The application of proteins as therapeutic agents is hindered by their chemical and physical instability, diminished oral bioavailability resulting from enzymatic breakdown in the gastrointestinal system, restricted permeability across the epithelial cells of the small intestine, and fast removal from the bloodstream. This section examines the significant challenges that must be surmounted to successfully deliver protein medicines.

2.1. Chemical and Physical Instabilities

Peptide and protein drugs although generally formulated in solid state still undergo multiple degradative reactions [6]. Chemical degradation involves covalent modification of the primary protein structure via bond cleavage or formation, while physical degradation refers to changes in higher-order structure by denaturation and noncovalent aggregation or precipitation. Physical and chemical types of reactions do not necessarily occur in isolation, but rather one may cause or facilitate the other [7]. Prominent mechanisms of chemical degradation in the solid state include deamidation, oxidation, and the Maillard reaction. Chemical instability due to deamidation has been observed for a number of important proteins, including human growth hormone, recombinant human interleukin-1 receptor antagonists, and recombinant bovine somatotropin [8]. A common deamidation reaction in peptides and proteins in drug formulations is the nonenzymatic intramolecular deamidation reaction of Asn residues. The use of peptide model VYPNGA has led to a better understanding of the Asn deamidation degradative process [8]. By examining the amino acid sequence of a particular peptide or protein with therapeutic potential, residues, which may be susceptible to deamidation, can be identified and formulation decisions made to minimize this type of degradation. The potential for degradative oxidation reactions can be found at various stages of production, packaging, and storage. For instance, peroxide contamination has been found in formulation excipients such as polytethylene glycols and surfactants leading to oxidation of these products [9]. The activation of molecular oxygen to more reactive species requires light or presence of a reducing agent and trace levels of transition metal ions, which can then convert molecular oxygen into more reactive oxidizing species such as superoxide radicals (O2-*), hydroxyl radical (*OH), or hydrogen peroxide (H_2O_2) [9]. Transition metal ions are often present in excipients, and processing in stainless steel equipment can lead to significant iron contamination [9] and thus represent potential sources, which may contribute to degradative oxidation of peptide or protein drugs. After formulation, the final packaging decision can also have an effect on drug stability. It was demonstrated that even low levels of oxygen (1%) in the vial headspace can result in complete oxidation of a particular product [9]. By understanding the potential sources of contaminants leading to oxidation at all stages of drug production, and the mechanisms by which oxidation reactions take place, formulation strategies can be adopted to minimize these events. For instance, in the process of developing the PTH (1-34) microprojection patch for transdermal delivery, oxidation was identified as the major chemical degradation pathway [10]. It was determined that the addition of 0.03% EDTA to the drug formulation could effectively delay oxidation, which was measured using RP-HPLC. Further, stability testing in the presence and absence of antioxidizing agents and other excipients was performed to assess the compatibility of the patch with packaging components. Indeed, several of the patch components were shown to contribute to volatile compounds, which were chemically and/or physically incompatible with the coated PTH (1-34) formulation. Overall, the selection of appropriate packaging materials and the use of a desiccant sachet in the package appeared to make it possible to achieve the target of 95% PTH (1-34) purity at the end of a two-year shelf life at ambient storage temperature [11]. In some protein formulations, reducing sugars (e.g., fructose, maltose, lactose, glucose, and xylose) react with basic protein residues such as lysine, arginine, asparagine, and glutamine [9]. In a stability study of recombinant human relaxin, it was discovered that the use of glucose as an excipient in a liophilized formulation resulted in covalent adducts of glucose with amino groups on the side chains of the protein formed by

Maillard reaction [12]. In this case, switching to the nonreducing sugar (trehalose), or a polyhydric alcohol (mannitol), resulted in greater relaxin stability.

Protein drugs very often undergo physical changes that may result in change of pharmacological effect and potency. Physical instability involves changes in the three-dimensional conformational integrity of the protein and does not necessarily involve covalent modification. These physical processes include denaturation, aggregation, precipitation, and adsorption to surfaces [8]. Protein drugs may undergo these changes during manufacturing, shipping, storage, and administration. Earlier concerns focused on denaturation (unfolding), oxidation, and deamination of protein drugs. Recently, aggregation has emerged as the main problem with protein therapeutics [11]. Protein aggregation is a multistage process that involves unfolding or misfolding of monomeric units of protein along with one or more assembly steps of monomeric protein to form soluble or insoluble oligomers or higher-molecular-weight aggregates [13]. Protein aggregates are often considered ordered if they occur as long, rigid fibrils or filaments. The most characterized aggregation state is the amyloid fibril, associated with neurodegenerative diseases such as Alzheimer's disease, Parkinson's disease, and Huntington's disease [14, 15]. Protein aggregation can be problematic during drug manufacturing, especially if it is insoluble and tends to precipitate, and typically reduces drug stability and shelf life [15]. In worst-case scenarios, aggregation might have an undesirable impact on drug potency, pharmacokinetics, and immunogenicity [16]. Protein aggregation can be triggered by many factors such as shear stress, high temperatures, changes in pH, and high protein concentration [16]. Unfortunately, it is very difficult to predict if the protein drug will undergo aggregation because of the complexity of the mechanism involved in the aggregate formation.

2.2. Biopharmaceutical Challenges

Therapeutic activity of proteins is highly dependent on their conformational structure, which is flexible and sensitive to external conditions such as pH, temperature, and impurities in the excipients [15]. The detection of structural changes in protein is complex in pharmaceutical formulations and is a major challenge for the development and quality of protein drugs [16]. In addition, protein-based drugs have been shown to be immunogenic and in some cases the production of neutralizing antibodies have led to the inhibition of the therapeutic effect [16].

Until recently, injections (i.e., intravenous, intramuscular, or subcutaneous routes) remained the most common means for administering protein drugs. However, the bioavailability of protein drugs using these routes are low due to their rapid elimination from the circulation through renal filtration, enzymatic degradation and uptake by the reticuloendothelial system [17]. Oral dosage is the most attractive route of administration because of the accompanying decreased medical costs and improved patient compliance. However, oral administration of protein drugs results in even lower bioavailability [2]. The main reasons for the low oral bioavailability are the instability of these drugs in the low pH environment of the gastrointestinal tract as well as inactivation and digestion by proteolytic enzymes in the intestinal lumen. In addition, protein drugs have high molecular masses and are hydrophilic, with logP values <0. This means that these drugs are more difficult to transport via the paracellular route across the epithelial cells lining of the small intestine [2, 16].

3. STRATEGIES FOR MITIGATING DELIVERY CHALLENGES

3.1. Processing Strategies for Improving Protein Stability

Despite their many attractive features, protein drugs come with many complications with regards to formulation. Unlike their small molecule drug counterparts, they are often complex molecules with secondary, tertiary, and quaternary structures and generally contain side chains with various chemical properties. The disruption of this complexity can lead to loss of function of the drug. Thus, the formulation of these biological compounds for therapeutic use must maintain their shape and form thus maintaining their activity [2].

3.1.1. Spray-freeze Drying

Spray-freeze drying was first introduced in 1994, and it was at first classified as a variant of dry milling [18]. Since pharmacological therapeutics have limited stability in liquid solutions, several methods, such as spray-freeze drying and spray drying, have been developed for proper removal of liquids such as water. Spray-freezing involves spraying a solution containing the macromolecule of interest into a vessel containing cryogenic liquid such as oxygen, nitrogen, or argon, which results in freezing of the droplets due to the low boiling point of the cryogenic fluids used [19]. Spray-freeze drying is the sublimation of solid water (ice) following freezing of the solution, and despite its disadvantages, it has become quite an established method in the pharmaceutical industry [20]. The reason for this is quite clear, spray-freeze drying significantly increases the shelf life of pharmaceuticals, it is an extremely sterile process (compared to spray drying), and the product can be readily reconstituted at the time of use. Spray-freeze drying entails three major steps: (1) freezing, the crystallization of water; (2) primary drying, the removal of ice via sublimation; and finally (3) secondary drying, the desorption of residual water from product [19].

Even though this method is used for obtaining protein particles, stresses involved with freezing and drying have been shown to cause irreversible damage to the protein due to degradation, aggregation, and eventual loss of biological activity [19]. Similar to spray drying the majority of the damage occurs in the atomization and freezing of the droplets in the cold vapor phase of the lyophilization process [21].

3.1.2. Supercritical Fluid Methods

Supercritical fluids (SCF) are used in variety of extraction and analytical methods. They can also be used for the production of pharmaceutical powders, mainly those intended for inhalation such as inhalation steroids dexamethasone, flunisolide, and triamcinolone acetonide [22]. SCFs have properties of gases and liquids at temperatures and pressures above their critical point. Advantages of SCFs include density values resulting in high dissolving power, lower viscosity levels compared to other liquids, and higher diffusivity allowing high mass transfer [19]. Among present SCFs, CO_2 is the most commonly used due to its low critical temperature (31.2°C) and pressure (7.4 MPa); other advantages include nonflammability, nontoxicity, and cost-effectiveness [19].

There are two major principles for particle precipitation when using SCFs. SCFs can be used as (1) solvents (rapid expansion of supercritical solution (RESS) and particles from gas saturated solutions (PGSS)) and (2) antisolvents (gas antisolvent (GAS), aerosol solvent extraction system (ASES), supercritical fluid antisolvent (SAS), precipitation with compressed antisolvent (PCA), and solution enhanced dispersion by supercritical fluids (SEDS)). Since the early 2000s, solutions consisting of proteins along with a cosolvent, such as ethanol, have been precipitated using CO_2 [23]. The integrity of such proteins depends on the operating conditions such as temperature, pressure, flow rates, and the concentration of the ingredients used, and by properly optimizing such conditions, the precipitation of proteins using the SCFs, such as CO_2, has become a promising method for particle precipitation [24].

3.1.3. Fluidized-bed Spray Coating

Fluidized-bed spray coating is a commonly used method in the pharmaceutical industry for coating of small particles [25]. Coating of particles has several advantages, such as providing acid resistance [24], modifying the release of the particles [26], protecting the therapeutic agent from light, and moisture and masking the taste of a substance [27]. In this process, particles to be coated come in contact with droplets of coating solution after being fluidized via air currents and are then dried using heated air; thus, after several loops through the spraying and drying zones, a uniform coat is achieved [28]. Further, the uniformity and success of the coating is dependent on the spreading of the droplet on the surface of the particle [29].

As a result of recent advancements in fluidized-bed spray coating systems, particles as small as 50 μm can be coated. For instance, fluidized-bed spray coating was applied to recombinant human deoxyribonuclease (rhDNase), and the coating was examined via scanning electron microscopy [30]. The coating demonstrated strong integrity when introduced to mechanical force; however, the process resulted in aggregation of the proteins,, which may be mainly due to the thermal stress involved with the process [29]. Aggregation was significantly reduced however, when rhDNase was formulated with calcium ions, thus suggesting in presence of proper stabilizers fluidized-bed spray coating is a feasible method for coating and preparing dried pharmaceutical proteins [31].

3.1.4. Lyophilization

Protein instability is one of the major reasons protein drugs are still administered via injections and not orally. Therefore, in order to overcome this hurdle, proteins must be made into solid forms to achieve an acceptable shelf life [32]. Lyophilization has become one of the most commonly used methods for generating solid protein drugs

[33]. Lyophilization consists of three steps beginning with (1) freezing, where the solution that is to be dried is frozen at a controlled rate thus removing water from the protein as ice crystals, at this point ~20% of water remains in a unfrozen phase known as maximal freeze concentrate [31]. Freezing is followed by (2) primary drying, where frozen water is removed via sublimation resulting in significant desorption of water (~10%). The remaining water is removed at higher temperatures in the final stage, (3) secondary drying, via desorption which lowers the fluid moisture content to few tenth of a percent [34].

A variety of stresses caused by lyophilization, such as low temperatures, formation of dendritic ice crystals, pH changes, phase separations, increase in ionic strengths, and removal of protein hydration shell, can result in reversible [33] and irreversible [34] structural changes in the protein [33]. Thus, for proteins that are sensitive to the listed stresses, specific cryo-/lyo-protectants can be used, such as commonly used sugars/polyols, nonaqueous solvents, polymers, protein itself, surfactants, and amino acids [33]. Further, extra effort is made to fully customize the lyophilization cycles in order to avoid lyophilization cycle-related stresses such as freezing rate and temperature, thermal treatment conditions, drying rate and temperature, and final moisture content [33].

3.1.5. Jet Milling

Jet milling is a method used for particle size reduction using interparticle collisions and abrasion to produce particles ranging between 1 and 20 μm [19]. Although Jet milling is a great method for particles size reduction (1–20 μm), it does come with some drawbacks, such as lack of control over size, shape, surface properties, and morphology. Furthermore, the high energy input can be detrimental to proteins as it can lead to protein degradation [19]. In a study where horseradish peroxidase was coprecipitated with carbomer and jet milled for two different time points, it was demonstrated that the longer the jet milling process, the more significant the reduction in protein activity [35]. In fact, grinding the power for 10 min in a mortar almost completely eliminated the activity of peroxidase [36] However, pulmonary activity of salmon calcitonin along with a variety of absorption enhancers (oleic acid, lecithin, citric acid, taurocholic acid, dimethyl-beta-cyclodextrin, and octyl-beta-D-glucoside) micronized after freeze drying with lactose showed significant blood levels of calcitonin in rats [37]. Further, it has been suggested that microparticle preparation is possible via melting, pregrinding, and a final jet milling step for particle size reduction [36]. Lastly, as peptides fed into the machine have to be coarse enough to allow for free flow and fine enough not to block the hopper and pipe work, they are at times required to be lyophilized which can result in protein degradation if no lyoprotectant is used [36].

3.1.6. Spray Drying

Spray drying is a method used for forming protein particles in lower molecular range [38]. The solution is automatically fed into droplets that rapidly dry due to high surface area and large amount of air–water interfacial area. During the drying process, which can range from 100 milliseconds to seconds, the critical increase in temperature is prevented by the evaporation of the solvent, which results in the temperature of particles remaining significantly lower than the temperature of the gas and drying powder is quickly removed from the drying zone to prevent overheating [25]. Spray drying allows control over a variety of particle design features, including particle size and distribution, surface energy and rugoses, particle density, surface area, porosity, and microviscosity [39]. Since the average radius of particles obtained ranges between 2 and 6 μm, spray drying is generally used for pulmonary particle delivery [40] such as the protein insulin [41].

Although the air-drying process of spray drying prevents thermal degradation of proteins, the atomization process may present a different obstacle. The high shear rate required for the atomization process can lead to degradation of macromolecules. For instance, a study demonstrated degradation of human growth hormone (hGH) during the air–liquid interface following atomization, while the tissue-type plasminogen activator (t-PA) remained intact [42]. There have been several proteins that have been successfully air-dried. Niven et al. spray dried formulations of recombinant human granulocyte colony-stimulating factor (rhG-CSF) [43], and Dalby et al. produced fine protein particles in a process where they combined nebulization, air drying, and electrostatic collection [44].

4. STRATEGIES FOR FORMULATING SOLUTIONS TO PROTEIN DELIVERY CHALLENGES

4.1. Nanotechnology Approaches

A promising method to improve the stability of therapeutic peptides and proteins is encapsulation within micro- or nanoparticles, designed to shield the medicine from adverse conditions in the body [45]. Biodrugs are often released from the particle at their target area through diffusion, swelling, erosion, or degradation [46]. Biological systems are typically safeguarded by nanometer-scale barriers that exhibit high specificity in the movement of biological substances. The permeation across these barriers and their access to particular biological compartments is determined by the chemical characteristics, size, and shape of biological molecules [47]. Nanotechnology, characterized by the development and use of materials, structures, devices, and systems through the modeling and fabrication of matter at the nanoscale (1–100 nm), can be employed to safeguard against the degradation of biological agents [48]. Due to their comparable scale to biological molecules, nanoparticles possess numerous medical applications and can be created for diverse activities. Due to their ability to traverse biological barriers, nanoparticles can facilitate the delivery of therapeutic compounds to targeted locations, enabling access to specific molecules and so influencing molecular interactions [48, 49].

A primary issue affecting the efficacy of certain existing medicines is their inadequate delivery to the necessary locations, often attributable to insufficient solubility.

Suboptimal efficacy may necessitate higher dosages, thereby leading to an escalation in side effects [50]. Nanocarriers can assist in surmounting certain challenges. The surface of nanocarriers typically comprises polymers or biodegradable compounds that are tailored to provide biocompatibility and specific targeting [48]. Nanocarriers provide several advantages over free drugs, including safeguarding the drug from premature interactions with undesirable biological entities and degradation, enhancing drug absorption in targeted tissues (such as cancers or tumors), improving pharmacokinetics, and facilitating intracellular penetration of the drug.

Nanoparticles and nanocarriers facilitate the targeted delivery of peptide medicines to specific locations, circumventing degradation in the gastrointestinal tract and first-pass metabolism through the hepatic pathway. Peptides have indeed been delivered via nanocarriers. Hyaluronic acid–Fe_2O_3 hybrid magnetic nanoparticles were designed to deliver peptides to HEK293 and A529 cells at a 100% level [52]. Further, functionalized gold nanoparticles consisting of a drug peptide ligand and a targeting peptide were shown to be both effective and enhance the activity and selectivity of such peptide multifunctionalized conjugates [53]. Furthermore, carrier molecules have been shown to increase membrane permeability of protein therapeutics such as insulin, interferon α2b, and human growth hormone through epithelial membrane of small intestine thus increasing the bioavailability of listed protein therapeutics [54].

4.2. PEGylation

Proposed in 1970s [55], PEGylation is the attachment of polyethylene glycol to drug molecules as a method of transforming proteins, peptides, small molecules, and oligonucleotides into more potent drugs [56]. PEGylated molecules tend to be more clinically useful compared to their unmodified counterparts as they tend to have higher stability and solubility, longer half-life in the systemic circulation, reduced renal clearance, reduced immunogenicity and antigenicity [57], and higher potency [58].

Protein drugs, such as enzymes, cytokines, and antibodies, have been shown to be significantly improved as a result of PEGylation [59]. Although it is common to see improvements in retention within circulation and reduction of immune response and degradation, the loss of biological activity due to PEGylation is quiet common [60]. The loss of biological activity is however compensated with improved pharmacokinetics as seen in α-interferon Pegasys® [61]. Currently, there are several PEGylated drugs available for public use, including PEG–adenosine deaminase (Adagen®) [62], PEG–asparaginase (Oncaspar®) [63], PEG–interferon α2b (PEG–Intron®) [64], PEG–interferon α2a (Pegasys®) [63], and PEG–growth hormone receptor antagonist (Pegvisomant, Somavert®) [65]. Before PEGylated drugs are made available to public use, they must undergo biological tests to ensure that the advantage of PEGylation does not result in increased toxicity [62].

5. STRATEGIES FOR REDUCING PROTEIN AGGREGATION AND IMPROVING BIOAVAILABILITY

A multitude of ways has been created and implemented to regulate or avert protein aggregation. Protein aggregation can be mitigated by using disulfide bonds, salt bridges, and metal ions to stabilize and solidify areas prone to local unfolding. Nonetheless, comprehensive clinical trials will be necessary to ascertain any deleterious effects linked to these alterations [15, 16]. A relatively straightforward method is to modify the protein's formulation. One method to diminish aggregation is to utilize protein solutions at reduced concentrations and proportionately greater volumes. Various excipients have been employed with differing degrees of efficacy to mitigate protein aggregation; yet, each possesses distinct limits [14]. Nonionic detergents may mitigate aggregation caused by shear and thermal effects. Cyclodextrins may also be employed to mitigate aggregation. Cyclodextrins inhibit the aggregation of insulin. One alternative method to diminish aggregation is the utilization of lyophilized dosage forms [16]. Lyophilization is often considered an excellent method for stabilizing proteins [13, 14]. Proteins can have reversible structural alterations in the lyophilized condition, rendering them more vulnerable to unfavorable side reactions. The aggregation of lyophilized insulin can be improved by the addition of trace moisture [15, 16].

Numerous techniques have been devised to enhance the oral bioavailability of protein therapeutics. One technique entails the alteration of the physiochemical characteristics of the gastrointestinal system. The incorporation of protease inhibitors as an adjuvant may diminish the rate of enzymatic degradation [18]. The enzymatic degradation of insulin in the intestine is mediated by the serine proteases trypsin, α-chymotrypsin, and thiol metalloproteinase insulin-degrading enzymes. Additives that inhibit these enzymes were shown to enhance the intestinal absorption of insulin by 10% in rats [66]. The manipulation of tight-junction permeability to enhance paracellular transport of protein molecules has been investigated. This method necessitates additional research prior to implementation [18].

A further technique to enhance the bioavailability of protein drugs entails the chemical alteration of the protein. This encompasses the production of a protein analog exhibiting enhanced enzymatic stability and/or membrane permeability. Insulin typically self-associates to form hexamers. The absorption of hexameric insulin is inferior to that of the monomeric insulin analog [2]. The alteration of amino acids involved in self-association leads to the creation of the monomeric insulin analog, insulin lispro (Humalog®, Eli Lilly), which is distinguished by its quick commencement of action after subcutaneous injection. Chemical modification may be employed to generate a prodrug, which can safeguard the medications from enzymatic breakdown [18]. The incorporation of new functional groups into protein medicines that are identifiable by transporters can enhance their absorption. Incorporating a dipeptide that is acknowledged by peptide-influx transporters in the gastrointestinal system with a protein medicine markedly enhances its oral bioavailability [16, 18]. Another method to enhance protein stability is through the acylation of the protein medication, which entails the attachment of fatty acids to the exposed residues on the protein's surface. This change enhances the protein's affinity for serum albumin, hence prolonging its half-life. The acetylation of insulin resulted in the creation of insulin detemir (Levemir®, Nova Nordisk), a long-acting insulin analog. The conjugation of protein pharmaceuticals with polymers is a method employed to enhance the bioavailability of protein medicines. At now, poly(ethylene glycol) (PEG) is the most extensively utilized polymer. Protein conjugation with PEG diminishes the plasma clearance rate by decreasing metabolic degradation [67].

Pharmaceutical technology can also enhance the bioavailability of protein medicines. The mucoadhesive delivery system was observed to extend the residence time of protein drugs at the absorption site and enhance the concentration gradient between the delivery system and intestinal membrane, ultimately leading to an increased rate of drug absorption [18]. Moreover, protein delivery systems constitute an efficient means of administering protein therapeutics. The most often utilized delivery techniques comprise liposomes, micelles, microspheres, and hydrogels. The utilization of carriers offers enhanced protection against enzymatic degradation and other detrimental influences, as the carrier wall entirely isolates drug molecules from their surroundings [18]. Liposomes exhibit optimal properties for protein encapsulation. Encapsulating insulin in liposomes enhances its oral absorption. A synthesis of these methodologies may be employed to construct an effective technique for the administration of protein therapeutics, such as a multifunctional smart polymer with pH-sensitive drug release, calcium ion deprivation capability, and mucoadhesive properties. This system's oral administration of insulin yields a bioavailability of 10% [18].

6. EXPLORATION OF VARIOUS DELIVERY ROUTES

The predominant approach for delivering protein and peptide molecules is parenteral administration of liquid formulations. This strategy has gained widespread acceptance among pharmaceutical corporations as the most expedient route to commercialization [69]. As the therapeutic range of protein and peptide molecules expands, the necessity for enhanced formulations concurrently rises. Although the design of innovative drug delivery methods is not critical for the success of these medicines, it is significant for enhancing efficacy, ensuring patient compliance, and minimizing errors in drug administration [20]. Consequently, in addition to parenteral administration of protein/peptide molecules, other delivery routes such as oral, nasal, pulmonary, ophthalmic, and transdermal methods have been investigated [69].

6.1. Parenteral Delivery

Parenterally administered protein drugs are most likely to be commercially successful since most animal studies and early clinical trials are performed via direct injections, thus making parenteral drug delivery one of the most popular forms of delivery assuming that injections meet the desired safety and efficacy targets [17]. Drugs delivered parenterally, whether intravenously or intramuscularly, gain full access to the systemic circulation due to rapid drug absorption. The short half-life of peptide drugs within the bloodstream results in repeat doses which correlate with oscillating drug concentrations within the blood [69].

There are numerous injection devices available for patients. For patients with daily injection requirements such as insulin, there are small diameter needle and syringes available. In fact, to improve patients' quality of life, the patient is now provided with prefilled syringes, syringe injectors, injectors, and pen devices, which may be preloaded with the drug of interest, and autoinjectors are regularly utilized as patients require more flexible and convenient injection devices moving away from the traditional syringe and vial [70]. For instance, insulin is now available in a variety of syringe injectable forms, infusion pumps, jet injectors (a needleless system that transports insulin transcutaneously), and reusable and prefilled pens [70]. All injectable devices must undergo stringent testing to ensure that the patient receives the proper dose of the drug in its expected form. For instance, in needleless systems that depend on high velocity liquid injection, which is dependent on compressed gas, the sheer stress can compromise the configuration of the protein [71, 72].

The rapid absorption of parenterally delivered drug is quickly followed by a rapid decline in the drug levels in the systemic circulation, which can be problematic in cases of chronic conditions where daily or weekly injections may be required for years. The requirement for numerous injections can result in decreased patient compliance, thus resulting in the development of prolonged release parenteral drug delivery systems [71]. These drug delivery systems include use of implants, which are biodegradable drug delivery systems mainly composed of either polylactic acid (PLA) or polyglycolic acid (PLGA) to control the release of the therapeutic drug [73]. However, since implants often require surgery and have been shown to have poor content uniformity in lower drug doses, in situ microparticle systems have been shown to be more advantageous due to the presence of an external oil phase [74]. ISM showed comparable drug release profile to drug release of microparticles prepared by solvent evaporation method, thus potentially becoming an alternative to more complicated microencapsulation methods [75].

6.2. Oral Delivery

One of the major challenges for protein drug delivery via the oral route is the susceptibility of the protein drug to proteolytic degradation in the gastrointestinal tract (GIT), which is at its highest in the stomach and the duodenum of the small intestines and is significantly lower in the mouth, pharynx, esophagus, ileum, and the colon. Another challenge is the bioavailability of the drug, which is dependent on two major factors, the molecular weight (MW) of the drug and its solubility. Bioavailability is essentially independent of MW for drugs less than 700 Da; however, with increasing MW passed this threshold, there is a decrease in the bioavailability of the drug. Drug compounds also need to meet a certain level of hydrophobicity criteria as they are required cross biological membranes. However, most biological drug compounds considered for therapeutic use are frequently greater than 700 Da and are hydrophilic [76]. Thus, degradation and poor absorption are the main bioavailability barriers.

There are however suggested methods for increasing the survival of the peptides as it moves through the GIT [75].

There are current methods for increasing the bioavailability of peptidic drugs such as (1) modifying the N- or C-terminus to increase half-life (encephalin, conversion of C-terminal methionine to methioniol group [77]); (2) altering the terminal amino acids from L-amino acid to a D-amino acid (arginine-vasopressin analog 1-deamino-8-D-arginine [77, 78]); (3) converting the linear peptide into a cyclic analog to avoid degradation by carboxy- and amino-peptidases (successfully performed in a model hexapeptide [77]); (4) use of peptidomimetics, which are molecules that mimic the action of peptides but are no longer peptidic in nature and prodrugs, which can be metabolized in the body releasing the therapeutic agent in return; and (5) coadministration of the peptide drug with digestive enzyme inhibitors [79]. The GIT presents both physical and chemical challenges for oral delivery of protein drugs; however, recent developments have made progress in facing each of those challenges and obstacles. Even though the development of new formulation methods, which have shown to improve bioavailability of protein drugs, are still costly, the progress in this field is still quite promising [20].

6.3. Nasal Delivery

The use of the nasal cavity as a site for systemic peptide drug delivery has several benefits, such as (1) rapid absorption rate, which in some cases have been shown to be as effective as intravenous injections and require lower doses; (2) high permeability due to the nasal epithelium (up to 1 kDa) [80]; along with (3) high total blood flow; (4) avoidance of first-pass metabolism; and (5) accessibility. The combination of such characteristics allows for a faster onset of pharmacological activity and lower side effects [81]. The olfactory nerves also allow for the direct transport of drug to the brain as the blood–brain barrier provides a challenging obstacle for numerous drugs such as antibiotics, antineoplastic agents, and other drugs that are active in the central nervous system [82].

There are a variety of formulation factors that can affect the absorption of drugs within the nasal cavity. Such factors include dose and volume, pH, osmolarity of the solution which the drug is dissolved in, viscosity, excipients used (such as absorption enhancers), dosage form (spray, powder, or drops), administration techniques (inhalation or mechanically assisted), and devices used to administer the drug [83]. Further, despite the fact that nasally administered drugs are able to avoid first-metabolism, bioavailability of peptide drugs is still limited due to the presence of broad range of metabolic enzymes that reside in the nasal mucosal cavity and the epithelial cell lining [84].

Currently, drugs ranging from small to large macromolecules such as protein drugs, hormones, and vaccines are delivered through the nasal cavity [85]. For instance, in the presence of absorption enhancers, which aid in modulating the nasal epithelium permeability, insulin can be effectively administered through the nasal cavity [84].

6.4. Pulmonary Delivery

The extensive surface area of the lung, combined with its highly vascularized thin epithelial lining, facilitates a noninvasive approach to drug delivery, enables direct access to systemic circulation, and permits the circumvention of first-pass metabolism and gastrointestinal degradation [86]. Successful pulmonary medication delivery necessitates that the drug reaches the alveoli or deep lung; hence, the particle size should be between 1–2 µm for optimal absorption [87]. Inhalation of medicines is an efficient method for administering treatments for respiratory conditions and various other ailments.

Although animal studies indicate that the bioavailability of medications administered through the pulmonary route varies between about 10% and 50% based on the protein type, comparable success rates have not been observed in human trials [70]. Pulmonary insulin administration exhibited approximately 50% bioavailability in animals [90], however in humans, it is only 10–15% [70]. The results indicate that the bioavailability of a medicine in animals does not reliably predict its bioavailability in humans. A further challenge related to pulmonary administration is the clinical toxicity of the lungs, especially with cytokines and growth hormones that may exert a localized impact on the tissue [70]. The drug's particle size significantly influences its absorption in the lungs [91]. As previously mentioned, smaller particle sizes reach the lungs more deeply, resulting in increased bioavailability. For larger molecular drugs, patients may require varying dosages and multiple administrations to attain the desired therapeutic effect. Additionally, a challenge in the pulmonary delivery of protein drugs is the swift elevation of drug levels in the serum, which may not pose an issue when the drug possesses a substantial margin of safety. While this may be advantageous in situations necessitating rapid medication delivery, such as insulin administration prior to a meal, it may lead to adverse side effects and necessitate more doses to attain and sustain the desired serum levels. Nevertheless, innovative technologies, including rapid-acting, slow-release analogs of medications like insulin, have been created to enhance pulmonary peptide drug delivery [91].

7. CONCISE SUMMARY

To design a medically effective analog of a protein medicine, several criteria must be considered. A rational initial step would be to get a comprehensive grasp of the physiological and chemical hurdles that the protein medicine will face. Despite being a relatively recent field, considerable advancements have been achieved in numerous domains. There has been a heightened comprehension of the benefits and drawbacks associated with various methods of protein medication administration. Consequently, through appropriate modifications—such as alterations to the N- or C- terminus, changes in terminal amino acids, transformation of protein conformation from linear to circular, utilization of peptidomimetics, enzyme inhibitors, or PEGylation—protein therapeutics can be designed based on the established understanding of proteolytic enzymes encountered in systemic circulation. Moreover, recent breakthroughs in nanomedicine have facilitated the encapsulation of proteins, leading to enhanced bioavailability. Advancements and innovations in formulation technology have enabled the feasible synthesis of protein pharmaceuticals, formerly deemed uneconomical for large-scale manufacturing. The effective formulation of the drug product relies on selecting the most stable protein drug form and comprehensively studying the compound's chemical and physical properties, as well as its stability under various situations in both short-term and long-term research.

AT A GLANCE

Proteins are recognized for their significant physiological importance, hence offering substantial potential for therapeutic applications. There is heightened interest in the delivery of protein and peptide therapeutics owing to recent enhancements in analytical techniques, progress in molecular biology and genetic engineering, and an improved comprehension of the regulatory functions of proteins and peptides. Significant obstacles must be addressed for the systemic administration of these biological substances. The primary obstacles that lead to diminished biological activity include low stability, immunogenicity, and toxicity. A multifaceted approach can be employed to address these difficulties and enhance the bioavailability of protein therapeutics. Alternative delivery pathways (e.g., nasal and pulmonary) and the advancement of novel techniques to surmount delivery obstacles (e.g., nanomedicine and PEGylation), coupled with the creation of innovative formulation strategies (e.g., spray-freeze drying, supercritical fluid methods, fluidized-bed spray coating, lyophilization, jet milling, and spray drying), have led to enhanced pharmacokinetics of protein therapeutics and, in certain instances, heightened patient adherence.

REFERENCES

1. M. S. Chang and B. Yeung, Eds., Formulation and Process Development Strategies for Manufacturing Biopharmaceuticals. Hoboken, NJ, USA: John Wiley & Sons, Inc., 2010.
2. J. Shaji and V. Patole, "Protein and peptide drug delivery: oral approaches," Indian J. Pharm. Sci., vol. 70, no. 3, pp. 269–77, Jan. 2008.
3. M. C. Manning, D. K. Chou, B. M. Murphy, R. W. Payne, and D. S. Katayama, "Stability of protein pharmaceuticals: an update," Pharm. Res., vol. 27, no. 4, pp. 544–75, Apr. 2010.
4. G. Hu, "Understanding the basics of peptide and protein production," Bioprocess Int., vol. 8, pp. 22–25, 2010.
5. L. R. Brown, "Commercial challenges of protein drug delivery," Expert Opin. Drug Deliv., vol. 2, no. 1, pp. 29–42, Jan. 2005.
6. M. A. H. Capelle, R. Gurny, and T. Arvinte, "High throughput screening of protein formulation stability: practical considerations," Eur. J. Pharm. Biopharm., vol. 65, no. 2, pp. 131–48, Feb. 2007.
7. M. Werle and A. Bernkop-Schnürch, "Strategies to improve plasma half life time of peptide and protein drugs," Amino Acids, vol. 30, no. 4, pp. 351–67, Jun. 2006.
8. M. C. Lai and E. M. Topp, "Solid-state chemical stability of proteins and peptides," J. Pharm. Sci., vol. 88, no. 5, pp. 489–500, May 1999.

9. L. (Lucy) Chang and M. J. Pikal, "Mechanisms of protein stabilization in the solid state," J. Pharm. Sci., vol. 98, no. 9, pp. 2886–2908, Sep. 2009.
10. A. A. Wakankar and R. T. Borchardt, "Formulation considerations for proteins susceptible to asparagine deamidation and aspartate isomerization," J. Pharm. Sci., vol. 95, no. 11, pp. 2321–36, Nov. 2006.
11. M. Ameri, P. E. Daddona, and Y.-F. Maa, "Demonstrated solid-state stability of parathyroid hormone PTH(1-34) coated on a novel transdermal microprojection delivery system," Pharm. Res., vol. 26, no. 11, pp. 2454–63, Nov. 2009.
12. R. Hamburger, E. Azaz, and M. Donbrow, "Autoxidation of polyoxyethylenic non-ionic surfactants and of polyethylene glycols," Pharm. Acta Helv., vol. 50, no. 1–2, pp. 10–7, Jan. 1975.
13. S. Li, T. W. Patapoff, D. Overcashier, C. Hsu, T. H. Nguyen, and R. T. Borchardt, "Effects of reducing sugars on the chemical stability of human relaxin in the lyophilized state," J. Pharm. Sci., vol. 85, no. 8, pp. 873–7, Aug. 1996.
14. E. T. Maggio, "Novel excipients prevent aggregation in manufacturing and formulation of protein and peptide therapeutics," Bioprocess Int., vol. 6, no. 10, pp. 58–65, Nov. 2008.
15. W. F. Weiss, T. M. Young, and C. J. Roberts, "Principles, approaches, and challenges for predicting protein aggregation rates and shelf life," J. Pharm. Sci., vol. 98, no. 4, pp. 1246–77, Apr. 2009.
16. S. Frokjaer and D. E. Otzen, "Protein drug stability: a formulation challenge," Nat. Rev. Drug Discov., vol. 4, no. 4, pp. 298–306, Apr. 2005.
17. V. P. Torchilin and A. N. Lukyanov, "Peptide and protein drug delivery to and into tumors: challenges and solutions," Drug Discov. Today, vol. 8, no. 6, pp. 259–66, Mar. 2003.
18. M. Morishita and N. A. Peppas, "Is the oral route possible for peptide and protein drug delivery?," Drug Discov. Today, vol. 11, no. 19–20, pp. 905–10, Oct. 2006.
19. S. A. Shoyele, "Engineering protein particles for pulmonary drug delivery," Methods Mol. Biol., vol. 437, pp. 149–60, Jan. 2008.
20. R. Singh, S. Singh, and J. W. Lillard, "Past, present, and future technologies for oral delivery of therapeutic proteins," J. Pharm. Sci., vol. 97, no. 7, pp. 2497–523, Jul. 2008.
21. S. D. Allison, T. W. Randolph, M. C. Manning, K. Middleton, A. Davis, and J. F. Carpenter, "Effects of drying methods and additives on structure and function of actin: mechanisms of dehydration-induced damage and its inhibition," Arch. Biochem. Biophys., vol. 358, no. 1, pp. 171–81, Oct. 1998.
22. M. C. Heller, J. F. Carpenter, and T. W. Randolph, "Protein formulation and lyophilization cycle design: prevention of damage due to freeze-concentration induced phase separation," Biotechnol. Bioeng., vol. 63, no. 2, pp. 166–74, Apr. 1999.
23. W. Han, W. Bao, Z. Wang, and S. Nattel, "Comparison of ion-channel subunit expression in canine cardiac Purkinje fibers and ventricular muscle," Circ. Res., vol. 91, no. 9, pp. 790–7, Nov. 2002.
24. H. Okamoto and K. Danjo, "Application of supercritical fluid to preparation of powders of high-molecular weight drugs for inhalation," Adv. Drug Deliv. Rev., vol. 60, no. 3, pp. 433–46, Feb. 2008.
25. K. Johnson, "Preparation of peptide and protein powders for inhalation," Adv. Drug Deliv. Rev., vol. 26, no. 1, pp. 3–15, Jun. 1997.

26. M. Luštrik, R. Dreu, R. Šibanc, and S. Srčič, "Comparative study of the uniformity of coating thickness of pellets coated with a conventional Wurster chamber and a swirl generator-equipped Wurster chamber," Pharm. Dev. Technol., vol. 17, no. 3, pp. 268–76, Jan..

27. M. A. Rahman and J. Ali, "Development and in vitro Evaluation of Enteric Coated Multiparticulate System for Resistant Tuberculosis," Indian J. Pharm. Sci., vol. 70, no. 4, pp. 477–81, Jan..

28. A. Dashevsky, K. Wagner, K. Kolter, and R. Bodmeier, "Physicochemical and release properties of pellets coated with Kollicoat SR 30 D, a new aqueous polyvinyl acetate dispersion for extended release," Int. J. Pharm., vol. 290, no. 1–2, pp. 15–23, Feb. 2005.

29. E. Teunou and D. Poncelet, "Batch and continuous fluid bed coating—review and state of the art," J. Food Eng., vol. 53, no. 4, pp. 325–340, Aug. 2002.

30. N. Pearnchob, J. Siepmann, and R. Bodmeier, "Pharmaceutical applications of shellac: moisture-protective and taste-masking coatings and extended-release matrix tablets," Drug Dev. Ind. Pharm., vol. 29, no. 8, pp. 925–38, Sep. 2003.

31. Y. F. Maa and C. C. Hsu, "Feasibility of protein spray coating using a fluid-bed Würster processor," Biotechnol. Bioeng., vol. 53, no. 6, pp. 560–6, Mar. 1997.

32. Y. Fukumori, H. Ichikawa, K. Jono, Y. Takeuchi, and T. Fukuda, "Computer simulation of agglomeration in the Wurster process," Chem. Pharm. Bull. (Tokyo)., vol. 40, no. 8, pp. 2159–63, Aug. 1992.

33. W. Wang, "Lyophilization and development of solid protein pharmaceuticals," Int. J. Pharm., vol. 203, no. 1–2, pp. 1–60, Aug. 2000.

34. S. Luthra, J.-P. Obert, D. S. Kalonia, and M. J. Pikal, "Investigation of drying stresses on proteins during lyophilization: differentiation between primary and secondary-drying stresses on lactate dehydrogenase using a humidity controlled mini freeze-dryer," J. Pharm. Sci., vol. 96, no. 1, pp. 61–70, Jan. 2007.

35. K. Griebenow and A. M. Klibanov, "Lyophilization-induced reversible changes in the secondary structure of proteins," Proc. Natl. Acad. Sci. U. S. A., vol. 92, no. 24, pp. 10969–76, Nov. 1995.

36. W. Schlocker, S. Gschliesser, and A. Bernkop-Schnürch, "Evaluation of the potential of air jet milling of solid protein-poly(acrylate) complexes for microparticle preparation," Eur. J. Pharm. Biopharm., vol. 62, no. 3, pp. 260–6, Apr. 2006.

37. D. B. Volkin and A. M. Klibanov, "Alterations in the structure of proteins that cause their irreversible inactivation," Dev. Biol. Stand., vol. 74, pp. 73–80; discussion 80–1, Jan. 1992.

38. S. Kobayashi, S. Kondo, and K. Juni, "Pulmonary delivery of salmon calcitonin dry powders containing absorption enhancers in rats," Pharm. Res., vol. 13, no. 1, pp. 80–3, Jan. 1996.

39. G. Nykamp, U. Carstensen, and B. W. Müller, "Jet milling--a new technique for microparticle preparation," Int. J. Pharm., vol. 242, no. 1–2, pp. 79–86, Aug. 2002.

40. R. Vehring, "Pharmaceutical particle engineering via spray drying," Pharm. Res., vol. 25, no. 5, pp. 999–1022, May 2008.

41. J. G. Weers, T. E. Tarara, and A. R. Clark, "Design of fine particles for pulmonary drug delivery," Expert Opin. Drug Deliv., vol. 4, no. 3, pp. 297–313, May 2007.

42. M. Sakagami and P. R. Byron, "Respirable microspheres for inhalation: the potential of manipulating pulmonary disposition for improved therapeutic efficacy," Clin. Pharmacokinet., vol. 44, no. 3, pp. 263–77, Jan. 2005.

43. A. X. C. N. Valente, R. Langer, H. A. Stone, and D. A. Edwards, "Recent advances in the development of an inhaled insulin product," BioDrugs, vol. 17, no. 1, pp. 9–17, Jan. 2003.
44. M. Mumenthaler, C. C. Hsu, and R. Pearlman, "Feasibility study on spray-drying protein pharmaceuticals: recombinant human growth hormone and tissue-type plasminogen activator," Pharm. Res., vol. 11, no. 1, pp. 12–20, Jan. 1994.
45. R. W. Niven, F. D. Lott, A. Y. Ip, and J. M. Cribbs, "Pulmonary delivery of powders and solutions containing recombinant human granulocyte colony-stimulating factor (rhG-CSF) to the rabbit," Pharm. Res., vol. 11, no. 8, pp. 1101–9, Aug. 1994.
46. R. Dalby, V. Naini, and P. Byron, "Droplets drying and electrostatic collection a novel alternative to conventional comminution techniques," J. Biopharm. Sci., 1992.
47. U. Bilati, E. Allémann, and E. Doelker, "Strategic approaches for overcoming peptide and protein instability within biodegradable nano- and microparticles," Eur. J. Pharm. Biopharm., vol. 59, no. 3, pp. 375–88, Apr. 2005.
48. B. Y. S. Kim, J. T. Rutka, and W. C. W. Chan, "Nanomedicine," N. Engl. J. Med., vol. 363, no. 25, pp. 2434–43, Dec. 2010.
49. K. Uekama, F. Hirayama, and T. Irie, "Cyclodextrin Drug Carrier Systems," Chem. Rev., vol. 98, no. 5, pp. 2045–2076, Jul. 1998.
50. D. Peer, J. M. Karp, S. Hong, O. C. Farokhzad, R. Margalit, and R. Langer, "Nanocarriers as an emerging platform for cancer therapy," Nat. Nanotechnol., vol. 2, no. 12, pp. 751–60, Dec. 2007.
51. Y. Xia, Y. Xiong, B. Lim, and S. E. Skrabalak, "Shape-controlled synthesis of metal nanocrystals: simple chemistry meets complex physics?," Angew. Chem. Int. Ed. Engl., vol. 48, no. 1, pp. 60–103, Jan. 2009.
52. M. Cavadas, Á. González-Fernández, and R. Franco, "Pathogen-mimetic stealth nanocarriers for drug delivery: a future possibility," Nanomedicine Nanotechnology, Biol. Med., vol. 7, no. 6, pp. 730–743, Dec. 2011.
53. K. K. Jain, "Nanomedicine: application of nanobiotechnology in medical practice," Med. Princ. Pract., vol. 17, no. 2, pp. 89–101, Jan. 2008.
54. A. Kumar, B. Sahoo, A. Montpetit, S. Behera, R. F. Lockey, and S. S. Mohapatra, "Development of hyaluronic acid–Fe_2O_3 hybrid magnetic nanoparticles for targeted delivery of peptides," Nanomedicine, vol. 3, no. 2, pp. 132–7, Jun. 2007.
55. L. Hosta-Rigau, I. Olmedo, J. Arbiol, L. J. Cruz, M. J. Kogan, and F. Albericio, "Multifunctionalized gold nanoparticles with peptides targeted to gastrin-releasing peptide receptor of a tumor cell line," Bioconjug. Chem., vol. 21, no. 6, pp. 1070–1078, Jun. 2010.
56. B. R. Stoll, H. R. Leipold, S. Milstein, and D. A. Edwards, "A mechanistic analysis of carrier-mediated oral delivery of protein therapeutics," J. Control. Release, vol. 64, no. 1–3, pp. 217–28, Feb. 2000.
57. F. Davis, A. Abuchowski, and T. Van Es. Enzyme-polyethylene glycol adducts: modified enzymes with unique properties. In: Broun G, Manecke G, Wingard L Jr, editors. Enzyme Engineering. New York: Springer, 1978. pp. 169–7.
58. M. Hamidi, A. Azadi, and P. Rafiei, "Pharmacokinetic consequences of pegylation," Drug Deliv., vol. 13, no. 6, pp. 399–409, Jan. 2006.
59. A. Abuchowski, J. R. McCoy, N. C. Palczuk, T. van Es, and F. F. Davis, "Effect of covalent attachment of polyethylene glycol on immunogenicity and circulating life of bovine liver catalase," J. Biol. Chem., vol. 252, no. 11, pp. 3582–6, Jun. 1977.

60. P. Bailon and C.-Y. Won, "PEG-modified biopharmaceuticals," Expert Opin. Drug Deliv., vol. 6, no. 1, pp. 1–16, Jan. 2009.

61. G. Pasut, A Guiotto, and FM Veronese,"Protein, peptide and non-peptide drug PEGylation for therapeutic application," Expert Opin. Drug Deliv., vol. 14, no. 6, pp. 859-894, Jun. 2004.

62. F. M. Veronese and G. Pasut, "PEGylation, successful approach to drug delivery," Drug Discov. Today, vol. 10, no. 21, pp. 1451–8, Nov. 2005.

63. P. Bailon, A. Palleroni, C. A. Schaffer, C. L. Spence, W. J. Fung, J. E. Porter, G. K. Ehrlich, W. Pan, Z. X. Xu, M. W. Modi, A. Farid, W. Berthold, and M. Graves, "Rational design of a potent, long-lasting form of interferon: a 40 kDa branched polyethylene glycol-conjugated interferon alpha-2a for the treatment of hepatitis C," Bioconjug. Chem., vol. 12, no. 2, pp. 195–202, Jan. 2001.

64. Y.-S. Wang, S. Youngster, M. Grace, J. Bausch, R. Bordens, and D. F. Wyss, "Structural and biological characterization of pegylated recombinant interferon alpha-2b and its therapeutic implications," Adv. Drug Deliv. Rev., vol. 54, no. 4, pp. 547–70, Jun. 2002.

65. Y. Levy, M. S. Hershfield, C. Fernandez-Mejia, S. H. Polmar, D. Scudiery, M. Berger, and R. U. Sorensen, "Adenosine deaminase deficiency with late onset of recurrent infections: response to treatment with polyethylene glycol-modified adenosine deaminase," J. Pediatr., vol. 113, no. 2, pp. 312–7, Aug. 1988.

66. M. L. Graham, "Pegaspargase: a review of clinical studies," Adv. Drug Deliv. Rev., vol. 55, no. 10, pp. 1293–302, Sep. 2003.

67. P. J. Trainer, W. M. Drake, L. Katznelson, P. U. Freda, V. Herman-Bonert, A. J. van der Lely, E. V Dimaraki, P. M. Stewart, K. E. Friend, M. L. Vance, G. M. Besser, J. A. Scarlett, M. O. Thorner, C. Parkinson, A. Klibanski, J. S. Powell, A. L. Barkan, M. C. Sheppard, M. Malsonado, D. R. Rose, D. R. Clemmons, G. Johannsson, B. A. Bengtsson, S. Stavrou, D. L. Kleinberg, D. M. Cook, L. S. Phillips, M. Bidlingmaier, C. J. Strasburger, S. Hackett, K. Zib, W. F. Bennett, and R. J. Davis, "Treatment of acromegaly with the growth hormone-receptor antagonist pegvisomant," N. Engl. J. Med., vol. 342, no. 16, pp. 1171–7, Apr. 2000.

68. R. B. Shah, F. Ahsan, and M. A. Khan, "Oral delivery of proteins: progress and prognostication," Crit. Rev. Ther. Drug Carrier Syst., vol. 19, no. 2, pp. 135–69, Jan. 2002.

69. S. Stolnik and K. Shakesheff, "Formulations for delivery of therapeutic proteins," Biotechnol. Lett., vol. 31, no. 1, pp. 1–11, Jan. 2009.

70. J. L. Cleland, A. Daugherty, and R. Mrsny, "Emerging protein delivery methods," Curr. Opin. Biotechnol., vol. 12, no. 2, pp. 212–9, Apr. 2001.

71. H. Bari, "A prolonged release parenteral drug delivery system-an overview," Int J Pharm Sci Rev Res, vol. 3, no. 1, pp.1-11, Jul. 2010.

72. K. E. Robertson, N. B. Glazer, and R. K. Campbell, "The latest developments in insulin injection devices," Diabetes Educ., vol. 26, no. 1, pp. 135–8, 141–6, 149–52, Jan. 2000.

73. J. Oberyé, B. Mannaerts, J. Huisman, and C. Timmer, "Local tolerance, pharmacokinetics, and dynamics of ganirelix (Orgalutran) administration by Medi-Jector compared to conventional needle injections," Hum. Reprod., vol. 15, no. 2, pp. 245–9, Feb. 2000.

74. P. Mikkelsen Lynch, J. Butler, D. Huerta, I. Tsals, D. Davidson, and S. Hamm, "A pharmacokinetic and tolerability evaluation of two continuous subcutaneous infusion systems compared to an oral controlled-release morphine," J. Pain Symptom Manage., vol. 19, no. 5, pp. 348–56, May 2000.

75. H. Kranz and R. Bodmeier, "A novel in situ forming drug delivery system for controlled parenteral drug delivery," Int. J. Pharm., 2007.
76. L. Brannon-Peppas, "Recent advances on the use of biodegradable microparticles and nanoparticles in controlled drug delivery," Int. J. Pharm., 1995.
77. G. Pauletti, S. Gangwar, and G. Knipp, "Structural requirements for intestinal absorption of peptide drugs," J. Control...., 1996.
78. S. J. Shire, "Formulation and manufacturability of biologics," Curr. Opin. Biotechnol., vol. 20, no. 6, pp. 708–14, Dec. 2009.
79. A. Fjellestad-Paulsen, C. Söderberg-Ahlm, and S. Lundin, "Metabolism of vasopressin, oxytocin, and their analogues in the human gastrointestinal tract," Peptides, vol. 16, no. 6, pp. 1141–7, Jan. 1995.
80. S. Lundin, N. Pantzar, A. Broeders, M. Ohlin, and B. R. Weström, "Differences in transport rate of oxytocin and vasopressin analogues across proximal and distal isolated segments of the small intestine of the rat," Pharm. Res., vol. 8, no. 10, pp. 1274–80, Oct. 1991.
81. A. Bernkop-Schnürch, "The use of inhibitory agents to overcome the enzymatic barrier to perorally administered therapeutic peptides and proteins," J. Control. Release, vol. 52, no. 1–2, pp. 1–16, Mar. 1998.
82. M. I. Ugwoke, N. Verbeke, and R. Kinget, "The biopharmaceutical aspects of nasal mucoadhesive drug delivery," J. Pharm. Pharmacol., vol. 53, no. 1, pp. 3–21, Jan. 2001.
83. S. Türker, E. Onur, and Y. Ozer, "Nasal route and drug delivery systems," Pharm. World Sci., vol. 26, no. 3, pp. 137–42, Jun. 2004.
84. Z. Antosova, M. Mackova, V. Kral, and T. Macek, "Therapeutic application of peptides and proteins: parenteral forever?," Trends Biotechnol., vol. 27, no. 11, pp. 628–35, Nov. 2009.
85. M. I. Ugwoke, R. U. Agu, N. Verbeke, and R. Kinget, "Nasal mucoadhesive drug delivery: background, applications, trends and future perspectives," Adv. Drug Deliv. Rev., vol. 57, no. 11, pp. 1640–65, Nov. 2005.
86. C. Ehrhardt and K.-J. Kim, Eds., Drug Absorption Studies, vol. VII. Boston, MA: Springer US, 2008.
87. M. Hinchcliffe and L. Illum, "Intranasal insulin delivery and therapy," Adv. Drug Deliv. Rev., vol. 35, no. 2–3, pp. 199–234, Feb. 1999.
88. A. Martini, L. Muggetti, and M. P. Warchol, "Nasal and pulmonary drug delivery systems," Expert Opin. Ther. Pat., vol. 10, no. 3, pp. 315–323, Mar. 2000.
89. J. Patton, J. Bukar, and S. Nagarajan, "Inhaled insulin," Adv. Drug Deliv. Rev., vol. 35, no. 2–3, pp. 235–247, Feb. 1999.
90. P. Dames, B. Gleich, A. Flemmer, K. Hajek, N. Seidl, F. Wiekhorst, D. Eberbeck, I. Bittmann, C. Bergemann, T. Weyh, L. Trahms, J. Rosenecker, and C. Rudolph, "Targeted delivery of magnetic aerosol droplets to the lung," Nat. Nanotechnol., vol. 2, no. 8, pp. 495–9, Aug. 2007.
91. C. Friebel and H. Steckel, "Single-use disposable dry powder inhalers for pulmonary drug delivery," Expert Opin. Drug Deliv., vol. 7, no. 12, pp. 1359–72, Dec. 2010.

9 Chapter

MAGNETIC MANIPULATION OF CELL MOCKUPS AND MCF-7 HUMAN BREAST CANCER CELLS, BOTH CONTACT AND NON-CONTACT

1. INTRODUCTION: AN INTRODUCTION

Proteins and peptides are polymers composed of amino acids that vary in chain length. These substances constitute a diverse category of biological macromolecules defined by an amino acid sequence that exhibits a distinctive three-dimensional shape [1]. The three-dimensional structure is essential for biochemical reactions and is also beneficial for feedback mechanisms, transport, and solubility in physiological fluids. Proteins serve numerous critical physiological functions, attributable to their capacity for precise binding to corresponding biological entities.

Enzymes, hormones, antibodies, globulins, hemoglobin, myoglobin, and other lipoproteins are proteins and peptides that facilitate catalysis and transport of substances inside the body. In 2010, it was reported that around 20 antibody products and 150 protein-based products were approved for use in the US market alone [3]. In that same year, it was reported that >100 approved protein drugs were in use, and ~800 were being developed to treat numerous conditions, including cancer, Alzheimer's, Huntington's, and Parkinson's diseases [4], with worldwide sales figures estimated to be around $70 billion [5]. It is clear that the protein drug class is continuing its strong economic growth, with the global market for bioengineered protein drugs being valued at $151.9 billion in 2013 and expectations that the market could reach $222.7 billion by 2019 (http://www.bccresearch.com/pressroom/bio/global-market-for- bioengineered-protein-drugs-to-reach-$222.7-billion-in-2019). Most of these protein and peptide-based products are still administered by daily or weekly injections [5]. Besides administration route, shelf life imposes a major challenge to the pharmaceutical industry as there are no general rules on how to stabilize protein products and guarantee its safety and activity during the time it is supposed to be marketable [6].

Protein drugs are biopharmaceuticals, which include other biological drugs such as nucleic acid-based drugs, monoclonal antibodies, and recombinant proteins. Although recent advancements in genomics and proteomics have created a large number of protein drug candidates, most fail to be biologically promising *in vivo* [5]. Proteins by nature are prone to denaturation and structural modifications by heat and agitation once in aqueous environments or organic solvent [5].

Major obstacles that contribute to low biological activity are low stability, immunogenicity, and toxicity [7]. A combination of these factors results in low plasma half-life, ranging from minutes to several hours, which necessitates repeated administrations, which in turn leads to higher costs and lower patient compliance [7]. To overcome the challenges that protein drugs present, the development of strategies that focus on improving the bioavailability of the drugs by alternative routes of delivery (parenteral, oral, nasal, pulmonary, etc.) and innovative formulation strategies (spray-freeze drying, supercritical fluid methods, fluidized-bed spray coating, lyophilization, jet milling and spray drying) are trending topics in the protein delivery sphere. The aim of these strategies is to improve protein stability during manufacturing, storage and *in vivo*, following drug administration, allowing the drug to reach the intended biological target. Furthermore, the development of new strategies for overcoming drug delivery challenges such as the use of Nanomedicine and PEGylation can eventually lead to improved pharmacokinetics of some protein drug candidates. In this chapter, we will examine the major challenges facing noninvasive protein drug delivery and strategies for overcoming these problems.

2. MAJOR PROTEIN DELIVERY CHALLENGES

The use of proteins as therapeutic agents is hampered by their chemical/physical instabilities, low oral bioavailability due to enzymatic degradation in the gastrointestinal tract, low permeability across the epithelial cells lining of the small intestine, and rapid elimination from the circulation. In this section, major obstacles to be overcome in order to successfully deliver protein drugs are examined.

2.1 Chemical and Physical Instabilities

Peptide and protein drugs although generally formulated in solid state still undergo multiple degradative reactions [6]. Chemical degradation involves covalent modification of the primary protein structure via bond cleavage or formation, while physical degradation refers to changes in higher-order structure by denaturation and noncovalent aggregation or precipitation. Physical and chemical types of reactions do not necessarily occur in isolation, but rather one may cause or facilitate the other [7]. Prominent mechanisms of chemical degradation in the solid state include deamidation, oxidation, and the Maillard reaction. Chemical instability due to deamidation has been observed for a number of important proteins, including human growth hormone, recombinant human interleukin-1 receptor antagonists, and recombinant bovine somatotropin [8]. A common deamidation reaction in peptides and proteins in drug formulations is the nonenzymatic intramolecular deamidation reaction of Asn residues. The use of peptide model VYPNGA has led to a better understanding of the Asn deamidation degradative process [8]. By examining the amino acid sequence of a particular peptide or protein with therapeutic potential, residues, which may be susceptible to deamidation, can be identified and formulation decisions made to minimize this type of degradation. The potential for degradative oxidation reactions can be found at various stages of production, packaging, and storage. For instance, peroxide contamination has been found in formulation excipients such as polytethylene glycols and surfactants leading to oxidation of these products [9]. The activation of molecular oxygen to more reactive species requires light or presence of a reducing agent and trace levels of transition metal ions, which can then convert molecular oxygen into more reactive oxidizing species such as superoxide radicals (O2-*), hydroxyl radical (*OH), or hydrogen peroxide (H_2O_2) [9]. Transition metal ions are often present in excipients, and processing in stainless steel equipment can lead to significant iron contamination [9] and thus represent potential sources, which may contribute to degradative oxidation of peptide or protein drugs. After formulation, the final packaging decision can also have an effect on drug stability. It was demonstrated that even low levels of oxygen (1%) in the vial headspace can result in complete oxidation of a particular product [9]. By understanding the potential sources of contaminants leading to oxidation at all stages of drug production, and the mechanisms by which oxidation reactions take place, formulation strategies can be adopted to minimize these events. For instance, in the process of developing the PTH (1-34) microprojection patch for transdermal delivery, oxidation was identified as the major chemical degradation pathway [10]. It was determined that the addition of 0.03% EDTA to the drug formulation could effectively delay oxidation, which was measured using RP-HPLC. Further, stability testing in the presence and absence of antioxidizing agents and other excipients was performed to assess the compatibility of the patch with packaging components. Indeed, several of the patch components were shown to contribute to volatile compounds, which were chemically and/or physically incompatible with the coated PTH (1-34) formulation. Overall, the selection of appropriate packaging materials and the use of a desiccant sachet in the package appeared to make it possible to achieve the target of 95% PTH (1-34) purity at the end of a two-year shelf life at ambient storage temperature [11]. In some protein formulations, reducing sugars (e.g., fructose, maltose, lactose, glucose, and xylose) react with basic protein residues such as lysine, arginine, asparagine, and glutamine [9]. In a stability study of recombinant human relaxin, it was discovered that the use of glucose as an excipient in a liophilized formulation resulted in covalent adducts of glucose with amino groups on the side chains of the protein formed by Maillard reaction [12]. In this case, switching to the nonreducing sugar (trehalose), or a polyhydric alcohol (mannitol), resulted in greater relaxin stability.

Protein drugs very often undergo physical changes that may result in change of pharmacological effect and potency. Physical instability involves changes in the three-dimensional conformational integrity of the protein and does not necessarily involve covalent modification. These physical processes include denaturation, aggregation, precipitation, and adsorption to surfaces [8]. Protein drugs may undergo these changes during manufacturing, shipping, storage, and administration. Earlier concerns focused on denaturation (unfolding), oxidation, and deamination of protein drugs. Recently, aggregation has emerged as the main problem with protein therapeutics [11]. Protein aggregation is a multistage process that involves unfolding or misfolding of monomeric units of protein along with one or more assembly steps of monomeric protein to form soluble or insoluble oligomers or higher-molecular-weight aggregates [13]. Protein aggregates are often considered ordered if they occur as long, rigid fibrils or filaments. The most characterized aggregation state is the amyloid fibril, associated with neurodegenerative diseases such as Alzheimer's disease, Parkinson's disease, and Huntington's disease [14, 15]. Protein aggregation can be problematic during drug manufacturing, especially if it is insoluble and tends to precipitate, and typically reduces drug stability and shelf life [15]. In worst-case scenarios, aggregation might have an undesirable impact on drug potency, pharmacokinetics, and immunogenicity [16]. Protein aggregation can be triggered by many factors such as shear stress, high temperatures, changes in pH, and high protein concentration [16]. Unfortunately, it is very difficult to predict if the protein drug will undergo aggregation because of the complexity of the mechanism involved in the aggregate formation.

2.2 Biopharmaceutical Challenges

Therapeutic activity of proteins is highly dependent on their conformational structure, which is flexible and sensitive to external conditions such as pH, temperature, and impurities in the excipients [15]. The detection of structural changes in protein is complex in pharmaceutical formulations and is a major challenge for the development and quality of protein drugs [16]. In addition, protein-based drugs have been shown to be immunogenic and in some cases the production of neutralizing antibodies have led to the inhibition of the therapeutic effect [16].

Until recently, injections (i.e., intravenous, intramuscular, or subcutaneous routes) remained the most common means for administering protein drugs. However, the bioavailability of protein drugs using these routes are low due to their rapid elimination from the circulation through renal filtration, enzymatic degradation and uptake by the reticuloendothelial system [17]. Oral dosage is the most attractive route of administration because of the accompanying decreased medical costs and improved patient compliance. However, oral administration of protein drugs results in even lower bioavailability [2]. The main reasons for the low oral bioavailability are the instability of these drugs in the low pH environment of the gastrointestinal tract as well as inactivation and digestion by proteolytic enzymes in the intestinal lumen. In addition, protein drugs have high molecular masses and are hydrophilic, with logP values <0. This means that these drugs are more difficult to transport via the paracellular route across the epithelial cells lining of the small intestine [2, 16].

3. STRATEGIES FOR MITIGATING DELIVERY CHALLENGES

3.1 Processing Strategies for Improving Protein Stability

Despite their many attractive features, protein drugs come with many complications with regards to formulation. Unlike their small molecule drug counterparts, they are often complex molecules with secondary, tertiary, and quaternary structures and generally contain side chains with various chemical properties. The disruption of this complexity can lead to loss of function of the drug. Thus, the formulation of these biological compounds for therapeutic use must maintain their shape and form thus maintaining their activity [2].

3.1.1 Spray-freeze Drying

Spray-freeze drying was first introduced in 1994, and it was at first classified as a variant of dry milling [18]. Since pharmacological therapeutics have limited stability in liquid solutions, several methods, such as spray-freeze drying and spray drying, have been developed for proper removal of liquids such as water. Spray-freezing involves spraying a solution containing the macromolecule of interest into a vessel containing cryogenic liquid such as oxygen, nitrogen, or argon, which results in freezing of the droplets due to the low boiling point of the cryogenic fluids used [19]. Spray-freeze drying is the sublimation of solid water (ice) following freezing of the solution, and despite its disadvantages, it has become quite an established method in the pharmaceutical industry [20]. The reason for this is quite clear, spray-freeze drying significantly increases the shelf life of pharmaceuticals, it is an extremely sterile process (compared to spray drying), and the product can be readily reconstituted at the time of use. Spray-freeze drying entails three major steps: (1) freezing, the crystallization of water; (2) primary drying, the removal of ice via sublimation; and finally (3) secondary drying, the desorption of residual water from product [19].

Even though this method is used for obtaining protein particles, stresses involved with freezing and drying have been shown to cause irreversible damage to the protein due to degradation, aggregation, and eventual loss of biological activity [19]. Similar to spray drying the majority of the damage occurs in the atomization and freezing of the droplets in the cold vapor phase of the lyophilization process [21].

3.1.2 Supercritical Fluid Methods

Supercritical fluids (SCF) are used in variety of extraction and analytical methods. They can also be used for the production of pharmaceutical powders, mainly those intended for inhalation such as inhalation steroids dexamethasone, flunisolide, and triamcinolone acetonide [22]. SCFs have properties of gases and liquids at temperatures and pressures above their critical point. Advantages of SCFs include density values resulting in high dissolving power, lower viscosity levels compared to other liquids, and higher diffusivity allowing high mass transfer [19]. Among present SCFs, CO2 is the most commonly used due to its low critical temperature (31.2°C) and pressure (7.4 MPa); other advantages include nonflammability, nontoxicity, and cost-effectiveness [19].

There are two major principles for particle precipitation when using SCFs. SCFs can be used as (1) solvents (rapid expansion of supercritical solution (RESS) and particles from gas saturated solutions (PGSS)) and (2) antisolvents (gas antisolvent (GAS), aerosol solvent extraction system (ASES), supercritical fluid antisolvent (SAS), precipitation with compressed antisolvent (PCA), and solution enhanced dispersion by supercritical fluids (SEDS)). Since the early 2000s, solutions consisting of proteins along with a cosolvent, such as ethanol, have been precipitated using CO_2 [23]. The integrity of such proteins depends on the operating conditions such as temperature, pressure, flow rates, and the concentration of the ingredients used, and by properly optimizing such conditions, the precipitation of proteins using the SCFs, such as CO_2, has become a promising method for particle precipitation [24].

3.1.3 Fluidized-bed Spray Coating

Fluidized-bed spray coating is a commonly used method in the pharmaceutical industry for coating of small particles [25]. Coating of particles has several advantages, such as providing acid resistance [24], modifying the release of the particles [26], protecting the therapeutic agent from light, and moisture and masking the taste of a substance [27]. In this process, particles to be coated come in contact with droplets of coating solution after being fluidized via air currents and are then dried using heated air; thus, after several loops through the spraying and drying zones, a uniform coat is achieved [28]. Further, the uniformity and success of the coating is dependent on the spreading of the droplet on the surface of the particle [29].

As a result of recent advancements in fluidized-bed spray coating systems, particles as small as 50 μm can be coated. For instance, fluidized-bed spray coating was applied to recombinant human deoxyribonuclease (rhDNase), and the coating was examined via scanning electron microscopy [30]. The coating demonstrated strong integrity when introduced to mechanical force; however, the process resulted in aggregation of the proteins,, which may be mainly due to the thermal stress involved with the process [29]. Aggregation was significantly reduced however, when rhDNase was formulated with calcium ions, thus suggesting in presence of proper stabilizers fluidized-bed spray coating is a feasible method for coating and preparing dried pharmaceutical proteins [31].

3.1.4 Lyophilization

Protein instability is one of the major reasons protein drugs are still administered via injections and not orally. Therefore, in order to overcome this hurdle, proteins must be made into solid forms to achieve an acceptable shelf life [32]. Lyophilization has become one of the most commonly used methods for generating solid protein drugs [33]. Lyophilization consists of three steps beginning with (1) freezing, where the solution that is to be dried is frozen at a controlled rate thus removing water from the protein as ice crystals, at this point ~20% of water remains in a unfrozen phase known as maximal freeze concentrate [31]. Freezing is followed by (2) primary drying, where frozen water is removed via sublimation resulting in significant desorption of water

(~10%). The remaining water is removed at higher temperatures in the final stage, (3) secondary drying, via desorption which lowers the fluid moisture content to few tenth of a percent [34].

A variety of stresses caused by lyophilization, such as low temperatures, formation of dendritic ice crystals, pH changes, phase separations, increase in ionic strengths, and removal of protein hydration shell, can result in reversible [33] and irreversible [34] structural changes in the protein [33]. Thus, for proteins that are sensitive to the listed stresses, specific cryo-/lyo- protectants can be used, such as commonly used sugars/polyols, nonaqueous solvents, polymers, protein itself, surfactants, and amino acids [33]. Further, extra effort is made to fully customize the lyophilization cycles in order to avoid lyophilization cycle-related stresses such as freezing rate and temperature, thermal treatment conditions, drying rate and temperature, and final moisture content [33].

3.1.5 Jet Milling

Jet milling is a method used for particle size reduction using interparticle collisions and abrasion to produce particles ranging between 1 and 20 μm [19]. Although Jet milling is a great method for particles size reduction (1–20 μm), it does come with some drawbacks, such as lack of control over size, shape, surface properties, and morphology. Furthermore, the high energy input can be detrimental to proteins as it can lead to protein degradation [19]. In a study where horseradish peroxidase was coprecipitated with carbomer and jet milled for two different time points, it was demonstrated that the longer the jet milling process, the more significant the reduction in protein activity [35]. In fact, grinding the power for 10 min in a mortar almost completely eliminated the activity of peroxidase [36] However, pulmonary activity of salmon calcitonin along with a variety of absorption enhancers (oleic acid, lecithin, citric acid, taurocholic acid, dimethyl-beta-cyclodextrin, and octyl-beta-D-glucoside) micronized after freeze drying with lactose showed significant blood levels of calcitonin in rats [37]. Further, it has been suggested that microparticle preparation is possible via melting, pregrinding, and a final jet milling step for particle size reduction [36]. Lastly, as peptides fed into the machine have to be coarse enough to allow for free flow and fine enough not to block the hopper and pipe work, they are at times required to be lyophilized which can result in protein degradation if no lyoprotectant is used [36].

3.1.6 Spray Drying

Spray drying is a method used for forming protein particles in lower molecular range [38]. The solution is automatically fed into droplets that rapidly dry due to high surface area and large amount of air–water interfacial area. During the drying process, which can range from 100 milliseconds to seconds, the critical increase in temperature is prevented by the evaporation of the solvent, which results in the temperature of particles remaining significantly lower than the temperature of the gas and drying powder is quickly removed from the drying zone to prevent overheating [25]. Spray drying allows control over a variety of particle design features, including particle size and distribution, surface energy and rugoses, particle density, surface area, porosity, and microviscosity [39]. Since the average radius of particles obtained ranges between 2 and 6 μm, spray drying is generally used for pulmonary particle delivery [40] such as the protein insulin [41].

Although the air-drying process of spray drying prevents thermal degradation of proteins, the atomization process may present a different obstacle. The high shear rate required for the atomization process can lead to degradation of macromolecules. For instance, a study demonstrated degradation of human growth hormone (hGH) during the air–liquid interface following atomization, while the tissue-type plasminogen activator (t-PA) remained intact [42]. There have been several proteins that have been successfully air-dried. Niven et al. spray dried formulations of recombinant human granulocyte colony-stimulating factor (rhG-CSF) [43], and Dalby et al. produced fine protein particles in a process where they combined nebulization, air drying, and electrostatic collection [44].

4. FORMULATION STRATEGIES FOR OVERCOMING PROTEIN DELIVERY CHALLENGES

4.1 Nanotechnology Approaches

Another promising approach to enhance the stability of therapeutic peptides and proteins is encapsulation into a micro- or nanoparticle, with the aim of protecting the drug from the hostile environments in the body [45]. At their target location, biodrugs typically are released from the particle by diffusion, swelling, erosion, or degradation [46]. Biological systems are usually protected by nanometer-sized barriers, which are extremely specific with regards to transport of biological molecules. Permeation through such barriers and their access to specific biological compartments is dictated by chemical properties, size, and shape of biological molecules [47]. Nanotechnology, defined as development and application of materials, structures, devices, and systems by modeling and manufacturing of the matter in the nanoscale range (1–100 nm), can be used to provide protection against the degreadation of biological agents [48]. As nanoparticles are similar in scale to biological molecules, nanoparticles can have many medical applications and be engineered to have various functions. As their properties allow them to cross biological barriers, nanoparticles can be used to transport therapeutic molecules to sites of interest, providing access to molecules of interest and thus modulation of molecular interactions [48, 49].

One of the main issues for lack of efficacy for some current therapeutics is the inability to be fully delivered to the required sites, which can be due to their low solubility. Low efficacy may result in increasing dosage, thus correlating with increased side effects [50]. The use of nanocarriers can aid in overcoming some of these obstacles. The surface of nanocarriers usually consists of polymers or biodegradable molecules that are customized to ensure biocompatibility and selective targeting [48]. In fact, nanocarriers may offer numerous advantages over free drugs, such as protecting the drug from premature interaction with unwanted biological entities and degradation, enhancing the absorption of the drug into a specific tissue of interest (cancers or tumors), increasing the pharmacokinetics of the drug, and improving the intracellular penetration of the drug [51].

Nanoparticles and nanocarriers can be used for delivery of peptide drugs to specific sites of interest, avoiding degradation in the GIT and first-pass metabolism via the hepatic route. In fact, peptides have been transported using nanocarriers. Hyaluronic acid-Fe2O3 hybrid magnetic nanoparticles were designed to deliver peptides to HEK293 and A529 cells at a 100% level [52]. Further, functionalized gold nanoparticles consisting of a drug peptide ligand and a targeting peptide were shown to be both effective and enhance the activity and selectivity of such peptide multifunctionalized conjugates [53]. Furthermore, carrier molecules have been shown to increase membrane permeability of protein therapeutics such as insulin, interferon α2b, and human growth hormone through epithelial membrane of small intestine thus increasing the bioavailability of listed protein therapeutics [54].

4.2 PEGylation

Proposed in 1970s [55], PEGylation is the attachment of polyethylene glycol to drug molecules as a method of transforming proteins, peptides, small molecules, and oligonucleotides into more potent drugs [56]. PEGylated molecules tend to be more clinically useful compared to their unmodified counterparts as they tend to have higher stability and solubility, longer half- life in the systemic circulation, reduced renal clearance, reduced immunogenicity and antigenicity [57], and higher potency [58].

Protein drugs, such as enzymes, cytokines, and antibodies, have been shown to be significantly improved as a result of PEGylation [59]. Although it is common to see improvements in retention within circulation and reduction of immune response and degradation, the loss of biological activity due to PEGylation is quiet common [60]. The loss of biological activity is however compensated with improved pharmacokinetics as seen in α-interferon Pegasys® [61]. Currently, there are several PEGylated drugs available for public use, including PEG- adenosine deaminase (Adagen®) [62], PEG-asparaginase (Oncaspar®) [63], PEG-interferon α2b (PEG-Intron®) [64], PEG-interferon α2a (Pegasys®) [63], and PEG-growth hormone receptor antagonist (Pegvisomant, Somavert®) [65]. Before PEGylated drugs are made available to public use, they must undergo biological tests to ensure that the advantage of PEGylation does not result in increased toxicity [62].

5. APPROACHES FOR DECREASING PROTEIN AGGREGATION AND ENHANCING BIO-AVAILABILITY

Numerous strategies have been developed and applied to control or prevent protein aggregation. Protein aggregation can be reduced by introducing disulphide bonds, salt bridges, and metal ions to stabilize and rigidify regions involved in local unfolding. However, extensive clinical trials will be required to confirm if there are any adverse effects associated with these modifications [15, 16]. A more direct approach is to alter the formulation of the protein. One approach to reduce aggregation is to work with protein solutions at lower concentrations and correspondingly larger volumes. A number of excipients have been used with varying success to reduce protein aggregation; however, each has its own limitations [14]. Nonionic detergents can be used to reduce aggregation induced by shear and heat. Cyclodextrins can also be used to reduce aggregation. For example, cyclodextrins suppress the aggregation of insulin. Another approach to reduce aggregation is to use lyophilized dosage forms [16]. Lyophilization is generally regarded as an effective means to stabilize proteins [13, 14]. However, proteins can undergo reversible conformational changes in the lyophilized state, which makes them more susceptible to undesirable side reactions. For example, the aggregation of lyophilized insulin can be ameliorated by the presence of trace moisture [15,16].

To improve the oral bioavailability of protein drugs, many strategies have been developed. One strategy involves the modulation of the physiochemical properties of the gastrointestinal tract. This could be achieved by the use of protease inhibitors as an additive to reduce the rate of enzymatic degradation [18]. For example, the enzymatic degradation of insulin in the intestine is known to be mediated by the serine proteases trypsin, α-chymotrypsin, and thiol metalloproteinase insulin degrading enzymes. The use of additives that inhibit these enzymes was found to increase the intestinal absorption of insulin by 10% in rats [66]. Also, the modulation of the tight-junction permeability to increase paracellular transport of protein molecules has been studied. However, this approach requires further investigations before it can be applied [18].

Another strategy to improve protein drug bioavailability involves chemical modification of the protein. This includes the synthesis of a protein analog with an improved enzymatic stability and/or membrane penetration. For example, insulin tends to self-associate to form hexamers. The absorption of hexameric insulin is lower than that of the monomeric insulin analog [2]. Mutation of the amino acids that are involved in self-association results in the formation of the monomeric insulin analog known as insulin lispro (Humalog®, Eli Lilly), which is characterized by rapid onset of action following subcutaneous injection [16]. Chemical modification could also be used to produce a prodrug, which could be useful to protect the drugs against enzymatic degradation [18]. The introduction of novel functional groups to protein drugs that are recognized by transporters can also aid in their absorption. For example, adding a dipeptide that is recognized by peptide-influx transporters in the gastrointestinal tract to a protein drug results in significant improvement in its oral bioavailability [16, 18]. Another way to improve protein stability is acylation of the protein drug, which involves the attachment of fatty acids to the exposed residues on the protein surface. This kind of modification increases the affinity of the protein to the serum albumin resulting in an increase in its half-life. Acetylation of insulin led to the development of insulin detemir (Levemir®, Nova Nordisk), which is a long-acting insulin analog [16]. The conjugation of protein drugs with polymers is one of the approaches used to improve the bioavailability of protein drugs. Currently, poly (ethylene glycol) (PEG) is the most widely used polymer. Protein conjugation with PEG reduces the plasma clearance rate by reducing the metabolic degradation [67].

It is also possible to increase the bioavailability of protein drugs by using pharmaceutical technologies. For example, the use of the mucoadhesive delivery system was found to prolong the residence time of protein drug at the local site of absorption and to increase the concentration gradient between delivery system and intestinal membrane, which ultimately results in a higher rate of drug absorption [18]. In addition, protein delivery systems represent an effective method to effectively deliver protein drugs. The most often used delivery systems include liposomes, micelles, microspheres, and hydrogels. The use of carriers provides a higher degree of protection against enzymatic degradation and other destructive factors because the carrier wall completely isolates drug molecules from the environment [18]. Liposomes possess the most suitable characteristics for protein encapsulation. Encapsulating insulin in liposomes results in enhanced oral absorption of insulin [16], [18]. A combination of these approaches can also be used for the development of a successful [16], [18] approach for the delivery of protein drugs, for example, the multifunctional smart polymer that is equipped with a pH- dependent drug release, Ca+2 deprivation ability, and mucoadhesive characteristic. The use of this system to deliver insulin by the oral route results in 10% bioavailability [18].

6. EXPLORATION OF VARIOUS DELIVERY ROUTES

Currently, the most accepted method of delivery of protein/peptide compounds is the parenteral administration of liquid formulations [68]. This method has become widely accepted by the pharmaceutical companies as it is the fastest way toward achieving commercialization [69]. However, as the therapeutic range of protein/peptide compounds increases, so does the demand for improved formulations. Even though designing novel drug delivery systems is not essential for the success of such compounds, they are important for increased efficacy, patient compliance, and reduced errors in drug administration [20]. Thus, along with parenteral administration of protein/peptide compounds, other routes of delivery such as oral, nasal, pulmonary, ocular, and transdermal delivery have been explored [69].

6.1 Parenteral Delivery

Parenterally administered protein drugs are most likely to be commercially successful since most animal studies and early clinical trials are performed via direct injections, thus making parenteral drug delivery one of the most popular forms of delivery assuming that injections meet the desired safety and efficacy targets [17]. Drugs delivered parenterally, whether intravenously or intramuscularly, gain full access to the systemic circulation due to rapid drug absorption. The short half-life of peptide drugs within the bloodstream results in repeat doses which correlate with oscillating drug concentrations within the blood [69].

There are numerous injection devices available for patients. For patients with daily injection requirements such as insulin, there are small diameter needle and syringes available. In fact, to improve patients' quality of life, the patient is now provided with prefilled syringes, syringe injectors, injectors, and pen devices, which may be preloaded with the drug of interest, and autoinjectors are regularly utilized as patients require more flexible and convenient injection devices moving away from the traditional syringe and vial [70]. For instance, insulin is now available in a variety of syringe injectable forms, infusion pumps, jet injectors (a needleless system that transports insulin transcutaneously), and reusable and prefilled pens [70]. All injectable devices must undergo stringent testing to ensure that the patient receives the proper dose of the drug in its expected form. For instance, in needleless systems that depend on high velocity liquid injection, which is dependent on compressed gas, the sheer stress can compromise the configuration of the protein [71, 72].

The rapid absorption of parenterally delivered drug is quickly followed by a rapid decline in the drug levels in the systemic circulation, which can be problematic in cases of chronic conditions where daily or weekly injections may be required for years. The requirement for numerous injections can result in decreased patient compliance, thus resulting in the development of prolonged release parenteral drug delivery systems [71]. These drug delivery systems include use of implants, which are biodegradable drug delivery systems mainly composed of either polylactic acid (PLA) or polyglycolic acid (PLGA) to control the release of the therapeutic drug [73]. However, since implants often require surgery and have been shown to have poor content uniformity in lower drug doses, in situ microparticle systems have been shown to be more advantageous due to the presence of an external oil phase [74]. ISM showed comparable drug release profile to drug release of microparticles prepared by solvent evaporation method, thus potentially becoming an alternative to more complicated microencapsulation methods [75].

6.2 Oral Delivery

One of the major challenges for protein drug delivery via the oral route is the susceptibility of the protein drug to proteolytic degradation in the gastrointestinal tract (GIT), which is at its highest in the stomach and the duodenum of the small intestines and is significantly lower in the mouth, pharynx, esophagus, ileum, and the colon. Another challenge is the bioavailability of the drug, which is dependent on two major factors, the molecular weight (MW) of the drug and its solubility. Bioavailability is essentially independent of MW for drugs less than 700 Da; however, with increasing MW passed this threshold, there is a decrease in the bioavailability of the drug. Drug compounds also need to meet a certain level of hydrophobicity criteria as they are required cross biological membranes. However, most biological drug compounds considered for therapeutic use are frequently greater than 700 Da and are hydrophilic [76]. Thus, degradation and poor absorption are the main bioavailability barriers. There are however suggested methods for increasing the survival of the peptides as it moves through the GIT [75].

There are current methods for increasing the bioavailability of peptidic drugs such as (1) modifying the N- or C-terminus to increase half-life (encephalin, conversion of C-terminal methionine to methioniol group [77]); (2) altering the terminal amino acids from L-amino acid to a D-amino acid (arginine-vasopressin analog 1-deamino-8-D-arginine [77, 78]); (3) converting the linear peptide into a cyclic analog to avoid degradation by carboxy- and amino-peptidases (successfully performed in a model hexapeptide [77]); (4) use of peptidomimetics, which are molecules that mimic the action of peptides but are no longer peptidic in nature and prodrugs, which can be metabolized in the body releasing the therapeutic agent in return; and (5) coadministration of the peptide drug with digestive enzyme inhibitors [79]. The GIT presents both physical and chemical challenges for oral delivery of protein drugs; however, recent developments have made progress in facing each of those challenges and obstacles. Even though the development of new formulation methods, which have shown to improve bioavailability of protein drugs, are still costly, the progress in this field is still quite promising [20].

6.3 Nasal Delivery

The use of the nasal cavity as a site for systemic peptide drug delivery has several benefits, such as (1) rapid absorption rate, which in some cases have been shown to be as effective as intravenous injections and require lower doses; (2) high permeability due to the nasal epithelium (up to 1 kDa) [80]; along with (3) high total blood flow; (4) avoidance of first-pass metabolism; and (5) accessibility. The combination of such characteristics allows for a faster onset of pharmacological activity and lower side effects [81]. The olfactory nerves also allow for the direct transport of drug to the brain as the blood–brain barrier provides a challenging obstacle for numerous drugs such as antibiotics, antineoplastic agents, and other drugs that are active in the central nervous system [82].

There are a variety of formulation factors that can affect the absorption of drugs within the nasal cavity. Such factors include dose and volume, pH, osmolarity of the solution which the drug is dissolved in, viscosity, excipients used (such as absorption enhancers), dosage form (spray, powder, or drops), administration techniques (inhalation or mechanically assisted), and devices used to administer the drug [83]. Further, despite the fact that nasally administered drugs are able to avoid first-metabolism, bioavailability of peptide drugs is still limited due to the presence of broad range of metabolic enzymes that reside in the nasal mucosal cavity and the epithelial cell lining [84].

Currently, drugs ranging from small to large macromolecules such as protein drugs, hormones, and vaccines are delivered through the nasal cavity [85]. For instance, in the presence of absorption enhancers, which aid in modulating the nasal epithelium permeability, insulin can be effectively administered through the nasal cavity [84].

6.4 Pulmonary delivery

The large surface area of the lung along with its well vascularized thin epithelial lining provides a noninvasive method for drug delivery, direct access to systemic circulation, and allows for avoidance of first pass metabolism and GIT degradation [86]. It has been suggested that to achieve successful pulmonary delivery of drug, the drug must reach the alveoli or deep lung; thus, the particle size must range within 1–2 µm for optimum absorption [87]. The inhalation of therapeutics is an effective means for providing therapies for respiratory [88] and a wide range of other disorders [89].

Even though animal studies have shown the bioavailability of drugs delivered via the pulmonary route ranging from ~10% to 50% depending on the type of protein, similar success rates have not been seen in human studies [70]. For instance, pulmonary insulin delivery demonstrated just below 50% bioavailability in animals [90]; bioavailability in humans is merely 10–15% [70]. These findings suggest that the bioavailability of a drug in animals is not necessarily predictive of that of a human. Another obstacle associated with pulmonary delivery is the clinical toxicology of the lungs, particularly when dealing with cytokines and growth factors that may have a local effect on the tissue [70]. The particle size of the drug also plays a critical role in its bioavailability in the lungs [91]. As previously mentioned, a smaller particle size results in deeper lung penetration, hence increasing bioavailability. Nonetheless, for bigger molecular medicines, patients may require varying dosages and several administrations to attain the desired therapeutic effect [70]. A further obstacle in the pulmonary administration of protein therapeutics is the swift elevation of drug concentrations in the blood, which may not pose issues when the agent possesses a substantial safety margin [89]. While this may be advantageous in situations necessitating rapid medication delivery, such as insulin administration prior to a meal, it can lead to undesirable side effects and necessitate several doses to attain and sustain the requisite serum levels. Nonetheless, innovative technologies, including rapid-acting, slow-release analogs of medications like insulin, have been created to enhance pulmonary peptide drug delivery [91].

7. CONCISE SUMMARY

To design a medically effective analog of a protein medicine, several criteria must be considered. It is essential to thoroughly comprehend the physiological and chemical hurdles that the protein medicine will face. Despite being a very nascent field, considerable advancements have been achieved across various domains. There has been a heightened comprehension of the benefits and drawbacks of various methods of protein medication administration. Consequently, through appropriate modifications—such as alterations to the N- or C- terminus, changes in terminal amino acids, transformation of protein conformation from linear to circular, utilization of peptidomimetics, enzyme inhibitors, or PEGylation—protein therapeutics can be designed based on the established understanding of proteolytic enzymes encountered in systemic circulation. Moreover, recent breakthroughs in nanomedicine have facilitated the encapsulation of proteins, leading to enhanced bioavailability.

Advancements and innovations in formulation technology have enabled the feasible synthesis of protein pharmaceuticals, formerly deemed uneconomical for large-scale manufacturing. The appropriate formulation of the drug product relies on selecting the most stable form of the protein medication and comprehensively studying the chemical and physical properties, as well as the stability of the molecule under various settings in both short-term and long-term research.

REFERENCES

1. M. S. Chang and B. Yeung, Eds., *Formulation and Process Development Strategies for Manufacturing Biopharmaceuticals*. Hoboken, NJ, USA: John Wiley & Sons, Inc., 2010.
2. J. Shaji and V. Patole, "Protein and peptide drug delivery: oral approaches," *Indian J. Pharm. Sci.*, vol. 70, no. 3, pp. 269–77, Jan. 2008.
3. M. C. Manning, D. K. Chou, B. M. Murphy, R. W. Payne, and D. S. Katayama, "Stability of protein pharmaceuticals: an update," *Pharm. Res.*, vol. 27, no. 4, pp. 544–75, Apr. 2010.
4. G. Hu, "Understanding the basics of peptide and protein production," *Bioprocess Int.*, vol. 8, pp. 22–25, 2010.
5. L. R. Brown, "Commercial challenges of protein drug delivery," *Expert Opin. Drug Deliv.*, vol. 2, no. 1, pp. 29–42, Jan. 2005.
6. M. A. H. Capelle, R. Gurny, and T. Arvinte, "High throughput screening of protein formulation stability: practical considerations," *Eur. J. Pharm. Biopharm.*, vol. 65, no. 2, pp. 131–48, Feb. 2007.
7. M. Werle and A. Bernkop-Schnürch, "Strategies to improve plasma half life time of peptide and protein drugs," *Amino Acids*, vol. 30, no. 4, pp. 351–67, Jun. 2006.
8. M. C. Lai and E. M. Topp, "Solid-state chemical stability of proteins and peptides," *J. Pharm. Sci.*, vol. 88, no. 5, pp. 489–500, May 1999.
9. L. (Lucy) Chang and M. J. Pikal, "Mechanisms of protein stabilization in the solid state," *J. Pharm. Sci.*, vol. 98, no. 9, pp. 2886–2908, Sep. 2009.
10. A. A. Wakankar and R. T. Borchardt, "Formulation considerations for proteins susceptible to asparagine deamidation and aspartate isomerization," *J. Pharm. Sci.*, vol. 95, no. 11, pp. 2321–36, Nov. 2006.
11. M. Ameri, P. E. Daddona, and Y.-F. Maa, "Demonstrated solid-state stability of parathyroid hormone PTH(1-34) coated on a novel transdermal microprojection delivery system," *Pharm. Res.*, vol. 26, no. 11, pp. 2454–63, Nov. 2009.
12. R. Hamburger, E. Azaz, and M. Donbrow, "Autoxidation of polyoxyethylenic non- ionic surfactants and of polyethylene glycols," *Pharm. Acta Helv.*, vol. 50, no. 1–2, pp. 10–7, Jan. 1975.
13. S. Li, T. W. Patapoff, D. Overcashier, C. Hsu, T. H. Nguyen, and R. T. Borchardt, "Effects of reducing sugars on the chemical stability of human relaxin in the lyophilized state," *J. Pharm. Sci.*, vol. 85, no. 8, pp. 873–7, Aug. 1996.
14. E. T. Maggio, "Novel excipients prevent aggregation in manufacturing and formulation of protein and peptide therapeutics," *Bioprocess Int.*, vol. 6, no. 10, pp. 58–65, Nov. 2008.
15. W. F. Weiss, T. M. Young, and C. J. Roberts, "Principles, approaches, and challenges for predicting protein aggregation rates and shelf life," *J. Pharm. Sci.*, vol. 98, no. 4, pp. 1246–77, Apr. 2009.

16. S. Frokjaer and D. E. Otzen, "Protein drug stability: a formulation challenge," *Nat. Rev. Drug Discov.*, vol. 4, no. 4, pp. 298–306, Apr. 2005.

17. V. P. Torchilin and A. N. Lukyanov, "Peptide and protein drug delivery to and into tumors: challenges and solutions," *Drug Discov. Today*, vol. 8, no. 6, pp. 259–66, Mar. 2003.

18. M. Morishita and N. A. Peppas, "Is the oral route possible for peptide and protein drug delivery?," *Drug Discov. Today*, vol. 11, no. 19–20, pp. 905–10, Oct. 2006.

19. S. A. Shoyele, "Engineering protein particles for pulmonary drug delivery," *Methods Mol. Biol.*, vol. 437, pp. 149–60, Jan. 2008.

20. R. Singh, S. Singh, and J. W. Lillard, "Past, present, and future technologies for oral delivery of therapeutic proteins," *J. Pharm. Sci.*, vol. 97, no. 7, pp. 2497–523, Jul. 2008.

21. S. D. Allison, T. W. Randolph, M. C. Manning, K. Middleton, A. Davis, and J. F. Carpenter, "Effects of drying methods and additives on structure and function of actin: mechanisms of dehydration-induced damage and its inhibition," *Arch. Biochem. Biophys.*, vol. 358, no. 1, pp. 171–81, Oct. 1998.

22. M. C. Heller, J. F. Carpenter, and T. W. Randolph, "Protein formulation and lyophilization cycle design: prevention of damage due to freeze-concentration induced phase separation," *Biotechnol. Bioeng.*, vol. 63, no. 2, pp. 166–74, Apr. 1999.

23. W. Han, W. Bao, Z. Wang, and S. Nattel, "Comparison of ion-channel subunit expression in canine cardiac Purkinje fibers and ventricular muscle," *Circ. Res.*, vol. 91, no. 9, pp. 790–7, Nov. 2002.

24. H. Okamoto and K. Danjo, "Application of supercritical fluid to preparation of powders of high-molecular weight drugs for inhalation," *Adv. Drug Deliv. Rev.*, vol. 60, no. 3, pp. 433–46, Feb. 2008.

25. K. Johnson, "Preparation of peptide and protein powders for inhalation," *Adv. Drug Deliv. Rev.*, vol. 26, no. 1, pp. 3–15, Jun. 1997.

26. M. Luštrik, R. Dreu, R. Šibanc, and S. Srčič, "Comparative study of the uniformity of coating thickness of pellets coated with a conventional Wurster chamber and a swirl generator-equipped Wurster chamber," *Pharm. Dev. Technol.*, vol. 17, no. 3, pp. 268– 76, Jan..

27. M. A. Rahman and J. Ali, "Development and in vitro Evaluation of Enteric Coated Multiparticulate System for Resistant Tuberculosis," *Indian J. Pharm. Sci.*, vol. 70, no. 4, pp. 477–81, Jan..

28. A. Dashevsky, K. Wagner, K. Kolter, and R. Bodmeier, "Physicochemical and release properties of pellets coated with Kollicoat SR 30 D, a new aqueous polyvinyl acetate dispersion for extended release," *Int. J. Pharm.*, vol. 290, no. 1–2, pp. 15–23, Feb. 2005.

29. E. Teunou and D. Poncelet, "Batch and continuous fluid bed coating—review and state of the art," *J. Food Eng.*, vol. 53, no. 4, pp. 325–340, Aug. 2002.

30. N. Pearnchob, J. Siepmann, and R. Bodmeier, "Pharmaceutical applications of shellac: moisture-protective and taste-masking coatings and extended-release matrix tablets," *Drug Dev. Ind. Pharm.*, vol. 29, no. 8, pp. 925–38, Sep. 2003.

31. Y. F. Maa and C. C. Hsu, "Feasibility of protein spray coating using a fluid-bed Würster processor," *Biotechnol. Bioeng.*, vol. 53, no. 6, pp. 560–6, Mar. 1997.

32. Y. Fukumori, H. Ichikawa, K. Jono, Y. Takeuchi, and T. Fukuda, "Computer simulation of agglomeration in the Wurster process," *Chem. Pharm. Bull. (Tokyo).*, vol. 40, no. 8, pp. 2159–63, Aug. 1992.

33. W. Wang, "Lyophilization and development of solid protein pharmaceuticals," *Int. J. Pharm.*, vol. 203, no. 1–2, pp. 1–60, Aug. 2000.
34. S. Luthra, J.-P. Obert, D. S. Kalonia, and M. J. Pikal, "Investigation of drying stresses on proteins during lyophilization: differentiation between primary and secondary- drying stresses on lactate dehydrogenase using a humidity controlled mini freeze- dryer," *J. Pharm. Sci.*, vol. 96, no. 1, pp. 61–70, Jan. 2007.
35. K. Griebenow and A. M. Klibanov, "Lyophilization-induced reversible changes in the secondary structure of proteins," *Proc. Natl. Acad. Sci. U. S. A.*, vol. 92, no. 24, pp. 10969–76, Nov. 1995.
36. W. Schlocker, S. Gschliesser, and A. Bernkop-Schnürch, "Evaluation of the potential of air jet milling of solid protein-poly(acrylate) complexes for microparticle preparation," *Eur. J. Pharm. Biopharm.*, vol. 62, no. 3, pp. 260–6, Apr. 2006.
37. D. B. Volkin and A. M. Klibanov, "Alterations in the structure of proteins that cause their irreversible inactivation," *Dev. Biol. Stand.*, vol. 74, pp. 73–80; discussion 80–1, Jan. 1992.
38. S. Kobayashi, S. Kondo, and K. Juni, "Pulmonary delivery of salmon calcitonin dry powders containing absorption enhancers in rats," *Pharm. Res.*, vol. 13, no. 1, pp. 80– 3, Jan. 1996.
39. G. Nykamp, U. Carstensen, and B. W. Müller, "Jet milling--a new technique for microparticle preparation," *Int. J. Pharm.*, vol. 242, no. 1–2, pp. 79–86, Aug. 2002.
40. R. Vehring, "Pharmaceutical particle engineering via spray drying," *Pharm. Res.*, vol. 25, no. 5, pp. 999–1022, May 2008.
41. J. G. Weers, T. E. Tarara, and A. R. Clark, "Design of fine particles for pulmonary drug delivery," *Expert Opin. Drug Deliv.*, vol. 4, no. 3, pp. 297–313, May 2007.
42. M. Sakagami and P. R. Byron, "Respirable microspheres for inhalation: the potential of manipulating pulmonary disposition for improved therapeutic efficacy," *Clin. Pharmacokinet.*, vol. 44, no. 3, pp. 263–77, Jan. 2005.
43. A. X. C. N. Valente, R. Langer, H. A. Stone, and D. A. Edwards, "Recent advances in the development of an inhaled insulin product," *BioDrugs*, vol. 17, no. 1, pp. 9–17, Jan. 2003.
44. M. Mumenthaler, C. C. Hsu, and R. Pearlman, "Feasibility study on spray-drying protein pharmaceuticals: recombinant human growth hormone and tissue-type plasminogen activator," *Pharm. Res.*, vol. 11, no. 1, pp. 12–20, Jan. 1994.
45. R. W. Niven, F. D. Lott, A. Y. Ip, and J. M. Cribbs, "Pulmonary delivery of powders and solutions containing recombinant human granulocyte colony-stimulating factor (rhG-CSF) to the rabbit," *Pharm. Res.*, vol. 11, no. 8, pp. 1101–9, Aug. 1994.
46. R. Dalby, V. Naini, and P. Byron, "Droplets drying and electrostatic collection a novel alternative to conventional comminution techniques," *J. Biopharm. Sci.*, 1992.
47. U. Bilati, E. Allémann, and E. Doelker, "Strategic approaches for overcoming peptide and protein instability within biodegradable nano- and microparticles," *Eur. J. Pharm. Biopharm.*, vol. 59, no. 3, pp. 375–88, Apr. 2005.
48. B. Y. S. Kim, J. T. Rutka, and W. C. W. Chan, "Nanomedicine," *N. Engl. J. Med.*, vol. 363, no. 25, pp. 2434–43, Dec. 2010.
49. K. Uekama, F. Hirayama, and T. Irie, "Cyclodextrin Drug Carrier Systems," *Chem. Rev.*, vol. 98, no. 5, pp. 2045–2076, Jul. 1998.
50. D. Peer, J. M. Karp, S. Hong, O. C. Farokhzad, R. Margalit, and R. Langer, "Nanocarriers as an emerging platform for cancer therapy," *Nat. Nanotechnol.*, vol. 2, no. 12, pp. 751–60, Dec. 2007.

51. Y. Xia, Y. Xiong, B. Lim, and S. E. Skrabalak, “Shape-controlled synthesis of metal nanocrystals: simple chemistry meets complex physics?,” *Angew. Chem. Int. Ed. Engl.*, vol. 48, no. 1, pp. 60–103, Jan. 2009.

52. M. Cavadas, Á. González-Fernández, and R. Franco, “Pathogen-mimetic stealth nanocarriers for drug delivery: a future possibility,” *Nanomedicine Nanotechnology, Biol. Med.*, vol. 7, no. 6, pp. 730–743, Dec. 2011.

53. K. K. Jain, “Nanomedicine: application of nanobiotechnology in medical practice,” *Med. Princ. Pract.*, vol. 17, no. 2, pp. 89–101, Jan. 2008.

54. A. Kumar, B. Sahoo, A. Montpetit, S. Behera, R. F. Lockey, and S. S. Mohapatra, “Development of hyaluronic acid–Fe2O3 hybrid magnetic nanoparticles for targeted delivery of peptides,” *Nanomedicine*, vol. 3, no. 2, pp. 132–7, Jun. 2007.

55. L. Hosta-Rigau, I. Olmedo, J. Arbiol, L. J. Cruz, M. J. Kogan, and F. Albericio, “Multifunctionalized gold nanoparticles with peptides targeted to gastrin-releasing peptide receptor of a tumor cell line,” *Bioconjug. Chem.*, vol. 21, no. 6, pp. 1070–1078, Jun. 2010.

56. B. R. Stoll, H. R. Leipold, S. Milstein, and D. A. Edwards, “A mechanistic analysis of carrier-mediated oral delivery of protein therapeutics,” *J. Control. Release*, vol. 64, no. 1–3, pp. 217–28, Feb. 2000.

57. F. Davis, A. Abuchowski, and T. Van Es. Enzyme-polyethylene glycol adducts: modified enzymes with unique properties. In: Broun G, Manecke G, Wingard L Jr, editors. *Enzyme Engineering*. New York: Springer, 1978. pp. 169–7.

58. M. Hamidi, A. Azadi, and P. Rafiei, “Pharmacokinetic consequences of pegylation,” *Drug Deliv.*, vol. 13, no. 6, pp. 399–409, Jan. 2006.

59. A. Abuchowski, J. R. McCoy, N. C. Palczuk, T. van Es, and F. F. Davis, “Effect of covalent attachment of polyethylene glycol on immunogenicity and circulating life of bovine liver catalase,” *J. Biol. Chem.*, vol. 252, no. 11, pp. 3582–6, Jun. 1977.

60. P. Bailon and C.-Y. Won, “PEG-modified biopharmaceuticals,” *Expert Opin. Drug Deliv.*, vol. 6, no. 1, pp. 1–16, Jan. 2009.

61. G. Pasut, A Guiotto, and FM Veronese,“Protein, peptide and non-peptide drug PEGylation for therapeutic application,” *Expert Opin. Drug Deliv.*, vol. *14, no. 6, pp. 859-894*, Jun. 2004.

62. F. M. Veronese and G. Pasut, “PEGylation, successful approach to drug delivery,” *Drug Discov. Today*, vol. 10, no. 21, pp. 1451–8, Nov. 2005.

63. P. Bailon, A. Palleroni, C. A. Schaffer, C. L. Spence, W. J. Fung, J. E. Porter, G. K. Ehrlich, W. Pan, Z. X. Xu, M. W. Modi, A. Farid, W. Berthold, and M. Graves, “Rational design of a potent, long-lasting form of interferon: a 40 kDa branched polyethylene glycol-conjugated interferon alpha-2a for the treatment of hepatitis C,” *Bioconjug. Chem.*, vol. 12, no. 2, pp. 195–202, Jan. 2001.

64. Y.-S. Wang, S. Youngster, M. Grace, J. Bausch, R. Bordens, and D. F. Wyss, “Structural and biological characterization of pegylated recombinant interferon alpha-2b and its therapeutic implications,” *Adv. Drug Deliv. Rev.*, vol. 54, no. 4, pp. 547–70, Jun. 2002.

65. Y. Levy, M. S. Hershfield, C. Fernandez-Mejia, S. H. Polmar, D. Scudiery, M. Berger, and R. U. Sorensen, “Adenosine deaminase deficiency with late onset of recurrent infections: response to treatment with polyethylene glycol-modified adenosine deaminase,” *J. Pediatr.*, vol. 113, no. 2, pp. 312–7, Aug. 1988.

66. M. L. Graham, “Pegaspargase: a review of clinical studies,” *Adv. Drug Deliv. Rev.*, vol. 55, no. 10, pp. 1293–302, Sep. 2003.

67. P. J. Trainer, W. M. Drake, L. Katznelson, P. U. Freda, V. Herman-Bonert, A. J. van der Lely, E. V Dimaraki, P. M. Stewart, K. E. Friend, M. L. Vance, G. M. Besser, J. A. Scarlett, M. O. Thorner, C. Parkinson, A. Klibanski, J. S. Powell, A. L. Barkan, M. C. Sheppard, M. Malsonado, D. R. Rose, D. R. Clemmons, G. Johannsson, B. A. Bengtsson, S. Stavrou, D. L. Kleinberg, D. M. Cook, L. S. Phillips, M. Bidlingmaier, C. J. Strasburger, S. Hackett, K. Zib, W. F. Bennett, and R. J. Davis, "Treatment of acromegaly with the growth hormone-receptor antagonist pegvisomant," *N. Engl. J. Med.*, vol. 342, no. 16, pp. 1171–7, Apr. 2000.

68. R. B. Shah, F. Ahsan, and M. A. Khan, "Oral delivery of proteins: progress and prognostication," *Crit. Rev. Ther. Drug Carrier Syst.*, vol. 19, no. 2, pp. 135–69, Jan. 2002.

69. S. Stolnik and K. Shakesheff, "Formulations for delivery of therapeutic proteins," *Biotechnol. Lett.*, vol. 31, no. 1, pp. 1–11, Jan. 2009.

70. J. L. Cleland, A. Daugherty, and R. Mrsny, "Emerging protein delivery methods,"*Curr. Opin. Biotechnol.*, vol. 12, no. 2, pp. 212–9, Apr. 2001.

71. H. Bari, "A prolonged release parenteral drug delivery system-an overview," *Int J Pharm Sci Rev Res*, vol. 3, no. 1, pp.1-11, Jul. 2010.

72. K. E. Robertson, N. B. Glazer, and R. K. Campbell, "The latest developments in insulin injection devices," *Diabetes Educ.*, vol. 26, no. 1, pp. 135–8, 141–6, 149–52, Jan. 2000.

73. J. Oberyé, B. Mannaerts, J. Huisman, and C. Timmer, "Local tolerance, pharmacokinetics, and dynamics of ganirelix (Orgalutran) administration by Medi-Jector compared to conventional needle injections," *Hum. Reprod.*, vol. 15, no. 2, pp. 245–9, Feb. 2000.

74. P. Mikkelsen Lynch, J. Butler, D. Huerta, I. Tsals, D. Davidson, and S. Hamm, "A pharmacokinetic and tolerability evaluation of two continuous subcutaneous infusion systems compared to an oral controlled-release morphine," *J. Pain Symptom Manage.*, vol. 19, no. 5, pp. 348–56, May 2000.

75. H. Kranz and R. Bodmeier, "A novel in situ forming drug delivery system for controlled parenteral drug delivery," *Int. J. Pharm.*, 2007.

76. L. Brannon-Peppas, "Recent advances on the use of biodegradable microparticles and nanoparticles in controlled drug delivery," *Int. J. Pharm.*, 1995.

77. G. Pauletti, S. Gangwar, and G. Knipp, "Structural requirements for intestinal absorption of peptide drugs," *J. Control.* , 1996.

78. S. J. Shire, "Formulation and manufacturability of biologics," *Curr. Opin. Biotechnol.*, vol. 20, no. 6, pp. 708–14, Dec. 2009.

79. A. Fjellestad-Paulsen, C. Söderberg-Ahlm, and S. Lundin, "Metabolism of vasopressin, oxytocin, and their analogues in the human gastrointestinal tract," *Peptides*, vol. 16, no. 6, pp. 1141–7, Jan. 1995.

80. S. Lundin, N. Pantzar, A. Broeders, M. Ohlin, and B. R. Weström, "Differences in transport rate of oxytocin and vasopressin analogues across proximal and distal isolated segments of the small intestine of the rat," *Pharm. Res.*, vol. 8, no. 10, pp. 1274– 80, Oct. 1991.

81. A. Bernkop-Schnürch, "The use of inhibitory agents to overcome the enzymatic barrier to perorally administered therapeutic peptides and proteins," *J. Control. Release*, vol. 52, no. 1–2, pp. 1–16, Mar. 1998.

82. M. I. Ugwoke, N. Verbeke, and R. Kinget, "The biopharmaceutical aspects of nasal mucoadhesive drug delivery," *J. Pharm. Pharmacol.*, vol. 53, no. 1, pp. 3–21, Jan. 2001.

83. S. Türker, E. Onur, and Y. Ozer, "Nasal route and drug delivery systems," *Pharm. World Sci.*, vol. 26, no. 3, pp. 137–42, Jun. 2004.

84. Z. Antosova, M. Mackova, V. Kral, and T. Macek, "Therapeutic application of peptides and proteins: parenteral forever?," *Trends Biotechnol.*, vol. 27, no. 11, pp. 628–35, Nov. 2009.

85. M. I. Ugwoke, R. U. Agu, N. Verbeke, and R. Kinget, "Nasal mucoadhesive drug delivery: background, applications, trends and future perspectives," *Adv. Drug Deliv. Rev.*, vol. 57, no. 11, pp. 1640–65, Nov. 2005.

86. C. Ehrhardt and K.-J. Kim, Eds., *Drug Absorption Studies*, vol. VII. Boston, MA: Springer US, 2008.

87. M. Hinchcliffe and L. Illum, "Intranasal insulin delivery and therapy," *Adv. Drug Deliv. Rev.*, vol. 35, no. 2–3, pp. 199–234, Feb. 1999.

88. A. Martini, L. Muggetti, and M. P. Warchol, "Nasal and pulmonary drug delivery systems," *Expert Opin. Ther. Pat.*, vol. 10, no. 3, pp. 315–323, Mar. 2000.

89. J. Patton, J. Bukar, and S. Nagarajan, "Inhaled insulin," *Adv. Drug Deliv. Rev.*, vol. 35, no. 2–3, pp. 235–247, Feb. 1999.

90. P. Dames, B. Gleich, A. Flemmer, K. Hajek, N. Seidl, F. Wiekhorst, D. Eberbeck, I. Bittmann, C. Bergemann, T. Weyh, L. Trahms, J. Rosenecker, and C. Rudolph, "Targeted delivery of magnetic aerosol droplets to the lung," *Nat. Nanotechnol.*, vol. 2, no. 8, pp. 495–9, Aug. 2007.

91. C. Friebel and H. Steckel, "Single-use disposable dry powder inhalers for pulmonary drug delivery," Expert Opin. Drug Deliv., vol. 7, no. 12, pp. 1359–72, Dec. 2010.

10 Chapter

SWELLABLE HYDROGEL SYSTEMS FOR REGULATED DRUG DELIVERY

1. INTRODUCTION: AN OVERVIEW

Hydrogels are hydrophilic polymer networks that may absorb substantial quantities of water, resulting in an increase in volume, a phenomenon referred to as swelling. Networks may consist of homopolymers or copolymers, with their structural configuration and physical stability attributed to the existence of cross-links, which can be either chemical (tie-points, junctions) or physical (entanglements, crystallites). The hydrogel's durability is contingent upon the resilience of its cross-links, allowing it to endure water exposure; otherwise, it may disintegrate and dissolve after a specified duration.

The initial documented reference to the prospective application of hydrogels in medical science likely originates from Wichterle and Lim in 1960, who suggested the utilization of methacrylate polymers for biomedical purposes, such as ocular filling post-enucleation. Since then, numerous applications of hydrogels in pharmacy and medicine have been developed, evaluated, and, in several instances, adopted for common usage. Over the past five decades, numerous significant evaluations and reference texts have been produced regarding the accomplished work. A thorough compilation of these reviews/books nowadays could be extensive and exceeds the parameters of this study. Only a few instances are provided here. For information on the medicinal applications of hydrogels, the reader may consult the handbook by Peppas [5] and the reviews by Hoffman [1], Peppas et al. [3], and Cabral and Moratti [6]. For information on the applications of hydrogels in drug delivery, the reader may consult the reviews by Kamath and Park [7], Peppas [8], Peppas et al. [2], and Hoare and Kohane [9]. The scientific interest in hydrogels and their uses is substantial, as evidenced by the significant volume of published papers and the prominence of numerous highly referenced articles in bibliographic databases. In 2012, the journal Advanced Drug Delivery Reviews issued a special edition featuring the most cited publications (each over 1,000 citations) from its 25-year history, with four out of 32 papers particularly focused on hydrogels [1, 10-12].

1.1. Swelling Hydrogels: Nature and Classification

Hydrogels are interesting candidates for pharmaceutical and biomedical applications because of their characteristics such as:

1. Biocompatibility and bioabsorbable nature
2. Mechanical properties
3. Degradation properties
4. Compliance with sterilization protocols [7]

In particular, the balance between mechanical and degradation properties plays a relevant role in the design of a pharmaceuticals as well as a scaffold made of hydrogel to allow the desired release profile from the pharmaceutical in the time interval needed by the drug to perform the desired effect on the body or to ensure the structural function of the scaffold over the necessary time interval for the body to reconstruct the damaged part.

Several hydrophilic polymers can be used to produce hydrogels [1]:

1. Natural polymers, for example, alginate and carrageenan (anionic polymers); chitosan (cationic polymer); dextran, agarose, cellulose, and derivatives (neutral polymers); and pectin
2. Synthetic polymers, for example, PEG and PLA (polyesters), acrylates, and PVA
3. Combinations of natural and synthetic polymers, for example, alginate and Pluronics© (block copolymers PPO-PEO-PPO)

Hydrogels can be classified according to several criteria. The most widespread and used one is based on the nature (physical or chemical) of the gel [1, 7, 9]:

- Physical or "reversible" hydrogels:

1. Simple entanglement systems, in which the network is held together by molecular entanglements or crystallites
2. Ion-mediated or "ionotropic" networks, in which the network is stabilized by interaction between polyelectrolyte and multivalent ions of opposite charges (e.g., alginate)
3. Thermally induced networks, in which the heating (or the cooling) induces the structure formation (e.g., Pluronics© micelles which require heat to be formed)

- Chemical or "permanent" hydrogels, mainly covalently bounded

1. Cross-linked polymers (by radiation, by chemical cross-linkers, and by multifunctional reactive compounds)
2. Copolymers obtained from monomer + cross-linkers or monomer + multifunctional macromer
3. Conversion of hydrophobic polymer in a hydrophilic polymer
4. Polymerization of a monomer in the presence of a solid polymer to obtain an interpenetrating network (IPN)

Other possible classifications are based on the following:

Macromolecular structure [1]:

1. Cross-linked or entangled networks of linear homopolymers, linear copolymers, and block or graft copolymers
2. Polyion–multivalent ion and polyion–polyion or H-bonded complexes
3. Hydrophilic networks stabilized by hydrophobic domains
4. Interpenetrating networks (IPNs) or physical blends

Final form of the system [1]:

1. Solid molded forms (e.g., soft contact lenses)
2. Pressed powder matrices (e.g., tablets for oral delivery)
3. Microparticles (e.g., bioadhesive carriers)
4. Coatings (e.g., on pills and capsules)
5. Membranes (e.g., in transdermal drug delivery patches)
6. Encapsulated solids (e.g., in osmotic pumps)
7. Liquids (e.g., solutions that form gels on heating or on cooling)

1.2. Swelling Hydrogels: Nanostructure Characterization

The three most important parameters, useful in order to characterize the nanostructure of the hydrogel network, are [2, 3]:

1. The polymer volume fraction in swollen state, ϕ2,sϕ2,s
2. The number-average molecular weight of the polymer chain between two neighboring cross-linking points, M¯¯¯¯¯CM¯C
3. The corresponding mesh size, ξξ

In this paper, the notation convention will be 1, solvent (water); 2, polymer; 3, solute (drug); and higher numbers for other components (e.g., ions).

1.2.1. Polymer Volume Fraction in Swollen State

The polymer volume fraction in swollen state, $\phi_{2,s}$, is a measure of the amount of water which can be retained in hydrogel, and it is given by the ratio between the dry polymer volume, V_p, and the swollen gel volume, V_G. It can be seen also as the reciprocal of the volumetric swelling ratio [13], Q:

$$\phi_{2,s} = \frac{V_P}{V_G} = \frac{1}{Q} \tag{1}$$

1.2.2. Molecular weight between two consecutive cross-links

The molecular weight between two consecutive cross-links (of chemical or physical nature), $\overline{M}_C$, is an average measure of the degree of polymer cross-linking. In order to estimate its value, the Gibbs free energy of the system has to be evaluated in terms of the elastic and the polymer/water mixing contributions ($\Delta G_{total}=\Delta G_{elastic}+\Delta G_{mixing}$). The equilibrium condition is achieved once the change of chemical potential due to the polymer/water mixing, $\Delta\mu_{mixing}$ (expressed on the basis of entropy and heat of mixing), and the change of chemical potential due to the elastic forces, ΔμelasticΔ$\mu elastic$, are equal. The change of chemical potential due to the elastic forces can be estimated on the basis of the theory of rubber elasticity [14, 15]. Equating these two terms, an expression for determining the molecular weight between two consecutive cross-links has been derived by Flory and Rehner [16] for a polymer network swollen by absorption of solvent:

$$\frac{1}{\bar{M}_C} = \frac{2}{\bar{M}_n} - \frac{\bar{\upsilon}}{V_1} \frac{\left[ln\left(1-\phi_{2,s}\right)+\phi_{2,s}+\chi_{12}\phi_{2,s}^2\right]}{\left[\phi_{2,s}^{1/3}-\phi_{2,s}/2\right]} \tag{2}$$

where $\bar{M}_n$ is the number-average molecular weight of the polymer, $\bar{\upsilon}$ is the polymer-specific volume, V_1 is the molar volume of the solvent, and χ_{12} is the Flory polymer-solvent interaction parameter. For a network obtained starting from a polymer in solution, in a "relaxed" state, with a volume fraction $\phi_{2,r}$, by swelling with further solvent molecules, Flory [17] and Bray and Merrill [18] derived another equation able to estimate the molecular weight between two consecutive cross-links:

$$\frac{1}{\bar{M}_C} = \frac{2}{\bar{M}_n} - \frac{\bar{\upsilon}}{V_1} \frac{\left[ln\left(1-\phi_{2,s}\right)+\phi_{2,s}+\chi_{12}\phi_{2,s}^2\right]}{\phi_{2,r}\left[\left(\frac{\phi_{2,s}}{\phi_{2,r}}\right)^{1/3}-\left(\frac{\phi_{2,s}}{2\phi_{2,r}}\right)\right]} \tag{3}$$

The relaxed state is the state of the polymer immediately after the cross-linking but before the swelling. The use of equation 3 has been assessed by Merrill and Peppas [19, 20] working with PVA hydrogels, and it has been used to estimate the interaction parameter, χ_{12}, and its dependence upon polymer concentration and temperature [21]. For ionic hydrogels, i.e., hydrogels in which ionic moieties are present, the theoretical treatment has to take into account the Gibbs free energy change due to the ionic nature of the network. Therefore, the change of chemical potential due to the ionic character of the hydrogel has to be taken into account. The problem has been faced out and solved by Brannon-Peppas and Peppas [22], who had derived the following two equations, to describe the swelling of anionic and cationic hydrogels, respectively, prepared in the presence of the solvent:

$$\begin{aligned} \frac{V_1}{4IM_r}\left(\frac{\phi_{2,s}}{\bar{\upsilon}}\right)^2\left(\frac{K_a}{10^{-pH}+K_a}\right)^2 &== \left[ln\left(1-\phi_{2,s}\right)+\phi_{2,s}+\chi_{12}\phi_{2,s}^2\right]_{1/3} \\ &+\left(\frac{V_1}{\bar{\upsilon}\bar{M}_C}\right)\left(1-\frac{2\bar{M}_C}{\bar{M}_n}\right)\phi_{2,r}\left[\left(\frac{\phi_{2,s}}{\phi_{2,r}}\right)^{1/3}-\left(\frac{\phi_{2,s}}{2\phi_{2,r}}\right)\right] \end{aligned} \tag{4}$$

$$\begin{aligned} \frac{V_1}{4IM_r}\left(\frac{\phi_{2,s}}{\bar{\upsilon}}\right)^2\left(\frac{K_b}{10^{pH-14}+K_b}\right)^2 &== \left[ln\left(1-\phi_{2,s}\right)+\phi_{2,s}+\chi_{12}\phi_{2,s}^2\right]_{1/3} \\ &+\left(\frac{V_1}{\bar{\upsilon}\bar{M}_C}\right)\left(1-\frac{2\bar{M}_C}{\bar{M}_n}\right)\phi_{2,r}\left[\left(\frac{\phi_{2,s}}{\phi_{2,r}}\right)^{1/3}-\left(\frac{\phi_{2,s}}{2\phi_{2,r}}\right)\right] \end{aligned} \tag{5}$$

where I is the ionic strength; K_a and K_b are the dissociation constants for the acid and the base, respectively; and M_r is the molecular weight of the repeating unit. The molecular weight between two consecutive cross-links $\overline{M}_C$ can be obtained for the two cases solving the suitable equation for the given value of pH.

1.2.3. Mesh Size

The mesh size, ξ, also known as the correlation length between two cross-links, is a measure of the space available between the macromolecular chains. Therefore, it is related to the ability of a drug molecule to diffuse through the network to be released. It can be calculated by [23]:

$$\xi = \alpha\left(\bar{r}_0^2\right)^{1/2} \tag{6}$$

where α is the elongation ratio (which for isotropically swollen hydrogels is given by $\alpha = \phi_{2,s}^{-1/3}$) and $\left(\bar{r}_0^2\right)^{1/2}$ is the unperturbed root-mean-square of the end-to-end distance for polymer chains between two neighboring cross-links. The last one can be evaluated as follows:

$$\left(\bar{r}_0^2\right)^{1/2} = l\left(C_n N\right)^{1/2} = l\left(C_n \frac{2\overline{M}_C}{M_r}\right)^{1/2} \tag{7}$$

where l is the length of the bond along the polymer backbone (for vinyl polymers is 0.154 nm), C_n is the Flory characteristic ratio (actually, eq. 7 is the definition of Flory's characteristic ratio: $C_n = \bar{r}_0^2 / N l^2$), and $N = (2\overline{M}_C / M_r)$ is the number of links for the chain. Therefore, the mesh size for isotropically swollen hydrogels can be calculated as follows:

$$\xi = l\phi_{2,s}^{-1/3}\left(C_n \frac{2\overline{M}_C}{M_r}\right)^{1/2} \tag{8}$$

All these three parameters $\{\phi_{2,s}, \overline{M}_C, \xi\}$ are important for the drug delivery processes, since they determine the kinetics of drug diffusion and release. They, which are related to one another, can be determined theoretically or by means of experimental techniques. The ability to tailor the molecular structure of hydrogels (i.e., to design hydrogels with desired values of the three parameters) allows to tailor the hydrogels' mechanical and diffusive properties.

1.2.4. Structure-properties Relationships: Mechanical Behavior

From the mechanical point of view, the rubber elasticity theory [24], applicable also to hydrogels for relatively small deformation (less than 20 %), allows to evaluate the tensile stress τ, expressed as the force per unit area of an unstretched sample, swollen by absorption of solvent (analogous to eq. 2):

$$\tau = \frac{RT}{\bar{\upsilon}\overline{M}_C}\left(\alpha - \frac{1}{\alpha^2}\right)\left(1 - \frac{2\overline{M}_C}{\overline{M}_n}\right)\phi_{2,s}^{1/3} \tag{9}$$

For the case in which the polymer is initially in solution at mass concentration $\rho_{2,r}$, the tensile stress can be calculated as follows [19]:

$$\tau = \rho_{2,r}\frac{RT}{\overline{M}_C}\left(\alpha - \frac{1}{\alpha^2}\right)\left(1 - \frac{2\overline{M}_C}{\overline{M}_n}\right)\left(\frac{\phi_{2,s}}{\phi_{2,r}}\right)^{1/3} \tag{10}$$

To characterize the hydrogel, the cross-linking concentration, c_x (sometimes defined as cross-linking density), can be used. The cross-linking concentration is defined as the mole of cross-links for unit volume, and thus, it can be calculated as follows [19]:

$$c_x = \frac{1}{\overline{v}\overline{M}_C} = \frac{\rho}{\overline{M}_C} \tag{11}$$

where ρ is the polymer density (the inverse of polymer-specific volume). Using the cross-linking concentration and the rubber elasticity theory, the elastic shear modulus at rest, G_0, can be evaluated (e.g., equation 4.9c in [15]), in which $\overline{M}_C$ can be calculated by eq. 2, 3, 4, or 5:

$$G_0 = c_x RT = \frac{\rho}{\overline{M}_C} RT \tag{12}$$

It is worth noticing that, according to the "equivalent network theory," in which the network is represented as a collection of spherical "blobs," whose diameters represent the network mesh size ξ of the entangled structure, it is possible to relate the cross-linking concentration, c_x, with the mesh size:

$$\xi = \left(\frac{1}{N_A}\frac{6}{\pi c_x}\right)^{1/3} = \left(\frac{1}{N_A}\frac{6}{\pi \rho}\overline{M}_C\right)^{1/3} \tag{13}$$

A comparison between eq. 8 and eq. 13 is not straightforward, since eq. 13 predicts a one-third power dependence of ξ from $\overline{M}_C$, whereas eq. 8 requires the knowledge of $\phi_{2,s}$ (plus, if necessary, of $\phi_{2,r}$ and of pH) dependence upon $\overline{M}_C$ (given by eq. 2, 3, 4, or 5), and thus, it is not possible to clearly identify the dependence of ξ from $\overline{M}_C$. Generally, the equivalent network theory (eq. 13) predicts mesh size smaller than the swelling theory (eq. 8).

1.2.5. Structure-properties Relationships: Mass-Transport Behavior

The release of an active ingredient (AI, a drug molecule) from a hydrogel-based system takes place mainly by diffusion. These systems are prepared by dissolution or dispersion of the drug within the polymer matrix, which is initially dry. Under this condition, the mass transport of the drug through the matrix is negligible; therefore, no release kinetics is observable. When the matrix comes into contact with water (or biological fluids mainly composed of water), the polymer gives origin to a swollen hydrogel network, within which the drug can diffuse and then it can be released (see also section 1.3). The diffusion in hydrogel networks can be concentration gradient-driven (Fickian diffusion) or polymer relaxation-driven (non-Fickian, or viscoelastic, diffusion). The non-Fickian diffusion is known as *anomalous transport*, and its limiting case has been defined by Alfrey et al. [25] as *Case-II transport*. The Case-II transport is characterized by a sharp front between the rubbery and the glassy region of the network (see also section 1.3), advancing at a constant velocity, and the rubbery region is a swollen network at equilibrium with the solvent. Because of the constant-velocity advancement of the front, in principle the Case-II diffusion can give rise to a constant mass-flow-rate release of the drug, i.e., a zero-order release kinetics [26].

Vrentas et al. [27, 28] have suggested a simple way to establish the regions in which Fickian and non-Fickian transports take place, on the basis of the *diffusional Deborah number*, $N_{De.D}$, defined according to eq. 14, in which λ_m is the characteristic stress-relaxation time of the polymer–solvent system and θ_D is the characteristic time for the diffusion of the solvent in the polymer:

$$N_{De.D} = \frac{\lambda_m}{\theta_D} = \frac{\int_0^\infty sG(s)ds / \int_0^\infty G(s)ds}{L_{Ch}^2 / D_{1.s}} \tag{14}$$

The stress-relaxation time, λ_m, can be evaluated by integrals of the shear relaxation modulus, $G(t)$, over the entire relaxation time spectrum; the diffusion time, θ_D, is given by the ratio between the second power of a characteristic diffusional path length (for the solvent), L_{Ch}, and the diffusion coefficient of the solvent in the swollen network, $D_{1.s}$ [29]. If the change in solvent concentration during the swelling process is limited, average values for each characteristic time have to be used, and then the full process can be characterized by a single value of the Deborah number. If the change in solvent concentration is large, the Deborah number have to be calculated for both the initial and final stages, and their order of magnitude will be used to characterize the behavior of the system.

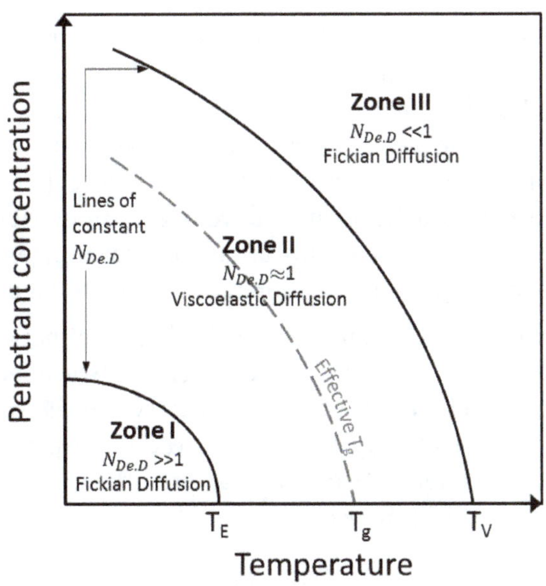

Figure 1. Schematic illustrating the different zones of diffusion, function of the temperature, and penetrant concentration. The solid lines represent lines at

constant diffusional Deborah number, $N_{De.D}$; the dashed gray line represents the effective glass transition temperature, T_g. The temperatures T_E and T_V represent the temperatures at which the polymer behaves like an elastic solid and viscous fluid, respectively. Figure redrawn on the basis of the suggestions in [27, 29].

The value of the diffusional Deborah number, $N_{De.D}$, discriminates the nature of the diffusive phenomena, as schematized in Figure 1:

Large values of the Deborah number ($N_{De.D} \gg 1$) identify **Zone I**, where the characteristic relaxation time, λ_m, is long with respect to characteristic diffusion time, θ_D: the polymer structure does not change during the water diffusion process, i.e., the polymer remains in its glassy state. The diffusion phenomenon is usually described by the conventional Fick's law, using coefficients of diffusion constant and independent from water/polymer concentrations.

Small values of the Deborah number ($N_{De.D} \ll 1$) identify **Zone III**, where the relaxation phenomenon is much faster than the diffusion phenomenon. Practically, it is a diffusion through a viscous mixture (the swollen, rubbery hydrogel), a process which can be described by again the conventional Fick's law, using coefficients of diffusion which are a strong function of water/polymer concentrations.

Intermediate values of the Deborah number ($N_{De.D} \approx 1$) identify **Zone II**, when the two characteristic times are of the same order of magnitude, i.e., the relaxation and the diffusion phenomena take place on the same time scale. This is the transition zone in which the polymer experiences its glass–rubber phase change, the mixture has a viscoelastic nature, and the diffusion is an *anomalous* transport (and its limit, the *Case-II* transport), which is non-Fickian.

Several models have been proposed to describe the deviation from the Fickian behavior, among which is the Camera-Roda and Sarti equation [30] that was proven [31] to be able to catch the *Case-II* and the *anomalous* transport behaviors with a minimum number of additional parameters. However, despite some experimental evidences of *Case II/anomalous* transport in polymers used for swellable hydrogel-based delivery systems [32-34], none of the mechanistic models developed to describe drug release have included this feature, considering an instantaneous rearrangement of the polymer chains and therefore limiting their attention to the Zone III (Figure 1) behavior.

Another way to characterize the behavior of the hydrogel network, with particular reference to drug diffusion, requires to consider the so-called swelling interface number, $N_{Sw.I}$, defined [35] by eq. 15, as the ratio between the velocity of the solvent penetration, v, and the rate of diffusion, i.e., the ratio between the diffusivity of the solute (the drug) in the swollen network, $D_{3.s}$, and the thickness of the swollen region through which the solute diffusion occurs, δ :

$$N_{Sw.I} = \frac{v}{D_{3.s} / \delta} \tag{15}$$

The analysis of diffusional Deborah number, $N_{De.D}$, and of swelling interface number, $N_{Sw.I}$, allows to identify the nature of the mass transport. In order to get a zero-order release kinetics, two conditions are expected to be satisfied [29]:

1. The movement of the solvent has to be controlled by polymer relaxation, i.e., $N_{De.D}$ has to be close to unity.
2. The solute diffusion has to be faster than the front movement (solvent movement), i.e., $N_{Sw.I}$ has to be lower than unity.

1.2.6. Modeling of the Diffusion Behavior

In order to model the diffusive phenomena which take place in hydrogel networks, several models have been proposed and they have been thoroughly reviewed [36-39], and the reader should refer to these reviews in order to have a better view of the problem. Generally, the models useful to predict the diffusivity of a solute "3" in a swollen network "s," $D_{3.s}$, with respect to the diffusivity of the same solute in the solvent "1," have the following general form [13] (the ratio $D_{3.s}/D_{3.1}$ is sometimes called "the retardation effect"):

$$\frac{D_{3.s}}{D_{3.1}} = f(\xi, \phi_2, r_s) \tag{16}$$

where ξ and ϕ_2 have been already defined and they are, respectively, the network mesh size and the polymer volume fraction, while the parameter r_s is the size of the diffusing solute. The mechanistic theories which are used in order to build the left-hand side of eq. 16 are known as hydrodynamic theories, obstruction theories, and theories based on free volume. In the following, the basics of each approach are reported along with the most common models.

Hydrodynamic theories

The hydrodynamic theory assumes that the solute molecules, depicted as hard spheres, move through the liquid phase of the network, the diffusion coefficient being dependent upon the drag force exerted by the liquid molecules on the spheres. The binary diffusive coefficient is given by the Stokes–Einstein equation, i.e., $D_{3.1}=k_{BT/f}$, where ff is the frictional draw coefficient (for hard spheres of radius R in a liquid of viscosity η, the frictional draw coefficient is $f=6\pi\eta R$), and the focus of the hydrodynamic theories is on the estimation of the frictional draw coefficient. Cukier [40] proposed eq. 17 for strongly cross-linked networks (rigid polymeric chains, chemical gels) and eq. 18 for weakly cross-linked networks (flexible polymeric chains, physical gels):

$$\frac{D_{3.s}}{D_{3.1}} = exp\left[-\left(\frac{3\pi L_c N_A}{M_f ln(L_c / 2r_f)}\right) r_s \phi_2^{0.5}\right] \tag{17}$$

$$\frac{D_{3.s}}{D_{3.1}} = exp\left[-k_c r_s \phi_2^{0.75}\right] \tag{18}$$

In eq. 17, L_c is the length of the polymeric chain, N_A is the Avogadro number, M_f is the molecular weight of the polymeric chain, and r_f is the polymer fiber radius. In eq. 18, k_c is a parameter depending on the polymer–solvent system. On the basis of the flow through a porous network, Phillips et al. [41] have obtained eq. 19:

$$\frac{D_{3,s}}{D_{3,1}} = \left[1 + \left(\frac{r_s^2}{k}\right)^{0.5} + \frac{1}{3}\frac{r_s^2}{k}\right]^{-1} \quad (19)$$

$$k = (0.31) r_s^2 \phi_2^{-1.17}$$

where k is the hydraulic permeability of the medium, considered to be made of straight and rigid fibers oriented in a random three-dimensional way.

Obstruction theories

The obstruction theories are based on the sieve effect due to the presence of an impenetrable polymer network. The diffusion takes place through the holes in the network; therefore, the path length is increased with respect to the diffusion in pure solvent. The retardation effect is thus calculated on the basis of the sieve effect. Different equations are obtained on the basis of the different model for the polymer network. A useful parameter is given by eq. 20, in which r_f is the polymer fiber radius:

$$\alpha = \left(\frac{r_s + r_f}{r_f}\right)^2 \phi_2 \quad (20)$$

Most of the models based on obstruction theories have the same mathematical structure, given by eq. 21. The two parameters $\{a,b\}$ are listed in Table 1 for different models (for Amsden's model, k_1 is a further parameter depending from the polymer–solvent system).

$$\frac{D_{3,s}}{D_{3,1}} = exp\left[-a \cdot \alpha^b\right] \quad (21)$$

Table 1. Obstruction theory-based models

Model		a	b
Ogston et al.	[42]	1.00	0.50
Johansson et al.	[43]	0.84	1.09
Amsden	[38]	$\frac{\pi}{(k_1 + 2\phi_2^{0.5})^2}$	1.00

By analogy with electrical conduction, Tsai and Strieder [44] proposed a different model, given by eq. 22:

$$\frac{D_{3.s}}{D_{3.1}}=\left(1+\frac{2}{3}\alpha\right)^{-1} \tag{22}$$

Obstruction theories are better applicable to heterogeneous networks made of rigid polymeric chains.

Combined (hydrodynamic and obstruction) theories

To improve the predictive capability of hydrodynamic and obstruction models, their retardation effects can be multiplied with each other. For example, Johansson et al. [45] combined their obstruction model [43] with the hydrodynamic model by Phillips et al. [41], obtaining eq. 23 which is a better predictor than the two parent models:

$$\frac{D_{3.s}}{D_{3.1}}=\frac{exp\left(-0.84\alpha^{1.09}\right)}{\left[1+\left(\frac{r_s^2}{k}\right)^{0.5}+\frac{1}{3}\frac{r_s^2}{k}\right]} \tag{23}$$

Another example is given by Clague and Phillips [46], who proposed a structure for the hydrodynamic term, and then they coupled this last with the obstruction model proposed by Tsai and Streider [44]. The resulting model is given here as eq. 24:

$$\frac{D_{3.s}}{D_{3.1}}=\left(1+\frac{2}{3}\alpha\right)^{-1} exp\left[-\pi\phi_2^{(0.174)ln\left(59.6r_f/r_s\right)\left(r_f/r_s\right)}\right] \tag{24}$$

Free volume theory

According to the free volume theory, a molecule of solute diffuses through the hydrogel by “jumping” into void which is present in the network. The free volume is the volume of the holes, formed on statistical bases due to random thermal motions. The total free volume is due to the water (solvent, index “ w ” or “ 1 ”) and to the polymer (index “ p ” or “ 2 ”), neglecting the presence of the drug, i.e., $v_f=\phi_1 v_{f.w}+\phi_2 v_{f.p}$. Assuming that the free volume in the polymer, $v_{f.p}$, is negligible, $v_f\approx(1-\phi_2)v_{f.w}$. The retardation effect can be evaluated on the basis of statistical reasoning, accounting for the probabilities of finding holes in the water free volume, $v_{f.w}$, close enough to the molecule which is moving, accounting that such holes are big enough and accounting for the sieving effects by the polymeric chains. Different estimations for these probabilities give different results for the retardation effect; however, the general structure of models for retardation effect, based on free volume theory, is always given by eq. 25. The two parameters $\{a,b\}$ are listed in Table 2 for the most common models. The parameter “ a ” plays the role of a sieving factor of the polymer network on the solute molecule, and for drug size smaller than the mesh size ($r_s \ll \xi$), aa is unity.

$$\frac{D_{3.s}}{D_{3.1}}=a\cdot exp\left[-b\left(\frac{\phi_2}{1-\phi_2}\right)\right] \tag{25}$$

Table 2. Free volume theory-based models

		a	b
Yasuda et al.	[47]	P_0	$\frac{Ba^*}{v_{f.w}}$
Peppas and Reinhart	[48]	$k_1\left(\frac{\overline{M}_c-\overline{M}_c^*}{\overline{M}_n-\overline{M}_c^*}\right)$	$k_2r_s^2$
Lustig and Peppas	[49]	$\left(1-\frac{r_s}{\xi}\right)$	$\frac{\gamma\pi\lambda}{v_{f.w}}r_s^2\cong 1$
Hennink et al.	[50]	Ψ	$k_2r_s^2$

In Table 2, the meanings of the parameters are P_0 is the probability of finding an opening between the polymer chains (sieve effect); a^* is the effective cross-sectional area of the solute molecule; B is a model parameter; k_1 and k_2 are two structural constants, different for each polymer–solvent system; $\overline{M}_c^*$ is a critical molecular weight between cross-links to allow solute passage; γ is a numerical factor ($0.5\le\gamma\le1.0$) used to correct overlapping of free volume between more than one solute molecule; λ is the jump length, which is roughly equivalent to the solute diameter ($\lambda\approx2r_s$) ; and Ψ is the sieving factor.

All the models listed in equations 17 to 25 are useful to have an idea of the retardation effect, but still there is not a single approach able to describe the behavior of all the hydrogels. Therefore, for modeling purposes, a phenomenological approach, based on simple equations, with a limited number of fitting parameters, is highly desirable. As a result of the free-volume approach, a simple equation useful to predict the diffusive coefficient for a given molecule specie "i" in hydrogel, with respect to the diffusive coefficient of the same molecule in the swollen network (at equilibrium conditions), $D_{i.H}/D_{i.s}$, has been proposed by Fujita [51], used firstly by Korsmeyer et al. [52], to describe the transport of both the solvent (i=1) and the solute (i=3) within the polymeric network:

$$\frac{D_{i.H}}{D_{i.s}}=exp\left[-\beta_i\left(1-\frac{\phi_1}{\phi_{1.s}}\right)\right] \tag{26}$$

where β_i is the single parameter of the equation, and the effect of this parameter on the predictions has been extensively tested by Korsmeyer et al. [53].

1.3. Phenomenology of Drug Release from Swelling Hydrogels

In controlled drug delivery, the main goal is to design systems able to give tailored release profiles, as function of the time as well as in response to external stimuli (sensitive systems) and/or in a certain environment (targeted delivery systems). One of the main goals of controlled drug delivery is a system able to give a zero-order release kinetics, i.e., a constant-rate release, for which the mass flow rate of drug released is designed to be equal to the rate of consumption of the drug by the body (by metabolism, excretion, and reactions with its targets), causing a constant plasma concentration of the active principle. Graham and McNeill [54] were the first to prove that by combination of the device geometry, nature of hydrogel, and initial concentration profile of the drug, a zero-order release kinetics is possible working with hydrogel-based systems (morphine release from pessaries shaped as hollow cylinders made of PEO, with a U-shaped initial concentration of the drug through the cylinder wall). This was the starting point for several studies, development, and applications of hydrogel-based pharmaceutical systems for drug delivery. Several pharmaceuticals based on this approach have made their way up to the market.

A full understanding of the phenomena involved, and their detailed mathematical description (modeling), is an objective still unfulfilled. The detailed knowledge of the transport phenomena involved is the key prerequisite in developing a reliable mathematical model useful for the prediction of the release kinetics as function of the formulation parameters or of the external conditions [55]; on the other hand, the availability of a reliable mathematical model of the drug release process could allow to theoretically predict the drug release profile for a given, newly designed, pharmaceutical product, reducing the number of necessary experiments and facilitating the development of new pharmaceuticals [11].

The basics of release mechanisms from swellable hydrogel-based pharmaceuticals are summarized in the following and they are schematized in Figure 2.

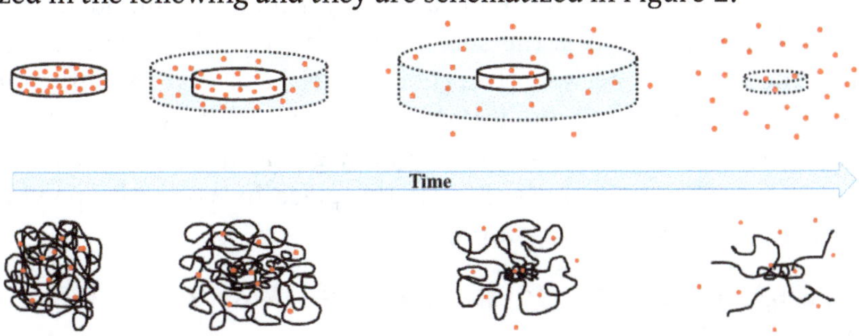

Figure 2. Drug release from a matrix (tablet) made of swellable hydrogel. The phenomena (described in the text) of water uptake, swelling, polymer chain relaxation, drug diffusion, polymer chain disentanglement, and polymer erosion are graphically depicted.

When swellable hydrogel-based matrix comes into contact with water, the following are observed:

1. The water diffuses into the matrix.
2. The water acts as a plasticizer, lowering the polymer glass transition temperature, TgTg, thus causing the glass–rubber transition, the gel formation, and polymer swelling (polymer chain relaxation).
3. The (soluble) drug dissolves and diffuses through the gel layer.

4. The drug can be released in the dissolution medium.
5. Finally, the polymer dissolves (erodes) at the matrix surface. In case of insoluble drugs, erosion is the main mechanism which allows drug release in the external medium.

This sequence of steps, suggested by Siepmann et al. [56], is coherent with a space distribution of the polymer chains as described by Ju et al. [57, 58], who identified several regions in a hydrogel-based matrix exposed to a water-based dissolution medium:

1. An inner *dry glassy core*, in which the polymer is practically un-hydrated
2. A *glassy gel layer*, in which the polymeric chains have very strong entanglements
3. A *rubbery gel layer*, with highly swollen hydrogels and strong entanglement
4. A *diffusion layer*, with weak entanglements within the few polymeric chains present
5. The external, or *bulk*, medium, in which the dissolved polymeric chains are found

These layers, which are not rigidly defined and thus not clearly identifiable, are characterized by a polymer concentration decreasing from the inner regions toward the outer regions, a water concentration decreasing from the outer regions toward the inner regions. Furthermore, they allow to identify several "fronts," i.e., interfaces which roughly locate the place in which most of the phenomena take place [59]. In particular, the interface between the diffusion layer and the bulk medium is known as the *erosion front* (because it is the surface on which most of the polymer erosion takes place), the interface between the rubbery gel layer and the diffusion layer is known as the *diffusion front* (because it is the place in which most of the drug diffusion takes place), and the interface between the glassy gel layer and the rubbery gel layer is known as the *swelling front* (because it is the place in which the polymer swells, experiencing the glass–rubber transition).

1.4. Swellable Hydrogels in Pharmaceutical Delivery: A Means to Comprehension

Once the general framework of the phenomena which take place during the drug release from a hydrogel-based pharmaceutical system has been clarified, there are still two needs:

1. The single phenomenon (e.g., the water uptake, the drug diffusion, the polymer dissolution, the shape deformation due to the swelling) has to be quantified, i.e., one or more experimental method(s) have to be pointed out, applied, and validated in order to gather quantitative data useful to confirm the hypothesized phenomenon and to know its extent.
2. Each single observed and quantified phenomenon has to be described by a mathematical sub-model, and all of them together should be collected in a comprehensive mathematical model, able to reproduce quantitatively all the

observed phenomena: at this level, the model can be seen as a *descriptive* tool. Once all the sub-models have been properly tuned using experimental data, the model could become *predictive*, i.e., able to describe the behavior of a novel system before it is tested or to describe the behavior of an existing system working outside the range of operative conditions within which it has been tested.

The road to the goal of a predictive model is pictorially depicted in Figure 3: on the right of the arrow, several experimental approaches published in literature have been listed (grouped by the main technique adopted in each paper); on the left of the arrow, the succession of modeling approaches proposed in literature is listed (grouped by similarity between the approaches). Of course, the lists are not exhaustive, since a huge number of papers on the topic have been published in the last years. In the remainder of the chapter, the experimental approaches (section 2) and the modeling approaches (section 3) will be reviewed in better details.

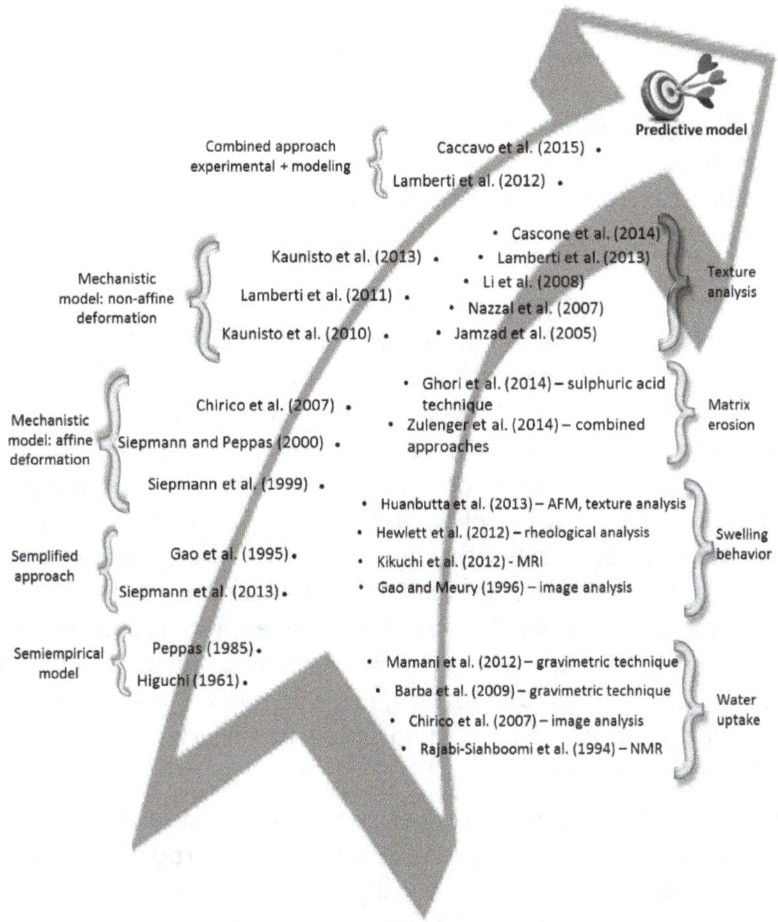

Figure 3. The evolution of experimental approaches (on the right of the arrow) and of theoretical approaches (on the left of the arrow) reported in literature with reference to the study of drug release from matrix made of swellable hydrogels.

2. EXPERIMENTAL METHOD

The study of hydrogel-based systems started on simplified systems (simple geometries such as cylinders or sheets, in which only 1D – for example, lateral – water uptake is allowed) and has been continued on more complicated systems (i.e., pharmaceutical forms composed of several units, each with a specific behavior). The complexity of the whole process which takes place during the drug release from hydrogel-based matrices has led to the development of several experimental techniques to deeply understand the behavior of these polymers.

2.1. Factors influencing the Drug Release

The factors influencing the drug release from hydrogel matrices have been studied for a long time to create a pharmaceutical form with the desired release profile both theoretically and experimentally. In fact, it has to be taken into account that, in addition to the phenomena which take place during a hydrogel hydration, the presence of a local drug concentration influences the polymer behavior [60]. As described in section 1.3, during the water uptake, the polymer chains are subjected to a relaxation, and the presence of an additional component (the drug) changes both the swelling osmotic pressure and the time-dependent relaxation process. Of course, not only the drug has an impact on the release rate from a hydrogel based matrix, but the entire formulation and its constituents influence the matrix behavior.

2.1.1. Influence of the formulation composition

Among these variables, the polymer concentration and its viscosity grade are the most used to control and modulate the drug release [61] due to the fact that the drug release profile is affected both kinetically and mechanistically by these two variables. For example, changes in HPMC (hydroxypropyl methylcellulose) percentages in the formulation can result in a wide range of release rate, but usually, faster drug release rate is obtained with lower HPMC content, as well as faster polymer release is obtained in these conditions. In the analysis of the influence of the HPMC viscosity grade on the drug release, it was demonstrated that the release rate decreases with the increase of the viscosity of the used polymer, but there is a "limiting HPMC viscosity grade" and beyond its value, no further decrease in the release rate is detected; usually, this value is 15000 cP [61]. These analyses can be performed only by evaluating the drug release in the dissolution medium; instead, more complex experimental methods are necessary to evaluate the microscopic variation in surface topography during the swelling such as the cryogenic SEM [62].

In the optimization of the matrix formulation, it is important to evaluate not only the composition of the matrix but even the micrometric properties such as the bulk density of the powders used. The true density of the powders can be measured using a pycnometer. The bulk density can be calculated pouring a pre-weighted amount of powder into a graduated cylinder and measuring the occupied volume. The tapped bulk density can be calculated by measuring the powder volume after tapping the cylinder three times from a defined height and with a constant frequency (i.e., from

2.5 cm height every 2 s); the ultimate tapped density can be calculated after continued tapping till no further volume decrease is observed [62]. The compressibility index was calculated using the bulk and ultimate tapped bulk density.

2.1.2. Influence of the polymer properties

In addition to the type of formulation, the drug release profile from a pharmaceutical form is affected by factors closely related to the polymer, such as its particle size distribution [63]. Studying the release rate of propranolol hydrochloride from HPMC K15M tablet, it was found that the release rate decreased as the particle size of polymer was reduced till about 180 μm. Further reduction caused no further decrease in dissolution rate. The different particle size fractions are usually obtained by sieving. This behavior is probably due to the fact that the larger-sized fraction of HPMC absorbs water faster than the smaller one [63]. These water uptake studies were performed by using DSC (differential scanning calorimetry). Of course, the behavior of the matrix strongly depends on the polymer chosen to constitute the pharmaceutical form. For example, Zuleger et al. [64] found that neither viscosity grade nor the particle size or the compaction pressure of methyl hydroxyethyl cellulose (MHEC) has a strong impact on the release rate of the drug embedded in these matrices. Thus, there is not a general rule from the matrix behavior; it depends on the formulation and drug used. Moreover, even the dissolution medium can influence the release kinetics, both in the case in which the polymer is sensitive to the medium pH and to the ionic strength of the medium.

A recent review on the factors affecting the drug release from hydrophilic matrices was published by Maderuelo et al. [65]. The authors analyzed the effect of different variables, which depend on drug (such as its solubility, particle size, and initial dose), on polymer (such as its particle size, viscosity, and the influence of the dissolution medium), or on formulation (such as manufacturing process) on the drug release kinetics.

2.2. Evaluation of the Water Uptake, Matrix Erosion, and Drug Release

The water uptake is a key parameter to determine the swelling phenomenon of a hydrogel and, as a consequence, the drug release from a matrix. For this reason, several scientists have developed different methods to quantify the water diffusion into the polymeric matrix.

The simplest technique used to evaluate the weight gain after a certain dissolution time, which is directly connected to the water uptake, is the gravimetrical method. According to this method, the weighted pharmaceutical form is immersed in the dissolution medium and, at predetermined time intervals, it is withdrawn from the medium, lightly patted, and weighted, and then it is dried until constant weight is reached [66]. The percent weight gain and the mass loss can be calculated according to the following equations:

$$\text{Weight gain}(\%) = \frac{\text{wet weight-dry weight}}{\text{dry weight}} \cdot 100 \tag{27}$$

$$\text{Mass loss}(\%) = \frac{\text{initial weight-dry weight}}{\text{initial weight}} \cdot 100 \tag{28}$$

The percent of mass loss is directly connected to the matrix erosion and drug release (if drug is contained in the polymer matrix) due to the fact that, after drying, only the polymer and drug remain in the matrix, meaning that all the weight loss during the dissolution is imputable to the dissolution of drug and polymer in the external medium. Investigation of matrix hydration and erosion is a fundamental approach to understand the mechanisms involved during the drug release and the parameters which influence the matrix behavior [67]. For example, if the mass loss follows an increasing kinetics with the dissolution time, probably the controlling mechanism in the pharmaceuticals is the erosion of the matrix; on the contrary, if the weight gain continuously increases, the controlling mechanism can be attributed to the swelling. On these bases, Mamani et al. [68] evaluated the influence of components ratio on the release kinetics varying the composition and pH of the dissolution medium.

Thus, the information which can be obtained by the estimation of the mass determination via gravimetrical analysis is the concentration profiles of water and polymer. If the matrix analyzed is composed also of a drug, with the aid of an analytical technique to determine the amount of drug released (i.e., the spectrometric method), all the macroscopic profiles can be measured [69]. Indeed, during the dissolution, the drug leaves the pharmaceutical form and dissolves in the dissolution medium. A typical dissolution test is performed using the standardized apparatuses approved by the USP (United States Pharmacopeia), which are numbered from 1 to 7 [70]. Withdrawing samples of the medium at certain time intervals, it is possible to know the amount of drug released and then, by the difference with the initial drug content, which is usually known by the manufacturer, the amount of drug still contained in the tablet. Repeating these tests for several dissolution times, the drug concentration profile can be evaluated. Usually, the percentage of drug release is evaluated according to the following expression:

$$\text{Drug release}(\%) = \frac{\text{drug released in the dissolution medium}}{\text{initial drug content}} \cdot 100 \tag{29}$$

The typical drug release profile from a matrix composed of a hydrogel (HPMC) and a drug (theophylline) is shown in Figure 4, red circles on the right axis [34]. As could be expected, the release kinetics is higher at the beginning of the dissolution (after 3 h of dissolution, about 30 % of the drug is released) and tends to decrease with time, till all of the drug contained into the matrix reaches the dissolution medium. On the contrary, the mass of the drug still contained in the matrix is shown in Figure 4 as green stars, on the left axis. It can be measured by the difference between the drug released and the initial amount of drug in the tablet or by a more direct measure. According to this method, after the chosen dissolution time, the tablet is removed from the medium, weighted, and dried. Then, the tablet is immersed into a medium till complete dissolution, and another spectrometric analysis can be performed on the medium to evaluate the concentration of the drug. Usually this technique is used to perform a check on the total amount of drug in the matrix, which can be different with respect to the theoretical one, i.e., due to manufacture errors.

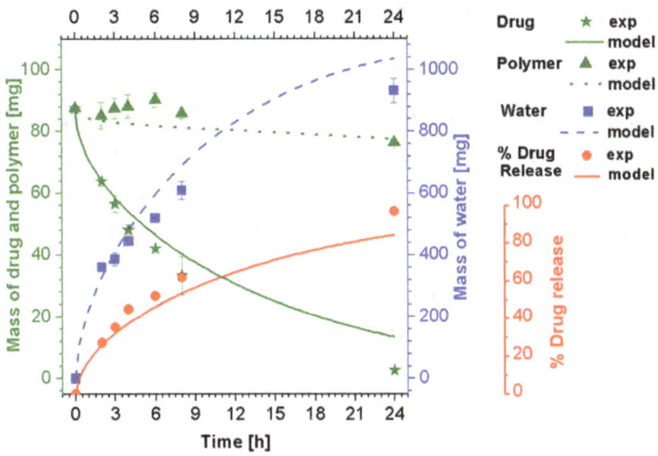

Figure 4. Mass evolution inside a swelling matrix during a dissolution test. Drug and polymer mass evolutions (in green) are reported on the left axis and water mass evolution (in blue) on the right axis. On the red axis, the percentage of drug released is shown.

Using the gravimetric technique to evaluate the total amount of water absorbed by the matrix, the method previously described to evaluate the weight gained by the pharmaceutical form can be used. After a certain dissolution time, the matrix can be removed from the dissolution medium, weighted, dried, and weighted again. By the difference between the wet and dry weights, the amount of water taken during the dissolution (after the predetermined time) can be evaluated. In Figure 4, the mass of water absorbed by the tablet is shown as blue squares, on the right axis. As could be seen from the graph, the amount of water which can be absorbed by a hydrogel is well beyond the initial amount of polymer, reaching ten times its value during the time interval shown. The last component which has to be quantified is the polymer. This can be done by a simple technique which provides that once the wet weight of the matrix after a certain dissolution time is known and once the drug and water amounts are quantified, the polymer mass can be calculated by the difference between these masses, according to the following expression:

$$\text{Polymer mass} = \text{wet weight}\left(\text{after dissolution}\right) - \left(\text{water} + \text{drug}\right)\text{ masses inside the matrix} \tag{30}$$

Another technique which allows to directly evaluate the amount of polymer dissolved in the dissolution medium and then of the polymer into the tablet is the sulfuric acid technique, recently re-proposed by Ghori et al. [71]. This method consists of taking from the dissolution medium samples of 1 mL at predetermined dissolution times and, after filtration, adding 1 mL of a solution of 5 % phenol in 0.1 M hydrochloric acid, followed by 5 mL of concentrated sulfuric acid. After 10 min of shaking, the solution is cooled (the reaction taking place is strongly exothermic), and a spectrometric analysis can be performed, at 490 nm of wavelength, due to the fact that the solution assumes an intense colored aspect. Besides, this method is more complicated than the measurement of the difference between components; it is a direct measurement of the polymer mass, which means a more reliable matrix characterization.

2.3. Mass Evolution Inside the Matrix

The described gravimetric technique has the practical advantage to be a very simple technique to determine the macroscopic behavior of a pharmaceutical matrix (i.e., the total water uptake, the total mass of polymer eroded by the dissolution medium) or films [72]. On the other hand, it is a destructive technique (different samples have to be removed from the dissolution medium and dried, one for each dissolution time) which gives no information about the concentration profiles inside the matrix and about how they vary with time. For this reason, it is clear that the macroscopic analyses described above are not sufficient to characterize the matrix behavior. Over the years, several experimental techniques have been developed to evaluate the mass evolution inside pharmaceutical matrices.

2.3.1. Image analysis technique

To evaluate the polymer concentration across the gel layer during the tablet hydration, a semiquantitative in situ technique based on the image analysis was developed [73]. According to this method, a HPMC matrix tablet was mounted on a weighted pin and inserted in a vessel filled with the dissolution medium. This stirred vessel was placed on top of a light box. Depending on the orientation of the tablet, the swelling along the radial or axial position can be observed and recorded by a black-and-white camera equipped with a macroscopic zoom lens mounted above the tablet. The light source was represented by a light box containing two fluorescent light tubes. The whole apparatus was closed to avoid the entrance of external sources of light. Each digitalized image had a gray level from 0 (black) to 255 (white) representing the relative scattered light intensity. To understand and explain the results obtained, it was necessary to correlate the scattered light intensity with the concentration of HPMC in the gel layer. This has been done in preparing a series of polymer solutions at known concentrations and evaluating their scattered light intensity, and, by the fitting of these data, a calibration curve to interpret the data was obtained. Due to the complexity involved in the simultaneous evaluation of what happen during the polymer matrix swelling, Bettini et al. [59] used the image analysis to evaluate the movement of the swelling front (as defined in section 1.3) of a tablet during the dissolution in a simplified system which allows the water penetration only in the lateral surface of the tablet. This system was obtained confining the tablet between two transparent Plexiglass disks; in this way, only the radial swelling is allowed, making the system simpler to analyze. Recording the swelling of the matrix during dissolution through the transparent disks, the obtained images were analyzed with image analysis software. Once more, this technique gives no information about the mass fraction evolutions inside the matrix.

On these bases, a nondestructive test to determine the water mass fraction along the radial profile of a pure HPMC tablet was developed by Chirico et al. [55]. Being the tablet composed only by the polymer, this work was focused only on the water penetration inside the matrix, and the tablet was confined between two glass slides to limit the water uptake only in the radial surface. The system composed of the tablet, confined between the glass slides was immersed in the dissolution medium, colored by adding trypan blue to enhance the visibility of the water penetration, and recorded with a camera. Both the camera and the dissolution chamber were closed in a dark room to avoid exposure to external light. Light intensity profiles were evaluated starting from the pictures by the image analysis technique. The analyses were performed, considering the picture as a matrix composed of pixels with intensity values ranging from 0 (white) to 255 (black). To relate the water mass fraction to the light intensity, a relation was adopted:

$$\left(\frac{I - I_0}{I_{max} - I_0}\right)^{\gamma} = \frac{\omega_1 - \omega_{10}}{\omega_{1eq} - \omega_{10}} \tag{31}$$

where ω_{10} and ω_{1eq} are the initial water mass fraction in the tablet (in case of a dry tablet, it is equal to 0) and the equilibrium water mass fraction in the hydrogel, respectively. Concerning the light intensity, it was varied between I_0, which is a plateau value observed at the matrix core, corresponding to the brightest image, and I_{max}, which is the maximum value observed at the fully hydrated gel, corresponding to the darkest image. Since both the variables (I and ω_1) vary from 0 to 1, the authors chose to apply the simplest relation between them, a linear one, which is realized when parameter γ is equal to 1.

A typical water mass fraction profile obtained via image analysis is reported in Figure 5, a) as gray dotted lines. Moreover, an image of the hydrate tablet after 1 day of dissolution is shown as an inset. Comparing the evolution of the water mass fraction calculated via image analysis and the appearance of the tablet, the correspondence is clear. In fact, in the picture, still visible is the glassy core, in which only a small amount of water is penetrated and the water fraction is the smallest; then it starts to increase due to the fact that the image becomes darker. Then, the swelling front (as defined in section 1.3) becomes visible with a decrease of the light intensity, which leads to an apparently inconsistent decrease of the water mass fraction; actually, this decrease is due to the presence of the swelling front. Then, the light intensity increases gradually, due to the fact that the gel is more hydrated as the radius increases, until the erosion radius is reached, which indicates the final dimension of the swollen tablet, corresponding to a light intensity and water fraction equal to 1. The main drawback of the described technique is the fact that only the water uptake inside the matrix can be evaluated due to the fact that the tablet is composed only of the hydrogel. In fact, the presence of the drug could disturb the image analysis, leading to mistakes in the evaluation of water concentration inside the pharmaceutical form. For this reason, a more complete method taking into account also the drug presence has to be developed.

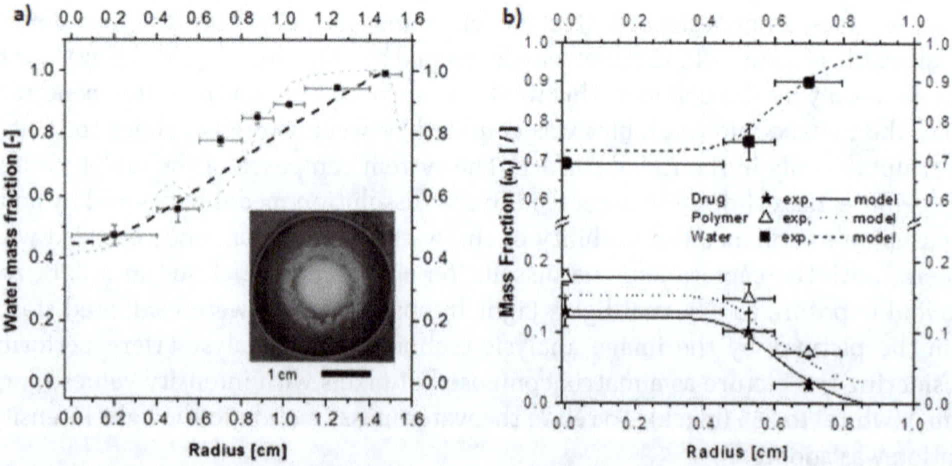

Figure 5. a) Water mass fraction along the radial direction after 48 h of dissolution of a radial system. The full squares are the experimental data obtained by the gravimetric analysis; the dotted gray curve is the result of the image analysis; the dashed black curve is the model prediction. In the inset, the real photo of the matrix used for the image analysis. b) Mass fraction evolutions along the radial direction for semioverall system after 6 h of dissolution (the values are averaged along the thickness direction). The scatters are the experimental data; the curves are the model predictions. In both the graphs, the vertical bars represent the standard deviation between the experimental runs, and the horizontal bars represent the extension of the section cut by the punch.

2.3.2. Gravimetric technique

In 2009, Barba et al. [69] proposed a method to quantify all the components inside a matrix at a given dissolution time. This approach, based on the gravimetric technique, was applied firstly on a simplified system, which allows the water uptake only from the lateral surface (the so-called radial system), and then to a more complex system in which the water can penetrate along the whole exchange area (the so-called semioverall system) [34]. The experimental procedure used to evaluate the mass evolutions (polymer, HPMC; drug, theophylline; and water) inside a swollen matrix is illustrated in Figure 6. In the case of the radial systems, the first step was to confine the matrix, containing a polymer, a drug, and eventually an initial water content, between two glass disks. Instead, in the case of the semioverall systems, the matrix was glued at the center of one glass slide, which represents the symmetry plane for the experiment; in fact, the tablet weighted the half part with respect to that used in the radial system. Then, the system was immersed in the dissolution medium until a predetermined time; at the end of this time, the swollen matrix was removed from the dissolution medium (step 2 in Figure 6) and the excess water was removed; in the case of the radial system, the superior slab was carefully removed. The swollen matrix was cut by a series of punches characterized by a thin wall centered in the matrix center (step 3 in Figure 6). The punches had a decreasing diameter: chosen the first punch and centered, all the matrix material external at the punch is recovered on a watch glass (step 4 in Figure 6) and weighted (step 5 in Figure 6). This material contained all the polymer, drug, and water in the wet tablet at greater radii than the punch one. Then, a punch with a small diameter was used for a second cut and, once more, the material recovered in another watch glass. These operations were repeated since a central core was reached, recovered, and weighted. All the samples collected were dried in oven at 45 °C (step 6 in Figure 6) until a constant weight was reached, meaning that all the water initially contained in the wet material was removed (step 7 in Figure 6). These last three phases can be combined together using an infrared moisture meter, as suggested by Tahara et al. [74]. Using this device, the wet material was weighted and dried simultaneously at a temperature of 120 °C, until the ratio of decreasing sample weights becomes less than 0.5 % for 5 min. In the last step of the gravimetrical analysis, each glass was immersed into a vessel containing distilled water till complete dissolution with the aim of quantifying, spectrometrically, the amount of drug still in the matrix.

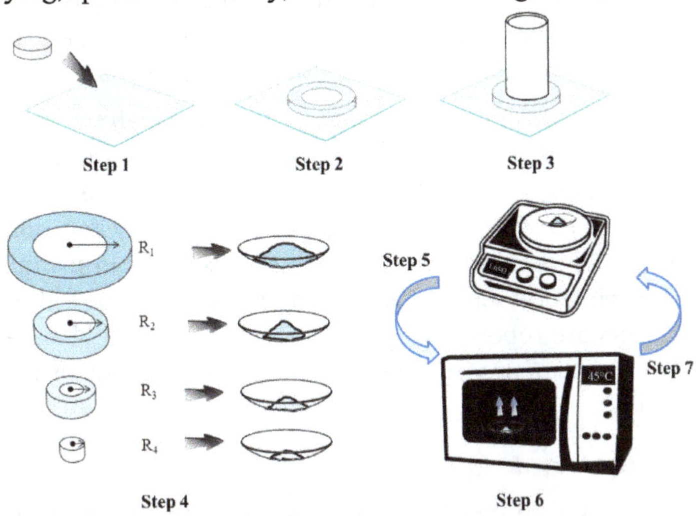

Figure 6. Experimental procedure used to evaluate the mass evolutions inside a swollen matrix by gravimetric technique.

Using this method, it is possible to evaluate how the amounts of drug, polymer, and water vary not only with the dissolution time but even with the matrix radius. A typical behavior of a matrix composed initially of 50 % wt of polymer and drug after 6 h of dissolution is reported in Figure 5, b). In this graph, the vertical bars represent the standard deviation between the experimental runs, and the horizontal bars represent the extension of the section cut by the punch. In fact, if the external section is considered, it ranges from 0.6 to 0.8 cm, which means that the punch used had a diameter of 0.6 cm and the wet matrix material recovered had a diameter greater than 0.6 cm and lower than 0.8 cm, which is the maximum radius reached by the swollen matrix. The experimental data were represented at the mean radius of the section of interest, as an average value of mass amount in that section. In Figure 5, the matrix was divided into three sections, two annuli and a central core, and the internal drug and polymer profiles are illustrated as full stars and empty triangles, respectively. As could be seen, both the polymer and drug tend to decrease with the radius; this is easily predictable because, due to the water penetration into the matrix, this tends to unfold the polymeric chains and the drug can easily diffuse outward in the dissolution medium. On the other hand, in the central glassy core, the water is not penetrated yet, and the fractions of the drug and polymer are higher. Concerning the polymer behavior, its fraction decreases with the matrix radius; this is due to the swelling phenomenon which takes place from the interface of the dissolution medium) toward the inner regions. Concerning the water profile in the swollen matrix, it is shown as full squares in Figure 5, b). The water mass fraction increases with the matrix radius, till it reaches a fraction equal to 1 at the interface with the dissolution medium, which is completely composed of water.

With the aid of this technique, the swollen tablet is completely characterized not only from a macroscopic point of view but also microscopically, because even the internal concentration profiles are known. As previously mentioned, the main drawback of this experimental method is that it is destructive for the sample analyzed.

The water profiles inside the matrix obtained via image analysis are compared with the gravimetric ones in Figure 5, a). To make comparable the results obtained by the gravimetric and the image analysis techniques, the γ value in eq. 31 was optimized to minimize the distance between the two sets of data for a system composed only of polymer and water. The found value is 0.425; thus, it is far from the unity [75], and it depends on the experimental setup. The gravimetric data are the full squares, and the image analysis results are reported as gray dotted line. As could be seen, in the most part of the profile, the data are in good agreement, even if they originate from very different techniques.

2.3.3. Magnetic resonance imaging

Nuclear magnetic resonance imaging (NMRI) is a technique used to produce a two-dimensional map of the density of nuclei inside a thin slice of a more complex object. Besides, the NMRI technique has been extensively used in various fields, such as medical diagnostic and polymer science; in recent years, it has been applied as a noninvasive method to study the behavior of hydrophilic matrices [76]. Usually the nucleus of interest is ^{1}H in water molecules; thus, the images show the spatial variation of the local water concentration inside the sample; for this reason, this technique is of great aid to characterize the water content inside a swollen matrix during the dissolution. Moreover, the NMRI technique provides an excellent method to evaluate the self-diffusion coefficients, a measure of transport due to the Brownian motion of molecules in the absence of a chemical concentration gradient [77]. The image experiments were usually carried out to measure the water diffusion inside a polymeric matrix and to observe the changing diameter of a tablet during the swelling [78].

Nuclear magnetic resonance imaging (NMRI) is a branch of NMR spectroscopy, usually used to study the swelling and diffusion phenomena of pharmaceutical forms under static conditions (without stirring). The extent of the swelling can be identified by this technique, identifying the position of the interface between the dry core of the tablet and the swollen region. On the other hand, the erosion front can be identified at the interface between the dissolution medium and the swollen region. A great improvement in the use of the MRI technique had been the development of a release cell where the images could be recorded directly at different times during the dissolution, happening in a stirred device [79]. The stirring of the medium was realized in a small release cell, which was equipped with a rotating disk. Gluing the tablet under the rotating disk, the relative movement of the tablet and the dissolution medium ensured the stirring. During the test, the MRI probe was placed at 1 mm below the rotating disk to optimize the tablet position. The release cell is connected to a vessel containing the dissolution medium, kept at constant temperature, which is continuously pumped in the cell by a peristaltic pump. The described setup was used to describe the water uptake into polyethylenoxide (PEO) matrices during a dissolution test [79]. The disk rotation was switched off 2 min before the start of imaging sequences, both in axial and radial directions, and samples of the dissolution medium were collected. The study of the water uptake in the tablet was performed using a multi-spin pulse sequence, in which the signal intensity is weighted on the bases of the proton spin–spin and spin–lattice relaxation times. Due to the very short proton spin–spin relaxation time, differences on the image intensity were mainly dependent on the properties of the dissolution medium. Once the experimental setup was built, it was possible to use this device to better understand the swelling and erosion phenomena happening during the dissolution of a complex matrix. For example, extended release tablets of HPMC were studied via this NMR microimaging technique, and the influence of additives solubility on the matrix behavior was analyzed [80]. By the use of this technique, the authors found that the rate of matrix erosion depends not only on the polymer fraction but even on the solubility of the additives used in the formulation and on the HPMC substituent heterogeneity [81].

In Figure 7, a), a typical example of the use of the NMRI technique to evaluate the water content of a matrix during dissolution is shown. The real picture was taken after 2.7 h of dissolution. At each pixel of the image (128x128) is associated a numerical value that, with the proper scaling factor (given by the instrument), can be related to the proton T2 relaxation. The proton T2 relaxation in turn is mainly attributed to water protons; therefore, it can be related to the amount of water through specific calibration curves. These calibration curves were obtained by analyzing water solutions with known concentrations of solutes. The calibration curve equation obtained with an exponential decay function of the second order was

$$H_2O\%_{(w/w)} = a_1 - a_2 \exp\left(-\frac{T2}{a_3}\right) - a_4 \exp\left(-\frac{T2}{a_5}\right) \tag{32}$$

where $a_1 \div a_5$ are specific parameters. The range of confidence of the calibration curve is 60–100% w/w of water content [34]. The experimental results were shown using different colors to indicate different hydration levels. For example, the blue color was used to indicate the layer of the matrix which showed a percentage of water, included between 60 and 65%. The results showed a water concentration profile along the " r " and " z " axes with the 97% w/w of water content on the erosion boundaries and with a decreasing trend going toward the tablet core. It is worth noting that in this system, the most hydrated layer, 90–97 % w/w, is extremely thin, due to the high system erosion.

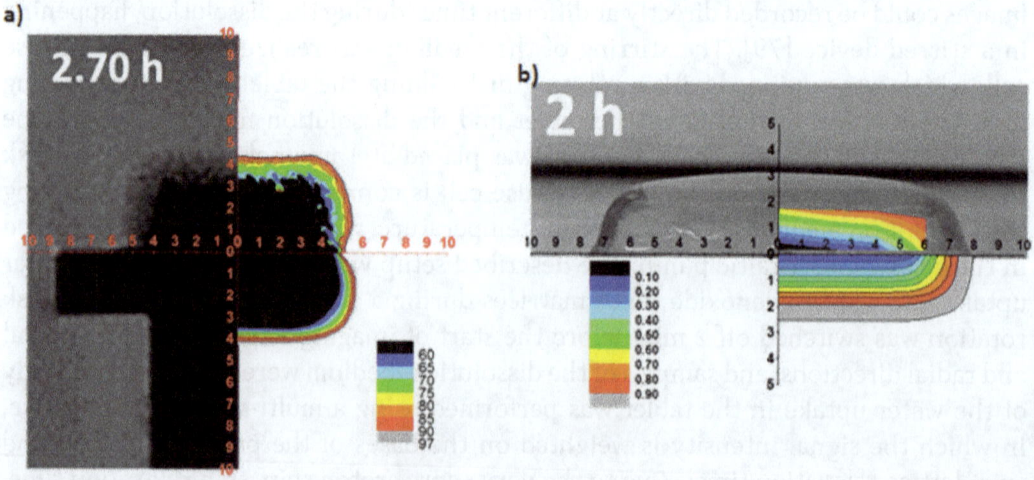

Figure 7. a) On the left, NMR image of a swollen matrix composed of HPMC after 2.7 h of dissolution. At the top, experimental water fraction distribution; at the bottom, calculated water fraction distribution. b) On the left top, photo of a semioverall system after 2 h of dissolution (the matrix was cut along its diameter). On the right top, experimental water mass fraction obtained by texture analysis; on the bottom right, model predictions. In both images, the dimensions are in mm; the color scale is referred to the water content fraction (black = lower water content; gray = fully hydrated matrix).

2.3.4. Texture analysis

A recent approach in pharmaceutical research and development consists of the study of the correlation between drug release and polymer hydration via texture analysis. In general, variation in the textural and physic-mechanical properties could be associated with changes in gel layer and glassy core [82]. One of the first approaches in using the texture analysis to correlate the mechanical properties of the polymeric gels and the water content was that of Yang et al. [82]. They proposed the use of a texture analyzer to evaluate the stress–strain behavior of the polymeric matrix. A matrix composed of HPMC and PEO at different compositions was subjected to dissolution tests. After predetermined time intervals, they were removed from the dissolution medium and subjected to a texture analysis. A probe of 2 mm in diameter was forced to penetrate inside the matrix and a transducer measured the resistance force opposed by the material to the probe penetration. The penetration was ended when a trigger force was reached (0.7 g), the value chosen in a manner in which it was possible to distinguish the glassy polymer from the polymer gel. From the slope of the force–displacement diagrams obtained, it was possible to establish the position of the gel layer; in fact, the resistance encountered by the texture probe is dependent on the gel strength; thus, in the inner part of the tablet, where the water was not penetrated and the gel was strong, the slope of the diagram was very high. On the contrary, in the external parts of the matrix, where the water was penetrated, the resistance encountered by the probe is lower, due to the fact that the gel was hydrated and the slope of the diagrams results to be less pronounced. Based on these considerations, the glassy core and rubbery gel interface can be determined, as well as the overall gel strength. To validate the reliability of these evaluations, the texture experimental data were compared with the position of the gel fronts measured by the NMRI technique. The main drawback of this method is the fact that it is not quantitative: in fact, only the position of the gel front can be quantified, not the water content in the matrix.

In addition to the determination of gel layer thickness and the movement of the erosion and swelling fronts, the texture analysis could be used to determine the total work of probe penetration inside the swollen matrix [66]. Using a method similar to that described previously, swollen thickness was determined by measuring the total probe displacement value (given by the instrument), the axial swelling can be determined by the force–displacement diagrams, and, finally, the work of penetration can be determined by the integration of the force–displacement curve (the area under the curve). The total work of penetration indicates the matrix stiffness or rigidity, and its evaluation can be helpful to understand the effect of an additive on a matrix formulation and how it affects its properties. Moreover, it has to be considered that the gel strength of a matrix system has a great relevance in vivo due to exposure to destructive forces in the gastrointestinal tract.

In 2008, a novel nondestructive probe equipped with a texture analyzer was developed [83], which can be used directly in the dissolution medium during the run. With the use of this probe, the swelling, the erosion, and the positions of the rubbery region and of the glassy core can be simultaneously measured. The probe is constituted by a body through which two supports can move. A circular plate with a central hole contains a fixed probe, which can be exposed outside when the plate is pushed upward. The plate is connected to the movable supports in the probe body. During the analysis, the body of the probe and the plate move downward in the dissolving tablet direction. The loading cell is calibrated in a manner that does not trigger the cell with the movement of the plate in the dissolution medium (the resistance is too low). On the contrary, when the plate reaches the surface of the swollen tablet, it is forced to stop its movement or to move upward if the tablet continues its expansion (due to the swelling). This movement forces the supports connected with the plate to slide into the probe body; this action triggers the load cell which starts to record the resistance force. This movement continues till the probe passes through the hole in the plate and reaches the swollen tablet. The probe is stopped when it reaches a maximum force of 150 g and returns in its original position. This procedure is repeated at preset time intervals and allows the evaluation of the relationship between the thickness of the glassy core and the swollen rubbery region with time. Using the texture analysis technique, various mathematical correlations can be obtained, such as the correlation between the drug dissolution and the polymer hydration obtained by Li and Gu [84]. Modified release tablets were subjected to a conventional dissolution test after their snapping into cylindrical caps, which had a diameter equal to the tablet time. The sample prepared allows the water penetration only along one direction (from the surface exposed to the dissolution medium); in this way, the analysis was significantly simplified. Then, these samples were subjected to a conventional dissolution test and then removed from the dissolution medium and subjected to a texture analysis. The relationship between polymer hydration and drug dissolution was obtained, correlating texture analysis parameters (such as the area under the force–displacement graph), drug release rate, and PEO proportion in the matrix by a mathematical fitting based on both linear and multiple regressions.

With the aim to quantify the amount of water penetrating into a hydrogel-based matrix, using a fast and simple technique, such as the texture analysis, a correlation between the percentage of water content and the penetration work resulting from an indentation test was developed [85]. In this case, matrices composed of HPMC and a model drug were confined between two glass slides, to allow the water uptake only by the radial direction and then immersed in the dissolution medium. After predefined times, the system (composed by the swollen matrix and the slabs) was withdrawn from the medium and the superior slab removed. Due to this sample preparation, the water amount in the matrix changes along the radius (at different radii, there is a different hydration level), but axially, the water content is the same. In particular, at the same radius, the water content is the same in all the matrix thickness. A texture analysis, in particular an indentation test, was performed on these swollen samples. A needle was used to penetrate, at a constant rate, into the matrix, and a diagram force–displacement was obtained. This procedure was repeated at several distances from the center of the matrix, to evaluate how the resistance force changes with the radius of the tablet. For each radius value, a force–displacement diagram was obtained, and, by the calculation of the area under the curve, the work of penetration of the needle to penetrate into the tablet was calculated. In parallel, a gravimetric analysis was performed on samples hydrated with the same procedure to obtain the water profiles inside the swollen matrix. The gravimetric data obtained were fitted using a Boltzmann-type equation to obtain a continuous trend of the water mass fraction inside the swollen matrix. Then, the results obtained in terms of water content (evaluated by the gravimetric technique) and the work of penetration (evaluated by the texture analysis) were compared to find a relation between them. A simple relation was obtained:

$$\omega_1(W_P) = \frac{b_1}{1+\left(b_2 W_p\right)^{b_3}} \tag{33}$$

where b_1,b_2, b_3 are equation parameters, ω_1 is the water mass fraction, and W_p is the penetration work. As expected, the penetration work decreases, increasing the water content; this is due to the fact that more hydrated is the matrix, more gel is formed, and less force is necessary to penetrate into the sample. The main drawback of this technique is the fact that this relation between the work and the water content is possible and reliable only if the water content along the matrix thickness is constant (the force–displacement curves are linear); in the cases where the matrix swells both in axial and radial directions, this relation is not so immediate.

Thus, this technique was improved to correlate the water content to the slope of the force–displacement diagrams [86]. This technique was calibrated firstly on the matrix which swells only in the radial direction, since the force increases linearly with the penetration of the matrix. The correlation obtained is

$$\omega_1(dF/ds) = c_1 Log\left(\frac{dF}{ds}\right) + c_2 \tag{34}$$

where c_1 and c_2 are equation parameters, ω_1 is the water percentage into the matrix, and d_F/d_s is the slope of the force–penetration curves. In this way, a calibration relation was obtained and, in each radius of the matrix, it is possible to know the water percentage. At this point, the method was extended to the matrix swollen both in the radial and in the axial direction, the so-called "semioverall" system. Concerning the texture analysis of these systems, the shape of the force–penetration curves was very different with respect to the previous one. In fact, being the water content variable even along the thickness (the water penetration happens both in the radial and axial directions), the measured force increases with the penetration of the needle in a nonlinear behavior. In fact, at the beginning of the test, the needle meets the gel layer formed on the top of the swollen tablet; thus, the force necessary to penetrate this layer is very low. Approaching the core of the tablet, where the water is not penetrated enough, the probe needs a higher force to penetrate the tablet, and the values measured by the texture analyzer increase exponentially. This test was repeated for several radii of the swollen matrix, to evaluate how the force necessary to penetrate varies not only with the thickness but even with the radius of the tablet. This behavior is characteristic of all the curves; the force magnitude varies depending on the radius where the penetration is carried on, since the hydration of the matrix occurs also along the radial direction, thus leaving the matrix center the water content increases; that means that the force necessary to penetrate the matrix decreases. Moreover, it has to be considered that also the thickness of the swollen matrix changes at the changing of the radius position. The experimental data are very well fitted by simple exponential curves. It is thus easy to obtain d_F/d_s which is, in this case, a function of the penetration distance rather than a single value for each test. Once it is evaluated how the d_F/d_s varies, for each radius, along the matrix thickness, it is possible to calculate the respective water content using eq. 34.

The measurement of water content in the axial direction can be repeated for each penetration point for all the hydration times considered. Thus, a contour plot can be drawn and compared with a real picture of the semioverall swollen tablet; in Figure 7, b) is shown a matrix after 2 h of dissolution. The picture taken is of a swollen tablet cut along a diameter, in such a way that the glassy core and the swollen gel are clearly distinguishable. The contour plot represents the water content in the tablet evaluated by the described technique, and it is shown in Figure 7, in the first quarter of the picture. Areas containing the same water amount are colored with the same filling, and, in general, the water content decreases while approaching the glass slide of the tablet. It can be noted that there are zones where it is not possible to evaluate the water content, due to both a water content higher than the limit imposed by the obtained relationship applicability (relationship between the force/displacement derivative and the water content) and the hydration in the more external zones, so high that the force opposed by the gel to the penetration is negligible and not easily detectable by the instrument. The legend of the color used and of the water percentage at which they correspond is shown in the third quarter of the picture.

2.4. Describe the Actions of the Swelling

In the description of the performances of delivery systems for controlled release, the swelling phenomenon has a central role. For this reason, over the years, several scientists tried to quantify and predict the capability of the matrices to swell and thus release the drug eventually contained inside, usually quantifying the so-called swelling ratio, which corresponds to the weight gain defined in section 2.2. One of the first attempts to describe the swelling phenomenon was that followed by Colombo and his coworkers [87]. The goal of their work was to quantify the matrix relaxation measuring the surface exposed during polymer swelling. To evaluate the influence of the swelling phenomenon on drug release, the amount of drug released was plotted versus the area of the system, at the same time, obtaining a linear relationship. This result indicates a direct dependence between the drug release and the tablet surface. Moreover, the authors proposed a new dimensionless number in order to correlate the matrix expansion during dissolution to the increase of the releasing area. This number is called the swelling area number, $N_{Sw.A}$, and it is defined as

$$N_{Sw.A} = \frac{1}{D_{3.s}} \frac{dA}{dt} \tag{35}$$

where d_A/d_t is the rate of the area change during the dissolution and $D_{3.s}$ is the drug diffusion coefficient in the swollen phase. Thus, this number represents the ratio between the matrix surface area expansion rate and the drug diffusion, weighting the contribution of the swelling and the diffusion phenomena on the drug release. The matrix swelling was determined by a measure of the releasing area from pictures of the matrix taken during the dissolution. By this technique, the influence of the presence of a hydrogel matrix coating on the swelling kinetics can be evaluated [88].

Later, the behavior of gel layer thickness in swellable matrices loaded with drugs was studied using a colorimetric technique [89]. This method was based on the dissolution of a radial system for predetermined intervals and the use of the image analysis technique to evaluate the position of the swelling, the diffusion, and the erosion fronts. This method is based on the fact that the used drug was light yellow in the dry state and became orange in solution, with a color intensity dependent on its concentration. These measures are able only to evaluate the radial position of the fronts, being a 1D analysis. Moreover, the water concentration at the glassy–rubber interface (c^*) (thus at the swelling front, as defined in section 1.3) was calculated starting from the glass transition temperature of the polymer (T_g) to the experimental temperature (T_{exp}), according to the following expression [29]:

$$c^* = \frac{T_g - T_{exp}}{\beta / \alpha_f} \tag{36}$$

where β is the contribution of water to the expansion of the polymer and α_f is the thermal linear expansion coefficient of the polymer. This equation is usually used in terms of volume fraction of the components because, due to the swelling of the polymer, the volume changes in the swollen tablet. Thus, the water volume fraction can be expressed as water volume per volume of polymer. Thus, from the image analysis, the position of the swelling front can be evaluated and by theoretical consideration, the water concentration at the interface calculated.

As seen in the previous paragraph, the NMRI technique is very useful to monitor the swelling and the erosion phenomena. Proton density- and diffusion-weighted images of the hydrating tablets can be acquired at different intervals, and apparent self-diffusion coefficient maps can be generated from the diffusion-weighted images [90]. The image intensities characteristic of the swollen tablets obtained from the NMRI analysis are usually evaluated by software, i.e., ImageJ.

During the swelling of a hydrogel, the mechanical properties of the gel, and then of the release formulation, change continuously. Thus, one of the analyses which can be performed to evaluate how the swelling influences the matrix behavior is the rheological characterization of the polymer. The effective elastic modulus and gel thickness during the swelling can be evaluated by indentation tests [91]. In a standard indentation test, the needle moves till it enters in contact with the sample and reaches a specified load target. The results in terms of load and displacement are used to compare the effective elastic modulus and gel thickness during the swelling. In particular, Hewlett et al. defined the effective modulus from the slope of the stress–displacement curve at a stress of 10 kPa at which corresponds the effective thickness, that is, the displacement at the point where the effective modulus was calculated. The definition of the effective elastic modulus allows to compare the behavior of different polymers. On the other hand, the viscoelastic materials are usually characterized in terms of dynamic mechanical behavior, when they are subjected to an oscillatory test. The authors performed an oscillatory indentation test to a swollen matrix. The indenter was advanced in contact with the sample. Once a specific load was reached, the indenter velocity was oscillated sinusoidally and the response of the material recorded. Higher loads were used at shorter hydration times and lower loads at longer hydration times because, dependent on the amount of water penetrated inside the matrix, the sample changes its characteristic, becoming harder or softer, respectively. Thus, the oscillatory indentation experiments can be used as a small-scale measure of the rheological behavior of polymers to evaluate the viscoelastic nature of the gel layer as it swells.

In general, for a full description of the swelling phenomenon, a single experimental approach cannot be sufficient to consider all the aspects involved. For this reason, a combined approach of four different methods was proposed [92]. In particular, four different methods can be used: determination of the expansion factor, texture analysis, visual swelling observation, and photomicroscopy. The determination of the expansion factor was performed by positioning the sample into a flat-bottomed test tube and adding a small volume of swelling medium. After the medium was penetrated into the sample, the axial expansion was calculated as the ratio between the measured heights of the swollen and dry tablet. Then, the expansion of the tablets and the development of the gel layer thickness were evaluated using a texture analysis. To evaluate visually the swelling phenomena and thus the water uptake, samples were confined between two disks (as in the radial system) and photographed after predetermined dissolution times using a digital camera to obtain the final dimensions of the tablets. Finally, the swelling of polymer slabs was analyzed by photomicrography with a microscope connected to a digital camera. The combination of all these methods allows a deep analysis of the swelling phenomenon.

As described in this section, a lot of experimental techniques which can be used to clearly understand the swelling kinetics of a polymer and the mobility of the water inside the matrix were developed over the years. Each technique described has its advantages and can be a valid aid for a study purpose. A complete review of all the techniques used to monitor the swelling–erosion behavior was proposed by Huanbutta et al. [93], and the pros and cons of each of them were elucidated.

3. VARIOUS MODELING APPROACHES

3.1. Introduction

As was already said, it is important to understand the processes that affect drug release in order to get a customized drug release. The mathematical modeling of these physical processes can help us understand them better and point out the most important parts of drug release from hydrogel-based delivery systems. It makes sense that modeling the physical processes involved could help with the creation and optimization of these systems, cutting down on the time and money needed for trial-and-error methods. The modeling is pretty complicated because there are a lot of different transport processes that work together and against each other. There are a lot of different mathematical models out there, ranging from simple empirical models to more complex mechanical models. Figure 3 shows the most important ones, and we'll talk about some of them below.

3.2. Empirical models

The first modeling attempt can be traced back to the semiempirical model of Higuchi [94], where the fractional drug release from an ointment (thin film) was related to the square root of the time:

$$\frac{M_t}{M_\infty} = k\sqrt{t} \tag{37}$$

Mt*Mt* is the cumulative amount of drug released at time t*t*. M∞*M∞* is the mass of drug released at infinite time (equal to the initial drug loading), and k*k* is a constant reflecting the design variables of the system.

In 1985, Peppas and coworkers [95] proposed a generalization of the Higuchi equation, in which the fractional drug release was related to the nth power of the time. The index "n" is an index function of the drug transport regime and of the shape of the delivery system.

$$\frac{M_t}{M_\infty} = k\ t^n \tag{38}$$

For example, for a thin film, the exponent "n" in eq. 38 is equal to 0.5 for Fickian diffusive process (Higuchi's equation), "n" is equal to 1 for the Case-II transport (swelling-controlled drug release), and it takes intermediate values for intermediate behaviors (anomalous transport).

To distinguish between the relative importance of the Fickian release and the swelling-controlled release, Peppas and Sahlin [96] proposed the model

$$\frac{M_t}{M_\infty} = k_1 t^m + k_2 t^{2m} \tag{39}$$

where k_1, k_2, and m are constants. The first term on the RHS represents the Fickian diffusional contribution, F, whereas the second term the swelling-controlled (case II) contribution, R. The relative importance of the two transport mechanisms can be highlighted by the ratio:

$$\frac{R}{F} = \frac{k_2 t^m}{k_1} \tag{40}$$

Bettini et al. [88] used this equation to investigate the effect of the HPMC molecular weight on the kinetics of drug release. No significant difference was found within the different grades of HPMC and the value of the ratio R/F was smaller than 0.1, suggesting that the drug transport is mainly Fickian diffusion driven.

Due to their simplicity, these equations have been used countless times to analyze the experimental results, often without taking into account that these equations are empirical in nature, and thus, they are useful only under some restrictions: constant diffusivities and negligible swelling (which is not the case of swellable systems [11, 97]). Thus, these equations should be used as simple fitting tools, giving limited information about the release mechanisms, in particular for complex systems such as the hydrogel-based ones.

3.3. The basics of the mechanistic modeling of the hydrogel-based systems

Let us consider a hydrogel-based system loaded with drug, submerged in a dissolution medium. The hydrogel "H" will be formed by the solvent (i=1), the polymer matrix (i=2), the drug (i=3), and the ions (i=4...N_C). To describe the movements of these species along with the hydrogel deformation, proper mass balance equations, coupled with the momentum conservation equation, are needed. Two different approaches can be used to describe this system: the multiphasic model and the multicomponent mixture model. With the first, the hydrogel is seen as constituted by different phases, each characterized by their own mass and momentum conservation equations. With the second approach, instead, the system is considered as made of one phase composed of several components. In Table 3 is depicted a general framework useful for the mechanistic modeling of hydrogel-based systems. Most of the literature works dealing with both the drug release from hydrogels and the hydrogel mechanics could be traced back to this scheme, as shown in the following. In the formulation of the multiphasic approach, it has been considered that the drug is already dissolved. The transient and the inertial terms in the momentum balance equations (Table 3 equations (G-I)) have been neglected.

3.3.1. Free energy of a hydrogel network

In Table 3, eq. (K), it is indicated that the stress tensor and the osmotic pressure of the hydrogel are functions of the Helmholtz free energy that in turn is divided in three terms: elastic, mixing, and ionic free energy. The Helmholtz and the Gibbs free energy for these systems are interchangeable since dG=dA+d(pV) and, at constant pressure, the pressure–volume product does not change significantly in swelling [98].

Table 3. A general framework for the mechanistic modeling of hydrogel-based systems

Multiphasic Approach	Multicomponent Approach
Mass Conversation: $\frac{\partial \rho_i}{\partial t} = -\nabla \cdot (\rho_i v_i) i = 1 \ldots N_C$ (A)	
$\begin{cases} \frac{\partial \phi_i}{\partial t} = -\nabla \cdot (\phi_i v_i) i = 1,\ 2 \\ \frac{\partial \phi_1 c_i}{\partial t} = -\nabla \cdot (\phi_1 c_i v_i) i = 3 \ldots N_C \end{cases}$ (B) $\phi_1 + \phi_2 \cong 1$ (C)	$\frac{\partial \rho_i}{\partial t} = -\nabla \cdot (\rho_i v_{mix}) - \nabla \cdot j_i i = 1 \ldots N_C$ (D) or $\rho \frac{\partial \omega_i}{\partial t} = -\rho v_{mix} \cdot \nabla \omega_i - \nabla \cdot j_i i = 1 \ldots N_C$ (E) $\sum_{i=1}^{N_C} \omega_i = 1$ (F)

<table>
<tr><th>Multiphasic Approach</th><th>Multicomponent Approach</th></tr>
<tr><td colspan="2">Momentum Conservation:
$\nabla \cdot (\sigma_H - p\delta) = 0$ (G)</td></tr>
<tr><td>$\begin{cases} 0 = \nabla \cdot (-\phi_1 p\delta + \mu_1 \dot{\gamma}) + \phi_1 RT \sum_{i=3}^{N_C} \nabla c_i + f_{12} + \sum_{i=3}^{N_C} f_{1i} & i=1 \\ 0 = \nabla \cdot (-\phi_2 p\delta + \sigma_2) - \phi_1 (z_F c_F F) \nabla \psi + f_{21} & i=2 \\ 0 = -\phi_1 RT \nabla c_i - \phi_1 (z_i c_i F) \nabla \psi + f_{i1} & i=3 \ldots N_C \end{cases}$ (H)</td><td>$\nabla \cdot (\sigma_{mix} - p\delta) = 0$ (I)</td></tr>
<tr><td colspan="2">Distribution of the iconic species:
$\nabla^2 \psi = -\frac{F}{\varepsilon \varepsilon_0} \left(\sum_{i=4}^{N_C} z_i c_i - z_F c_f \right), \quad \overset{electroneutrality}{\nabla^2 \psi = 0}$ (J)</td></tr>
<tr><td colspan="2">Constitutive Equations:
$\{p_{osm}, \sigma_H\} = g(A_{el}, A_{mix}, A_{ion})$ (K)
$p = p' + p^{osm}$ (L)</td></tr>
<tr><td>$f_{ij} = -f_{ji} = f_{ij}(\zeta, v_i, v_j)$ (M)</td><td>$j_i = -\rho_i (v_i - v_{mix}) \propto -$
$-\rho D_i g(\mu_i, \ x_i, \ \omega_i, \ M, \ p_{osm}, \ \psi, \ldots)$
$D_i = g(\rho_1 or \ \rho_2)$ (N)</td></tr>
<tr><td colspan="2">Unknows to solve for:</td></tr>
<tr><td>$\phi_1, \phi_2, c_3 \ldots c_{N_C}, \ v_1 \ldots v_{N_C}$</td><td>$\omega_i, \ v_{mix}$</td></tr>
<tr><td colspan="2">*Hydrogel (H) = Solvent (i=1) + Polymer (i=2) + Drug (i=3) + Ions (i=4...NC)</td></tr>
</table>

The hydrogel can be viewed as formed by an elastomeric network with solvent molecules and ions, and the overall free energy of the system will have to consider the presence and the interactions of these species.

Let us consider a dry elastomeric network in which the stress–strain relation is based on the concept of the finite elasticity theory. This theory relates the deformations of the material to the stresses needed to obtain that deformation through the so-called strain energy density function: $W=W(\lambda_1, \lambda_2, \lambda_3)$ where λ_i represents the stretch ratio in each direction (a material for which the stress–strain relationship derives from a strain energy density function is defined hyperelastic). The strain energy density function corresponds to the Helmholtz free energy per unit volume [99], and it can be derived from statistical theories of the elastomeric network. The aim of statistical models is to provide predictive relationships between the molecular structure and topology of the network and its macroscopic behavior.

Several molecular models for rubber networks have been proposed [98, 100], and the two limiting cases are the "affine" and the "phantom" models. Both these simplified network models give a strain energy density function of neo-Hookean type, i.e., in the following is reported the expression derived from the affine network:

$$W^{aff}(\lambda_1,\lambda_2,\lambda_3) = A_{el}^{aff}(\lambda_1,\lambda_2,\lambda_3) = \frac{1}{2}k_bT\left[\frac{\nu_{el}}{V_0}(\lambda_1^2+\lambda_2^2+\lambda_3^2-3) - 2\frac{\mu_{el}}{V_0}\ln(\lambda_1\lambda_2\lambda_3)\right] \quad (41)$$

where k_b is the Boltzmann constant, T is the temperature, V_0 is the volume of the dry polymer, ν_{el} is the number of elastic chains, and μ_{el} is the number of junctions in the network. Equation 41 can be reformulated in terms of Finger deformation tensor $B=FF^T$, where $F=dx/dX$ is the deformation gradient (in which x and X are the vectors representing a generic point P in the current and in the reference configuration, respectively):

$$A_{el}^{aff}(\boldsymbol{B}) = \frac{1}{2}k_bT\left[\frac{\nu_{el}}{V_0}(I_B-3) - \frac{\mu_{el}}{V_0}\ln(III_B)\right] \quad (42)$$

where $I_B=tr(B)$ and $II\ I_B=\det(B)$ are the first and the third invariants of B.

Since the hydrogel is characterized by the solvent present, the mixing contribution to the free energy has to be considered. As there is no explicit molecular model for the energy of mixing in gel (cross-linked polymer plus solvent), the functional dependence of the free energy of the mixing is generally assumed to be the same as in a polymer solution (linear polymer plus solvent). The classical treatment is based on the Flory–Huggins model, which is built on a lattice model with the assumption of uniform polymer segment concentration throughout the entire system. The free energy of mixing is given by

$$A_{mix} = \frac{RT}{V}\left[n_1\ln(\phi_1) + n_2\ln(\phi_2) + n_1\phi_2\chi_{12}\right] \quad (43)$$

where R is the gas constant, n_1 and ϕ_1 are the number of moles and the volume fraction of the solvent, n_2 and ϕ_2 are the number of moles and the volume fraction of the polymer, and χ_{12} is the Flory–Huggins interaction parameter.

When the network chains contain ionic groups (polyelectrolyte gels), there will be additional forces that affect their swelling properties, like the translational entropy of counterions, Coulomb interactions, and ion pair multiplets. It is evident that the mobile and fixed ions present contribute to the system free energy. Several expressions, based on different assumptions, have been used [101-104]. Quite commonly, the free energy due to ionic charges is divided into mobile ion contribution and fixed charge contribution:

$$A_{ion} = A_{ion}^{mob} + A_{ion}^{fix} \quad (44)$$

Following the Frenkel–Flory–Rehner approach, the free energy of a swelling cross-linked polymer is separable and additive, so that

$$A = A_{el} + A_{mix} + A_{ion} \quad (45)$$

This allows to consider singularly the free energy contributions and to derive constitutive equations for polymeric gels. It is quite common to relate the network stress only to the elastic Helmholtz free energy:

$$\sigma_2 = 2J^{-1}B\frac{\partial A_{el}(B)}{\partial B} \tag{46}$$

where J=det(F). The mixing and ionic free energy terms instead are often considered as contributing factors to the osmotic pressure (p^{osm}), despite some other approaches that are possible [105].

3.3.2. Multicomponent approach: Mass transfer

In 1999, Siepmann et al. [106] developed a mechanistic model based on purely diffusive mass transport equations (Table 3 equations (D) with $(\rho_i v_{mix}) \rightarrow 0$ and $j_i = -D_i \nabla \rho_i$) to calculate the drug release from HPMC-based matrices. The modeled system was made of three species, water "1", polymer "2", and drug "3", and the domain was the 2D axisymmetric representation of a cylindrical tablet (Figure 8). The water and drug transport equations were solved under the assumptions of:

- No volume contraction upon mixing
- Fast drug dissolution compared to drug diffusion
- Perfect sink condition for the drug
- Strong dependence of the diffusivities (of water and drug) on the hydration level
- Affine deformations

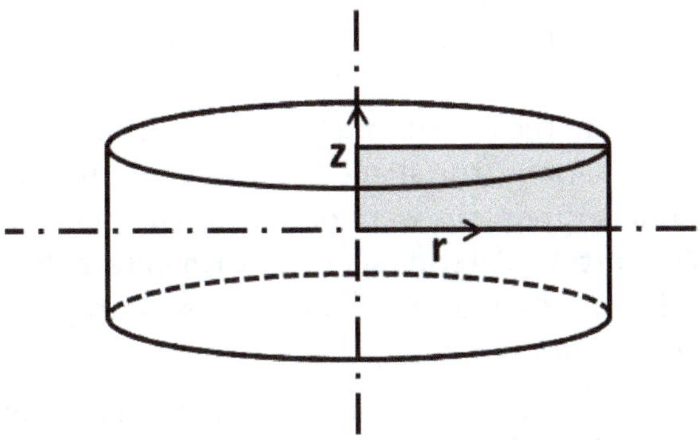

Figure 8. Schematic of the matrix, in light gray, the mathematical domain on which the transport equations were solved.

The mass transport equations (PDEs: partial differential equations) for water and drug in cylindrical coordinates were numerically (finite difference) solved along with the proper initial and boundary conditions:

$$\begin{cases} \dfrac{\partial \rho_i}{\partial t} = \dfrac{1}{r}\dfrac{\partial}{\partial r}\left(D_i \dfrac{\partial \rho_i}{\partial r}\right) + \dfrac{\partial}{\partial z}\left(D_i \dfrac{\partial \rho_i}{\partial z}\right) \quad i = 1,3 \\ @t = 0, \forall r, \forall z, \ \rho_i = \rho_{i,0} \\ @r = R(t), \forall t, \forall z \ \rho_i = \rho_{i,eq} \\ @z = Z(t), \ \forall t, \forall r \ \rho_i = \rho_{i,eq} \\ @r = 0, \ \forall t, \forall z \dfrac{\partial \rho_i}{\partial r} = 0 \\ @r = 0, \ \forall t, \forall z \dfrac{\partial \rho_i}{\partial r} = 0 \end{cases} \tag{47}$$

where ρ_i is the mass concentration of the ith species, $\rho_{i,eq}$ is the interface mass concentration of the ith species, and D_i is the diffusion coefficient of the ith species, described by a Fujita-type equation [51] (the general form given by eq. 26):

$$D_i = D_{i,eq} exp\left[-\beta_i\left(1 - \frac{\rho_1}{\rho_{1,eq}}\right)\right] \tag{48}$$

where $D_{i,eq}/\exp(\beta_i)$ are the values of the effective diffusion coefficients in the dry matrix ($\rho_1 = 0$) and $D_{i,eq}$ are the values of the effective diffusion coefficients in the fully swollen matrix ($\rho_1 = \rho_{1,eq}$). The polymer erosion/release was described with the following ordinary differential equation (ODE):

$$\begin{cases} \dfrac{dm_2}{dt} = -k_{er} A_{er}(t) \\ @t = 0 m_2 = m_{2,0} \end{cases} \tag{49}$$

where m_2 and $m_{2,0}$ are the polymer mass and the initial polymer mass, k_{er} is an erosion constant, and A_{er} is the erosion surface, that is, the surface exposed to the external medium. The system deformation was obtained, calculating at each time step the amount of water absorbed in the matrix and the released amount of drug and polymer. Considering affine deformations (the shape is conserved), the swelling and shrinking in the axial and the radial directions were obtained. The model parameters, $D_{i,eq}$, β_i, k_{er} were found from the fitting of a wide set of experimental data. The so-tuned model was able to describe the evolution of the global masses of drug, water, and polymer in the system at several dissolution times.

In 2003, Kiil and Dam-Johansen [107] proposed a 1D model able to describe the radial movements of swelling, diffusion, and erosion fronts along with the hydration and drug release, under the (main) assumptions of drug release only in the radial direction, negligible matrix erosion, and constant diffusivities. Even in this case, the system description was based on the mass transport equation (Table 3 equations (D) with $(\rho_i v_{mix}) \rightarrow 0$ and $j_i = -D_i \nabla \rho_i$) with the addition of physical constraints to model the deformation. In particular, the domain was divided radially in three zones individuated by the front radii: zone 1 (solid part) characterized by the swelling radius, zone 2 (gel plus solid drug) between the diffusion and swelling radii, and zone 3 (gel plus dissolved drug) between the erosion and the diffusion radii. The model was made of one ODE, one algebraic equation, and four PDEs to describe, respectively, the movement of the swelling radius, the erosion front, the diffusion front, the dissolved drug concentration, and the water concentration in zones 3 and 2. Most of the model parameters were taken from literature; others, i.e., diffusivities and dissolution kinetic constants, were adjusted by fitting the experimental data. Despite such a complete approach, the model was not able to describe the swelling that occurs when there is no more solid part (zone 1) and its complexity has downhearted from developing a 2D axisymmetric version.

Inspired by Siepmann's work, in the 2007, Chirico et al. [55] developed a 1D model to describe the hydration of pure HPMC tablets confined between two glass slabs (Figure 9).

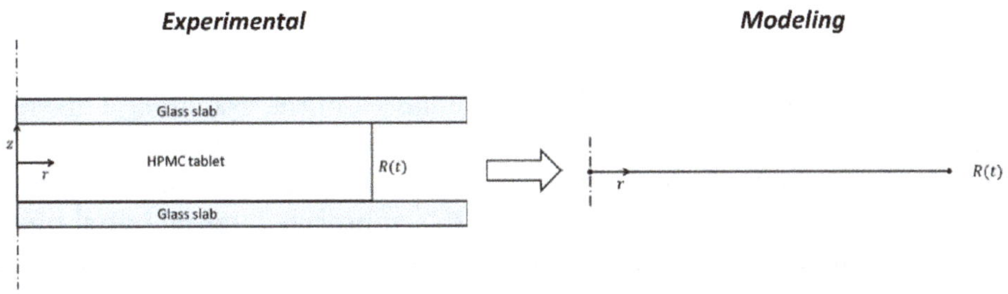

Figure 9. Experimental tablet dissolution scheme (left) and modeling domain (right)

Considering that the main transport phenomenon is the pseudo-diffusion of water from the medium ($r>R(t)$) into the tablet through the radial direction (Table 3 equations (E) with (v_{mix})→0), the water mass balance in cylindrical coordinates was solved numerically (with a finite difference method):

$$\begin{cases} \rho \dfrac{\partial \omega_1}{\partial t} = \dfrac{1}{r}\dfrac{\partial}{\partial r}\left(r\,\rho\,D_1 \dfrac{\partial \omega_1}{\partial r}\right) \\ @t=0, \forall r, \omega_1 = \omega_{1,0} \\ @r=0, \forall t, \dfrac{\partial \omega_1}{\partial r} = 0 \\ @r=R(t), \forall t, \omega_1 = \omega_{1,eq} \end{cases} \tag{50}$$

where ω_1 is the water mass fraction, $\omega_{1,eq}$ is the equilibrium water mass fraction in the gel (0.97 [55]), and D_1 is the diffusion coefficient of water in HPMC, modeled with a Fujita-type equation (the general form given by eq. 26) to account for the dependency of diffusivity on the water content:

$$D_1 = D_{1,eq} exp\left[-\beta_1\left(1-\frac{\omega_1}{\omega_{1,eq}}\right)\right] \tag{51}$$

where $D_{1,eq}$ is the diffusivity in the fully swollen gel (@ω_1=$\omega_{1,eq}$), and β_1 is a parameter that tunes the degree of dependency of D_1 on the water content.

The system swelling was described, considering the variation of the total mass due to the water inlet and the polymer erosion.

$$m_1 = \int \rho_{(\omega_1)}\ \omega_1\ dV$$

$$\begin{cases} \dfrac{dm_2}{dt} = -k_{er}A_{er}(t) \\ @t = 0\ m_2 = m_{2,0} \end{cases} \tag{52}$$

$$V(t) = \pi R^2 H = \frac{m_1 + m_2}{\langle \rho_{(\omega_1)} \rangle}$$

where m_1 and m_2 are the water and polymer masses in the system at a given time, k_{er} and A_{er} are the erosion constant and the erosion surface (surface exposed to the external medium), $V(t)$ and H are the system volume and the tablet thickness, and $\langle\rho(\omega_1)\rangle$ is the averaged system density. With this approach, after an initial tuning of the model parameters ($D_{1,eq}$, β_1, k_{er}), the macroscopic system swelling, the amount of water uptake, and the polymer dissolved were correctly described. In their work, the authors compared, satisfactorily, the model results with an extra experimental data: the water mass fraction profile along the radial direction obtained by analyzing the normalized light intensity of swollen tablet pictures; an example of this model application is shown in Figure 5a. The model abilities were later on improved [108] to describe the drug release kinetics from different shaped matrices, bringing back everything to a 1D model valid for slabs, spheres, infinite cylinders, and finite cylinders (where the approach proposed by Coviello et al. [109] was used).

Despite that these transport models were validated against a wide set of experimental data, they were limited by the strong assumption of affine deformation that impedes the use of such models in more geometrically complex systems where the non-affine deformation can sensibly affect the drug release.

In 2011, Lamberti et al. [110] proposed a 2D axisymmetric model, in some ways similar to the Siepmann's model but with a big step forward: the assumption of affine deformation was no longer needed.

The transport equations for water and drug were solved for the respective mass fraction with a finite element method (FEM), along with the proper initial and boundary conditions (Table 3 equations (E) with $\langle v_{mix}\rangle \rightarrow 0$):

$$\begin{cases} \rho \dfrac{\partial \omega_i}{\partial t} = \boldsymbol{\nabla} \cdot \left(\rho D_i \boldsymbol{\nabla} \omega_i \right) \; i = 1,3 \\ @t = 0, \forall r, \forall z, \omega_i = \omega_{i,0} \\ @r = R(t), \forall t, \forall z \, \omega_i = \omega_{i,eq} \\ @z = Z(t), \forall t, \forall r \, \omega_i = \omega_{i,eq} \\ @r = 0, \forall t, \forall z \dfrac{\partial \omega_i}{\partial r} = 0 \\ @z = 0, \forall t, \forall r \dfrac{\partial \omega_i}{\partial z} = 0 \end{cases} \tag{53}$$

where ω_i is the mass fraction of the ith species, $\omega_{i,eq}$ are the interface mass fraction of the ith species, and D_i is the diffusion coefficient of the ith species, described by a Fujita-type equation (see eqs. 48 and 51). The constitutive equation for the system density was obtained considering the summability of the specific volume of the single species:

$$\frac{1}{\rho} = \frac{\omega_1}{\rho_{10}} + \frac{(1-\omega_1-\omega_3)}{\rho_{20}} + \frac{\omega_3}{\rho_{30}} \tag{54}$$

where $\rho_{10}, \rho_{20}, \rho_{30}$ are the pure species densities.

The peculiarity of this approach was the decomposition of the inlet water flux to describe the system swelling. In particular, it was considered that part of the total inlet water mass flux was responsible for the tablet swelling, $j_{1,swe}$, whereas the rest ($j_{1,diff}$) was responsible for the inner layer hydration. Assuming that

$$j_{1,swe} = k_{swe} j_{1,diff}$$

and (55)

$$j_1 = j_{1,diff} + j_{1,swe} = (1 + k_{swe}) \rho \, D_1 \boldsymbol{\nabla} \omega_1$$

where k_{swe} is a new fitting parameter.

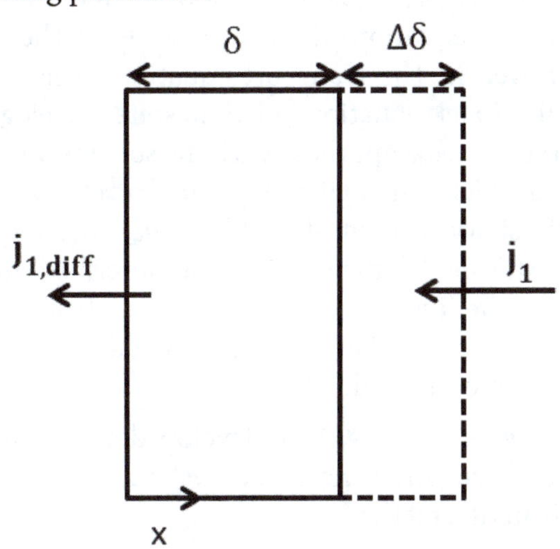

Figure 10. Representation of the water mass balance on a boundary element

The rate of deformation was obtained performing a water mass balance on a boundary element (Figure 10):

$$\rho \frac{d}{dt}\left(A\delta\omega_{1,eq}\right) = A \cdot j_{1,diff} - A \cdot j_1$$
$$v_{swe} = \frac{d\delta}{dt} = -\frac{j_{1,swe}}{\rho\ \omega_{1,eq}} = -\frac{k_{swe} j_{1,diff}}{\rho\ \omega_{1,eq}} \qquad (56)$$

where v_{swe} is the swelling velocity of the boundary element. On the other hand, the polymer erosion could lead to a volume decrease; therefore, an opposite constant velocity (the erosion velocity v_{eros}=-k_{eros}) was considered, so that the effective velocity of the boundary element was given by

$$v = v_{swe} + v_{eros} \qquad (57)$$

The application of this boundary velocity through an ALE (Arbitrary Lagrangian-Eulerian) moving mesh method was proved to describe the matrix non-affine swelling. The model, after an initial tuning of the parameters, was successfully compared to macroscopic results in terms of overall water, drug, and polymer masses, erosion radius, and semi-thickness as well as a picture of swollen tablets.

The approach used in this model overcame the affine deformation at the cost of an additional parameter: the k_{swe} (1° drawback). Moreover, the mass fraction constraint (Table 3 equation (F)) was not implemented along with the PDEs (as well as in Siepmann's model), possibly leading to unrealistic results in some domain points (2° drawback).

Kaunisto et al. developed a mechanistic model (in 2010 for the dissolution of pure poly(ethylene oxide) tablets [111], extended in 2013 [112] to HPMC matrices loaded with a poorly soluble drug) to analyze the drug release behavior in swellable systems. In this model (considered at constant density), the polymer mass fraction description was coupled with the transport equations for drug and water through the mass fraction constraint (Table 3 equations (E-F) with (v_{mix})→0), therefore overcoming the Lamberti model 2° drawback. The transport equations were based on a simplified version of the generalized Fick equation [113]. Despite the elegant approach, all the multicomponent interactions, except those with the solvent, were assumed to be zero, and the multicomponent Fick diffusivities were interpreted as "pseudo-binary." For the water–polymer diffusivity, a "Fujita-type" form was used (eqs. 48 and 51). Even in this case, like in Lamberti's model, the swelling was described through an ALE moving mesh method, but the swelling velocity was derived from a polymer/solid drug mass balance on the erosion boundaries, with zero additional parameters, therefore overcoming also the 1° Lamberti model drawback.

Recently, in 2015, Caccavo et al. [114, 115] developed a mechanistic model based on the diffusion of water and drug in a concentrate system, accounting for the molar mass gradient, coupled with an ALE method.

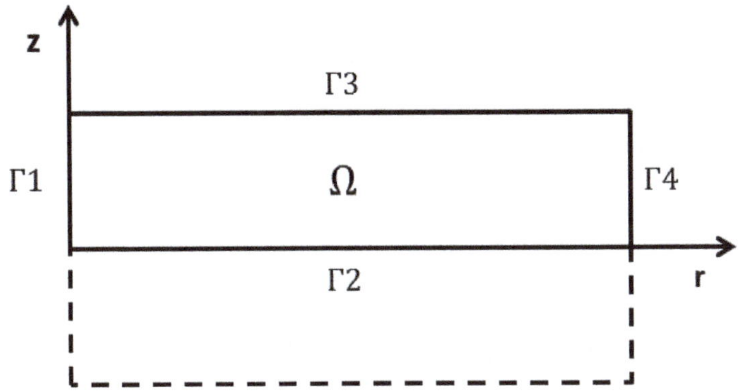

Figure 11. Computational domain for the model of Caccavo et al. [114, 115]

Under the assumption of:

- No volume change upon mixing.
- The drug dissolution within the matrix is fast compared to drug diffusion.
- Perfect sink conditions for drug and constant critical solvent concentration on the erosion front are maintained.
- The water convection contribution to mass transfer is negligible.
- The swelling is due to the water uptake and to the translocation of polymer. The polymer flow at the interface between the tablet and the external medium causes the swelling and the shape change, without polymer release.
- The erosion is due to external fluid dynamics and thus to interactions between the tablet surface and external fluid, which remains constant during the dissolution runs.

The water and drug balances (transport equations) (Table 3 equations (E-F) with $(v_{mix})\rightarrow 0$) in cylindrical coordinates (Figure 11) were:

$$\begin{cases} \rho\dfrac{\partial \omega_i}{\partial t} = \boldsymbol{\nabla}\cdot\left(\rho D_i \boldsymbol{\nabla}\omega_i + \rho\dfrac{\omega_i}{M} D_i \boldsymbol{\nabla} M\right) \\ \omega_2 = 1-(\omega_1+\omega_3) \\ @t=0\ \forall x \in \Omega\ \omega_i = \omega_{i0} \\ @x \in \Gamma 1\ \forall t>0\ j_i = 0 \\ @x \in \Gamma 2\ \forall t>0\ j_i = 0 \\ @x \in \Gamma 3\ \forall t>0\ \omega_i = \omega_{i,eq} \\ @x \in \Gamma 4\ \forall t>0\ \omega_i = \omega_{i,eq} \end{cases} \tag{58}$$

where M is the average molar mass. The ideal mixing rule (like in Lamberti's model) was used for the system density, and the diffusion coefficients were described with Fujita-type equations (eqs. 48 and 51). The domain deformation was described with the ALE method imposing the swelling and the erosion velocities on the erosion boundaries:

$$\begin{cases} \frac{\partial^2}{\partial R^2}\left(\frac{\partial r}{\partial t}\right)+\frac{\partial^2}{\partial Z^2}\left(\frac{\partial r}{\partial t}\right)=0 \\ \frac{\partial^2}{\partial R^2}\left(\frac{\partial z}{\partial t}\right)+\frac{\partial^2}{\partial Z^2}\left(\frac{\partial z}{\partial t}\right)=0 \\ @t=0 \;\; r=r_0; z=z_0 \\ @x\epsilon\Gamma 1 \forall t>0 \;\; dr=0 \\ @x\epsilon\Gamma 2 \forall t>0 \;\; dz=0 \\ @x\epsilon\Gamma 3 \forall t>0 \;\; \frac{\partial z}{\partial t}=\left(v_{swe}+v_{er}\right)\big|_z \\ @x\epsilon\Gamma 4 \forall t>0 \;\; \frac{\partial r}{\partial t}=\left(v_{swe}+v_{er}\right)\big|_r \end{cases} \quad (59)$$

where the uppercase and the lowercase indicate the domain coordinates in the reference and current configuration, respectively. The swelling velocity was derived through a polymer mass balance on the erosion front [114]. The polymer flow toward the erosion front was intended to be used to form new layers of gel, contributing in this way to the swelling phenomena.

$$v_{swe}=-\frac{(j_1+j_3)}{\rho\,\omega_2} \quad (60)$$

whereas the erosion velocity was accounted using a constant value $|v_{er}|=-k_{er}$.

Thanks to this approach, the evolution of the water, drug, and polymer masses was described, along with the mass fraction profiles inside the swollen tablets (Figure 5b) and the tablet shape evolution (Figure 12).

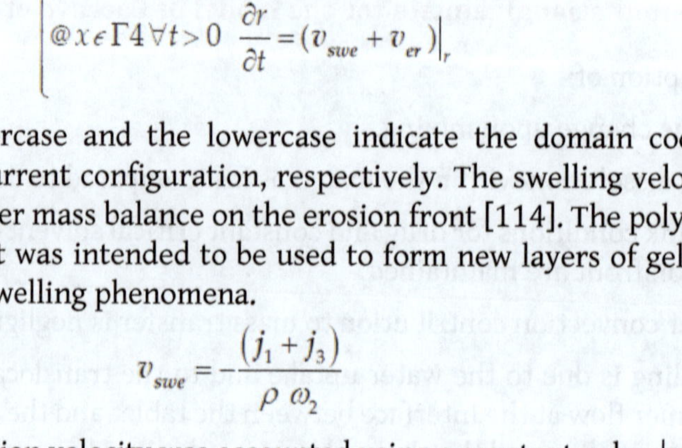

Figure 12. Calculated hydration level, in terms of water mass fraction, and swelling at several dissolution times. In the pictures is represented the half portion of the tablet.

Moreover, the model was successfully compared to experimental data of water mass fraction distribution obtained with the texture analysis (Figure 7b) [115]. A modified version of the model [34], with the inclusion of an excipient (lactose), was compared to hydration and swelling data obtained from an MRI technique, proving that in case of Fickian transport, the model is still reliable (Figure 7a) with some discrepancy at higher dissolution times where the fluid dynamic forces, in the specific testing tool, take over and deform the weak gel.

3.3.3. Multicomponent approach: Mass and momentum transfer

Achilleos et al. [101, 116] proposed a modified transport model for a polyelectrolyte gel made of four components (water "1", polymer "2", Na^+ "4", Cl^- "5"), where the volume transition of the hydrogel was still considered to be driven by the ionic diffusion, but the osmotic pressure is contributed by the mixing, elastic, and electrostatic free energies. Since the system is considered monophasic, with the presence of several species, this kind of formulation can be considered, according to the scheme of Table 3, a multicomponent approach.

Following the mixture theory approach, the mass and momentum balance equations can be written for the mixture, considering a mass average velocity (vmix$v$mix). The system is considered in isothermal conditions so that there is no need for an energy balance. Along with the momentum and mass balance for the mixture, the species mass balance has to be satisfied. All these equations were nondimensionalized and written in terms of polymer velocity (and not the mass average velocity), since it is the one that enters in the stress constitutive expression:

$$\begin{cases} \rho^* \dfrac{D^{(2)}\omega_i}{Dt} - \rho^* \dfrac{\omega_i}{\omega_2}\dfrac{D^{(2)}\omega_2}{Dt} + \boldsymbol{\nabla}\cdot\left(j_i^* - \dfrac{\omega_i}{\omega_2} j_2^*\right) = 0, i \neq 2 \\ \boldsymbol{\nabla}\cdot v_2^* + \dfrac{1}{\rho^*}\dfrac{D^{(2)}\rho^*}{Dt} + \dfrac{1}{\omega_2}\dfrac{D^{(2)}\omega_2}{Dt} = 0 \\ \boldsymbol{\nabla}\cdot\sigma_2^* - \boldsymbol{\nabla} p'^* = 0 \\ \nabla^2\psi^* \propto -\left(\displaystyle\sum_{i=4}^{N_C} \dfrac{z_i\omega_i M_1}{M_i} - \dfrac{z_2\omega_2 a M_1}{M_{2,m}}\right) = 0 \end{cases} \tag{61}$$

where ρ^*, v_2^*, p'^*, and ψ^* are the dimensionless mixture density, polymer velocity, hydrostatic pressure, and electrical potential, respectively. ω_i, j_i^*, M_i, and z_i are the weight fraction, the dimensionless diffusive flux, the molecular weight, and the charge of the ith species, respectively. The variable a and $M_{2,m}$ represent the polymer network ionization ($0 \leq a \leq 1$) and the molecular weight of a monomer. $D^{(2)}/Dt$ is the substantial derivative following the polymer velocity.

Equation 61 represents (in order) the species mass balances (N_C-1) (Table 3 eq. (E)), the continuity equation (Table 3 sum on N_C of eq. (D)), the momentum balance (Table 3 eq. (I)), and the electroneutrality condition (Table 3 eq. (J)). These equations solve for ω_i, p'^*, v_2^*, ψ^*, respectively. It is worth to specify that the mixture stress tensor, with this approach, is equal to the polymer network stress tensor: $\sigma_{mix}=\sigma_2$.

3.3.3.1. Constitutive equations

The diffusive flux of the ith components is given by (Table 3 eq. (N)):

$$j_i^* = -D_i^* \omega_i \left(\boldsymbol{\nabla} p_i^{osm^*} + \frac{M_i}{M_1} \boldsymbol{\nabla} \cdot \boldsymbol{\sigma}_2^* + z_i \boldsymbol{\nabla} \psi^* \right) \tag{62}$$

where $p_i^{osm^*}$ and D_i^* are the dimensionless osmotic pressure and diffusion coefficient (D_1 was considered function of the water concentration) of the ith components. The Helmholtz free energy of the mixture, consisting of mixing (A_{mix}), elastic (A_{el}), and electrostatic (A_{ion}) contributions, can be used to obtain the osmotic pressure and the network stress (Table 3 eq. (K)). The mixture and the electrostatic contribution were accounted in the osmotic pressure:

$$\begin{aligned} p_i^{osm^*} &= \left(ln(\omega_i) + \chi_{i,2}\omega_2 + 1 \right) - \omega_2 \sum_{\substack{\beta=1 \\ \beta \neq 2}}^{N_C} \frac{\chi_{\beta,2}\omega_\beta M_i}{M_\beta} - \sum_{\substack{\beta=1 \\ \beta \neq 2}}^{N_C} \frac{\omega_\beta M_i}{M_\beta} \\ &+ C_{DH} \left(I_s^{1.5} \frac{M_i}{M_1} - 3 z_i I_s^{0.5} \right) + C_{mf}\, a^2 \omega_2 \left(-\frac{z_i^2 M_1}{I_s M_i} + 1 \right) \end{aligned} \tag{63}$$

where $\chi_{i,2}$ is the Flory–Huggins interaction parameter and C_{DH} and C_{mf} are two determined constants. The osmotic pressure is therefore composed of a solvent–polymer mixing contribution, a mobile ions contribution, and fixed charges contribution. The elastic contribution of the Helmholtz free energy was used, according to eq. 46, to derive the network stress tensor:

$$\boldsymbol{\sigma}_2 = 2J^{-1} B \frac{\partial A_{el}(B)}{\partial B} = G_0 \frac{\phi_2}{\phi_{20}} (B - \boldsymbol{\delta}) = G(B - \boldsymbol{\delta}) \tag{64}$$

where G_0 is the hydrogel modulus and ϕ_2 and ϕ_{20} are the volume fraction of the polymer and the volume fraction of polymer at the gelation (stress-free state) so that the shear modulus is $G = G_0 \phi_2 / \phi_{20}$. The network stress was related to the polymer velocity v_2:

$$\frac{D^{(2)} \boldsymbol{\sigma}_2}{Dt} - \boldsymbol{\sigma}_2 \cdot \boldsymbol{\nabla} v_2 - \boldsymbol{\nabla} v_2^T \cdot \boldsymbol{\sigma}_2 + \boldsymbol{\sigma}_2 \boldsymbol{\nabla} \cdot v_2 = G_0 \frac{\phi_2}{\phi_{20}} \left(\boldsymbol{\nabla} v_2 + \nabla v_2^T \right) \tag{65}$$

These last equations, coupled with the momentum balance, allow to solve for σ_2. Applying the proper initial and boundary conditions, this model solution (obtained with a FEM method) provided the hydrogel water concentration, deformation, stress, and potential fields as functions of external and gel parameters: solution molarity, degree of polymerization, shear modulus, and problem geometry.

3.3.4. Multicomponent approach: Monophasic theory

On the basis of the poroelastic theory, Suo and his group developed a framework (the monophasic theory) for modeling the mass transport of small molecular species in a three-dimensional polymeric network coupled with large deformations [105, 117]. Once again, the model can be classified, according to the scheme of Table 3, as a multicomponent approach. Indeed, the system is monophasic and the solvent transport is modeled with a diffusive mass transport equation.

The basic idea is that because of its microstructure, a gel is capable of two basic modes of deformation. First, the stretching of polymer chains accompanied by local rearrangement of small molecules allows a gel to change its shape rapidly but maintain a constant volume. The gel behaves just like an incompressible elastomer in this mode, showing a viscoelastic nature. The second mode, which involves long-range transportation of the small molecules, is usually slow and size dependent. The deformation in the second mode allows the gel to swell or shrink in volume, emphasizing the poroelastic nature.

The first mode of deformation was neglected in the earliest publication [117], considering an instantaneous rearrangement of the polymer chain, therefore not considering the viscoelastic nature of the hydrogel. In the wake of this framework, several other works have been published [105, 118-122]. Later on, in seek of completeness, the viscoelastic nature of hydrogel has been then added to the framework [123].

In the following the viscoporoelastic model [123] will be reported, using the "index notation" and the summation convention (with the uppercase and with the lowercase are denoted the variables in the reference and current state, respectively). Let ΩΩ be the volume of each solvent molecule in the gel. Taking the dry state of the polymer network to be the reference, it is possible to relate the nominal solvent concentration CC to the volumetric expansion det$F$ as

$$\det \boldsymbol{F} := \frac{V_{tot}}{V_{dry}} = 1 + \frac{V_{solv}}{V_{dry}} = 1 + \frac{V_{solv}}{N_{solv\ molecules}} \frac{N_{solv\ molecules}}{V_{dry}} = 1 + \Omega C \tag{66}$$

As usual, the gel Helmholtz free energy is considered as the sum of the elastic (affine network) contribution and the polymer–solvent mixing contribution. A peculiarity of this approach is the reformulation of the Flory–Huggins $A_{mix}(C)$ as $A_{mix}(F)$, using eq. 66, therefore considering the strain energy density function given by the sum of the elastic and mixing free energy.

3.3.4.1. Nonequilibrium thermodynamics

The second law of thermodynamics dictates that the total free energy of a closed system keeps constant or decreases in any physical process. Assuming that the energy is dissipated mainly through two processes, solvent migration $\dot{W}_s$ and viscous deformation $\dot{W}_V$ ($\dot{W}_s$ being dependent on the true solvent flux j_1 and $\dot{W}_V$ being dependent on the deviatoric part of the strain rate tensor), it is possible to write

$$\frac{\partial \Phi}{\partial t} - \frac{\partial W}{\partial t} + \int_V \dot{W}_s dV + \int_V \dot{W}_V dV = 0 \tag{67}$$

where the first term is the rate of variation of the total free energy (Φ) of the hydrogel $\partial\Phi/\partial t = \int \partial A/\partial t \, dV$. The second term is the total work (W) done to the hydrogel, including the mechanical work by the surface traction and the chemical work via absorption of solvent molecules $\partial W/\partial t = \int_{\partial V} t_i \partial x/\partial t \, dS + \int_{\partial V} \bar{\mu}$, where t_i is the stress acting on the gel surface, $\bar{\mu}$ is the chemical potential of the solvent in the external medium, and I is the molecular flux. The third and fourth terms represent the free energy dissipation due to solvent migration ($\dot{W}_s$) and viscous deformation ($\dot{W}_V$).

Moreover, the system has to respect the solvent molecule conservation $\partial C/\partial t = -(\partial J_K)/(\partial X_K)$ that rewritten in terms of C=C(F) can be added (using a Lagrange multiplier (μ)) to eq. 67:

$$\int_V \frac{\partial A}{\partial F_{iK}}\frac{\partial v_i}{\partial X_K}dV - \int_{\partial V} t_i\frac{\partial x_i}{\partial t}dS - \int_{\partial V}\bar{\mu}\, IdS + \int_V \dot{W}_s dV + \int_V \dot{W}_V dV + \int_V \mu\left[\frac{detF}{\Omega}H_{Ki}\frac{\partial v_i}{\partial X_K} + \frac{\partial J_L}{\partial X_L}\right]dV = 0 \tag{68}$$

where the tensor H=F^{-1}. With the aid of integration by parts and the divergence theorem, it can be shown that to satisfy eq. 68,

$$\begin{cases} \dfrac{\partial P_{iK}}{\partial X_K} = 0 \\ P_{iK}N_K = t_i \\ \dfrac{\partial C}{\partial t} + \dfrac{\partial J_L}{\partial X_L} = \dfrac{detF}{\Omega}H_{Ki}\dfrac{\partial v_i}{\partial X_K} + \dfrac{\partial J_L}{\partial X_L} = 0 \\ J_K = -\dfrac{D}{k_b T}\dfrac{detF - 1}{\Omega\, detF}H_{Ki}H_{Li}\dfrac{\partial \mu}{\partial X_L} \\ \mu = \bar{\mu} \end{cases} \tag{69}$$

where P_{iK} is the nominal stress (first Piola–Kirchhoff stress that relates to the Cauchy stress by σ_{mix}=PF^T.) defined as

$$P_{iK} = Nk_b T(F_{iK} - H_{iK}) + \frac{k_b T}{\Omega}\left[\ln\left(1 - \frac{1}{detF}\right)detF + 1 + \frac{\chi}{detF}\right]H_{Ki} + \eta\, detF\, H_{Lj}\left(\frac{1}{2}H_{Kj}\frac{\partial v_i}{\partial X_L} + \frac{1}{2}H_{Ki}\frac{\partial v_j}{\partial X_L} - \frac{1}{3}H_{Ki}\frac{\partial v_i}{\partial X_L}\right) - \mu\frac{detF}{\Omega}H_{Ki} \tag{70}$$

Equation 70 represents the momentum (Table 3 eq. (I) in terms of nominal stress) and the solvent mass conservation equations (Table 3 eq. (D) in the reference configuration) in the hydrogel, derived from nonequilibrium thermodynamics considerations, along with their natural boundary conditions rising from the transformation from the strong to the weak form. The expression of the stress tensor in eq. 70 results in a more complex equation, i.e., with respect to Achilleos's model, since this accounts for the network elasticity, the polymer–solvent mixing, and the energy dissipations.

3.3.5. Multiphasic models

With the "multiphasic models," the hydrogel is divided into two (biphasic) or three (triphasic) phases, including a solid polymer network phase, a fluidic solvent phase, and a mobile ion phase for polyelectrolyte hydrogels. In the following will be analyzed the biphasic (polymer plus water) model of Birgersson and Kurnia [124-126]. It has to be said that with the multiphasic approach, unlike the multicomponent approach, some attempts have been made in coupling the drug release and the hydrogel mechanics

[127], treating the drug as a diffusant species, according to Table 3.

In 2008, an interesting work aiming to describe the transient analysis of temperature-sensitive neutral hydrogels was published [126] and improved in the years [128] until the last publication in 2012 [125]. The starting point was the mass and the momentum conservation of the phases, coupled with the energy conservation. It was demonstrated [126] that the energy transport is considerably quicker than the deformation; therefore, the system can be accurately described through an isothermal deformation based on the new equilibrium temperature [125].

Considering the conservation of the mass for the two phases (Table 3 equations (B)):

$$\begin{aligned} \frac{\partial \phi_1}{\partial t} &= -\boldsymbol{\nabla} \cdot (\phi_1 v_1) \\ \frac{\partial \phi_2}{\partial t} &= -\boldsymbol{\nabla} \cdot (\phi_2 v_2) \end{aligned} \tag{71}$$

where ϕ_2 and ϕ_1 are the polymer and the fluid volume fractions and v_2 and v_1 the polymer and fluid velocities. Summing these equations, the mixture mass conservation expression was derived:

$$0 = -\boldsymbol{\nabla} \cdot (\phi_2 v_2 + (1-\phi_2) v_1) = -\boldsymbol{\nabla} \cdot v_{vol} \tag{72}$$

where v_{vol} is the system volume average velocity. After some manipulations, it is possible to reformulate the polymer mass conservation in terms of the relative velocity ($v_R = v_1 - v_2$):

$$\boldsymbol{\nabla} \cdot v_2 = -\frac{\boldsymbol{\nabla} \cdot q}{\rho_{1,0}} \tag{73}$$

where $q = \phi_1 \rho_{1,0} v_R$ is the relative flow vector of the fluid phase with respect to the polymer phase.

Considering the momentum conservation for the polymer and fluid phases (Table 3 equations (H) for nonionic system and with $(\mu_1 \dot{\gamma}) \rightarrow 0$):

$$\begin{aligned} 0 &= \nabla \cdot (-\phi_1 p \boldsymbol{\delta}) + f_{12} \\ 0 &= \nabla \cdot (-\phi_2 p \boldsymbol{\delta} + \boldsymbol{\sigma}_2) + f_{21} \end{aligned} \tag{74}$$

In eq. 74, pp is the fluid pressure inside the hydrogel, σ_2 is the polymer stress tensor, and f_{12} and f_{21} are the reaction couple of the drag force between the two phases: $f_{12} = -f_{21} = p\nabla\phi_p + \zeta\, v_R$, where ζ is the friction coefficient defined as $\zeta = \mu_1 \phi_1^2 / \kappa$, function of the fluid viscosity μ_1, of the fluid volume fraction, and of the hydrogel permeability κ. From the momentum balance on the fluid phase, the pressure gradient can be related to q:

$$\boldsymbol{\nabla} p = -\frac{\mu_1}{\kappa} \frac{q}{\rho_{1,0}} \tag{75}$$

While summing both eq. 71, the mixture moment conservation can be obtained:

$$0 = \boldsymbol{\nabla} \cdot \left(-pI + \boldsymbol{\sigma}_2\right) \tag{76}$$

Equation 76 highlights that in the multiphasic approach, due to the preliminary assumptions, the stress tensor is the one of the polymer network, while the solvent-polymer interaction -- and eventually the ion effect -- influences the momentum of the hydrogel through the pressure term.

3.3.5.1. Constitutive equations

The Helmholtz free energy of a hydrogel is constituted by the elasticity-related term and by the polymer-solvent mixing-related term. As usual, the elastic contribution is attributed to the polymer chain through the Cauchy stress, and the mixing term is considered through the osmotic pressure.

The mixing term of the Helmholtz free energy was considered through the presence of an osmotic pressure with the expression [129]

$$p^{osm} = -\frac{k_b T}{V_m}\left[\phi_P + \chi\phi_P^2 + \ln\left(1-\phi_P\right)\right] \tag{77}$$

where χ is the polymer-solvent interaction parameter, k_b is the Boltzmann constant, T is the temperature, and V_m is the volume occupied by one monomer.

The Cauchy stress tensor for the polymer σ_2 was derived using eq. 46 and an affine elastic free energy:

$$\boldsymbol{\sigma}_2 = \mathrm{G}\left(\boldsymbol{B} - \frac{1}{2}\boldsymbol{\delta}\right) \tag{78}$$

Equation 78 is similar to eq. 64, a part from the factor 0.5 that multiplies the unit tensor. It is worth highlighting that in some cases, it might be useful to separate the concept of reference configuration (state of polymerization of the hydrogel) from the initial configuration to avoid singular behavior (i.e., for polymerization in gas where $\phi_2 \approx 1$, the osmotic pressure goes to infinity). However, this is not the case, and the reader is referred to [105, 119, 129] for further information.

At this point with the proper initial and boundary conditions, knowing the constitutive equations, the partial differential eqs. 73, 75, and 76 could be simultaneously solved for q, p, and v_2 that in conjunction with a moving mesh and the other algebraic equations previously defined, allow to completely characterize the hydrogel deformation due to a temperature variation. The authors, to avoid the use of a moving mesh, recast the equations in Lagrangian configuration; however, since this last step is not indispensable for the modeling approach comprehension, it will not show here, and the interested readers are referred to [125, 126].

4. NOMENCLATURE

A	Generic area	$[m^2]$
A	Helmholtz free energy per unit volume	$[J/m^3]$

A_{el}	Elastic contribution to the Helmholtz free energy	$[J/m^3]$
A_{ion}	Ionic contribution to the Helmholtz free energy	$[J/m^3]$
A_{mix}	Mixing contribution to the Helmholtz free energy	$[J/m^3]$
B	Finger tensor (left Cauchy–Green)	[-]
C	Solvent concentration in the reference configuration (see 3.3.4)	$[1/m^3]$
C_n	Flory's characteristic ratio	[-]
c^*	Solvent concentration at the glass–rubber interface (see 2.4)	$[kg_{solvent}/kg_{dry\ Polymer}]$
c_i	Concentration of the ith species	$[mol/m^3]$
c_x	Cross-linking concentration	$[mol/m^3]$
D_i	Diffusion coefficient of the ith species	$[m^2/s]$
$D^{(i)}/Dt$	Substantial derivative following the ith species velocity	$[1/s]$
dF/ds	Slope of the force–penetration curve	$[N/m]$
F	Faraday's constant	$[C/mol]$
F	Fickian contribution to drug release	[-]
F	Deformation gradient tensor	[-]
f	Frictional draw coefficient	$[(J\cdot s)/m^2]$
f_{ij}	Drag force per unit volume of the phase ii on the phase jj	$[N/m^3]$
G	Hydrogel shear modulus	$[Pa]$
G_0	Hydrogel initial shear modulus at the stress-free state (gelation condition)	$[Pa]$
H	Tablet height	$[m]$
H	Inverse of the deformation gradient tensor	[-]
I	Light intensity	[-]
I	Ionic strength	$[mol/m^3]$
I_0	Light intensity of the dry tablet	[-]
I_B	First invariant of the Finger tensor	[-]
III_B	Third invariant of the Finger tensor	[-]
I_{max}	Light intensity of the fully hydrated gel	[-]
J	Solvent flux in the reference configuration (see 3.3.4)	$[1/(m^2s)]$
j_i	Mass flux of the ith species	$[kg/(m^2s)]$
K_a	Acid dissociation constant	
K_b	Basic dissociation constant	
k	Hydraulic permeability	$[m^2]$
k	Generic constant	

k_b	Boltzmann's constant	$[J/K]$
k_{er}	Erosion constant	$[kg/(m^2s)]$
k_{eros}	Erosion constant velocity	$[m/s]$
k_{swe}	Constant of swelling	[-]
L_{Ch}	Characteristic diffusion path length	$[m]$
L_c	Length of the polymeric chain	$[m]$
l	Length of the bond along the polymer backbone	$[m]$
M	Average molecular weight	$[kg/mol]$
M_∞	Amount of drug released at infinite time	$[kg]$
M_f	Weight of the polymeric chain	$[kg]$
M_i	Molecular weight of the ith species	$[kg/mol]$
M_r	Molecular weight of the repeating unit	$[kg/mol]$
M_t	Cumulative amount of drug released at time tt	$[kg]$
$\overline{M}_C$	Molecular weight between two consecutive cross-links	[kg/mol]$[kg/mol]$
$\overline{M}_n$	Number-average molecular weight of the polymer	[kg/mol]$[kg/mol]$
m_i	Mass of the ith species	$[kg]$
N	Number of links for chain	[-]
N_A	Avogadro constant	$[1/mol]$
$N_{De.D}$	Diffusional Deborah number	[-]
$N_{Sw.A}$	Swelling area number	[-]
$N_{Sw.I}$	Swelling interface number	[-]
N_c	Number of species	[-]
n_i	Mole of the ith species	$[mol]$
P	First Piola–Kirchhoff stress tensor	$[Pa]$
p	Total intrinsic fluid pressure	$[Pa]$
p'	Total intrinsic fluid pressure minus osmotic pressure (eq. L)	$[Pa]$
p^{osm}	Osmotic pressure	$[Pa]$
Q	Volumetric swelling ratio	[-]
q	Relative flow vector of fluid phase with respect to the polymer phase	$[kg/(m^2s)]$
R	Gas constant	$[J/(K\ mol)]$
R	Swelling contribution to drug release	
r_f	Polymer fiber radius	$[m]$
r_s	Size of the diffusing solute	$[m]$

$\left(\bar{r}_0^2\right)^{1/2}$	Unperturbed root-mean-square of the end-to-end distance for polymer chains between two neighboring cross-links	$[m]$
T	Temperature	$[K]$
T2	Spin–spin relaxation time	$[s]$
T_{exp}	Experimental temperature	$[K]$
T_g	Glass transition temperature	$[K]$
t_i	Stress acting on the gel surface	$[Pa]$
V	System volume	$[m^3]$
V_0	Volume of the dry polymer	$[m^3]$
V_1	Molar volume of the solvent	$[m^3/mol]$
V_G	Volume of the swollen gel	$[m^3]$
V_p	Volume of the dry polymer	$[m^3]$
v	Velocity of the solvent penetration	$[m/s]$
v_f	Total free volume	$[m^3]$
$v_{f,p}$	Polymer free volume	$[m^3]$
$v_{f,w}$	Water free volume	$[m^3]$
v_R	Relative velocity of the fluid phase with respect to the polymer phase	$[m/s]$
v_{eros}	Erosion velocity	$[m/s\ ]$
v_i	Velocity of the ith species	$[m/s]$
v_{mix}	Mass average velocity of the mixture	$[m/s]$
v_{swe}	Swelling velocity	$[m/s]$
v_{vol}	System volume average velocity	$[m/s]$
W	Total work done to the hydrogel	$[J]$
W_p	Penetration work	$[J]$
W^{aff}	Strain energy density function from affine network theory	$[J/m^3]$
$\dot{W}_V$	Energy dissipation due to viscous deformation	$[W/m^3]$
$\dot{W}_s$	Energy dissipation due to solvent migration	$[W/m^3]$
x_i	Molar fraction of the ith species	[-]
z_i	ith species charge	[-]
Greek symbols		
α	Elongation ratio	[-]
α	Obstruction theory parameter	[-]
α_f	Thermal linear expansion coefficient of the polymer	$[1/K]$

β	Contribution of the water to the expansion of the polymer	$[kg_{dry\ Polymer}/kg_{solvent}]$
β_i	Diffusivity parameter for the ith species	[-]
γ	Parameters used to relate the light intensity to the weight fraction	[-]
$\dot{\gamma}$	Rate of strain tensor	$[1/s]$
δ	Thickness of the swollen region through which the solute diffuses (see 1.2.5)	$[m]$
δ	infinitesimal thickness of the boundary element (see 3.3.2)	$[m]$.
δ	Identity tensor	[-]
ε	Relative permittivity	[-]
ε_0	Vacuum permittivity	$[F/m]$
ζ	Friction coefficient	$[(Pa{\cdot}s)/m^2]$
θ_D	Characteristic time for the diffusion of the solvent in the polymer	$[s]$
λ_m	Characteristic stress-relaxation time	$[s]$
$\bar{\mu}$	Chemical potential of the solvent in the external medium	$[J]$
μ_{el}	Number of junctions in the network	[-]
μ_1	Fluid viscosity	$[Pa{\cdot}s]$
ν_{el}	Number of elastic chains	[-]
ξ	Gel mesh size	$[m]$
η	Viscosity	$[Pa{\cdot}s]$
π	Pi	
ρ_i	Density of the ith species	$[kg/m^3]$
σ	Cauchy stress tensor	$[Pa]$
τ	Tensile stress	$[Pa]$
$\bar{\upsilon}$	Polymer-specific volume	$[m^3/kg]$
Φ	Total Helmholtz free energy	$[J]$
ϕ_i	Volume fraction of the ith species	[-]
χ_{12}	Flory–Huggins solvent–polymer interaction parameter	[-]
ψ	Electric potential	$[V]$
Ω	Volume of each solvent molecule in the gel	$[m^3]$
ω_i	Mass fraction of the ith species	[-]

REFERENCES

1. A.S. Hoffman, Hydrogels for biomedical applications, Advanced Drug Delivery Reviews, 64 (2012) 18-23.
2. N. Peppas, P. Bures, W. Leobandung, H. Ichikawa, Hydrogels in pharmaceutical formulations, European Journal of Pharmaceutics and Biopharmaceutics, 50 (2000) 27-46.
3. N.A. Peppas, J.Z. Hilt, A. Khademhosseini, R. Langer, Hydrogels in biology and medicine: from molecular principles to bionanotechnology, Advanced Materials, 18 (2006) 1345.
4. O. Wichterle, D. Lim, Hydrophilic gels for biological use, Nature, 185 (1960) 117-118.
5. N.A. Peppas, Hydrogels in Medicine and Pharmacy, CRC Press, Boca Raton, 1987.
6. J. Cabral, S.C. Moratti, Hydrogels for biomedical applications, Future Medicinal Chemistry, 3 (2011) 1877-1888.
7. K.R. Kamath, K. Park, Biodegradable hydrogels in drug delivery, Advanced Drug Delivery Reviews, 11 (1993) 59-84.
8. N.A. Peppas, Hydrogels and drug delivery, Current Opinion in Colloid & Interface Science, 2 (1997) 531-537.
9. T.R. Hoare, D.S. Kohane, Hydrogels in drug delivery: progress and challenges, Polymer, 49 (2008) 1993-2007.
10. Y. Qiu, K. Park, Environment-sensitive hydrogels for drug delivery, Advanced Drug Delivery Reviews, 53 (2001) 321-339.
11. J. Siepmann, N.A. Peppas, Modeling of drug release from delivery systems based on hydroxypropyl methylcellulose (HPMC), Advanced Drug Delivery Reviews, 48 (2001) 139-157.
12. W.E. Hennink, C.F. van Nostrum, Novel crosslinking methods to design hydrogels, Advanced Drug Delivery Reviews, 54 (2002) 13-36.
13. C.-C. Lin, A.T. Metters, Hydrogels in controlled release formulations: network design and mathematical modeling, Advanced Drug Delivery Reviews, 58 (2006) 1379-1408.
14. P.J. Flory, Principles of Polymer Chemistry, Cornell University Press, Ithaca, 1953.
15. L.R.G. Treloar, The Physics of Rubber Elasticity, Oxford University Press, 1975.
16. P.J. Flory, J. Rehner Jr, Statistical mechanics of crosslinked polymer networks II. Swelling, The Journal of Chemical Physics, 11 (1943) 521-526.
17. P.J. Flory, Statistical mechanics of swelling of network structures, The Journal of Chemical Physics, 18 (1950) 108-111.
18. J.C. Bray, E.W. Merrill, Poly (vinyl alcohol) hydrogels. Formation by electron beam irradiation of aqueous solutions and subsequent crystallization, Journal of Applied Polymer Science, 17 (1973) 3779-3794.
19. N.A. Peppas, E.W. Merrill, Crosslinked poly (vinyl alcohol) hydrogels as swollen elastic networks, Journal of Applied Polymer Science, 21 (1977) 1763-1770.
20. N.A. Peppas, E.W. Merrill, Poly (vinyl alcohol) hydrogels: reinforcement of radiationcrosslinked networks by crystallization, Journal of Polymer Science: Polymer Chemistry Edition, 14 (1976) 441-457.
21. N.A. Peppas, E.W. Merrill, Determination of interaction parameter $\chi 1$, for poly (vinyl alcohol) and water in gels crosslinked from solutions, Journal of Polymer Science: Polymer Chemistry Edition, 14 (1976) 459-464.
22. L. Brannon-Peppas, N.A. Peppas, Equilibrium swelling behavior of pH-sensitive hydrogels, Chemical Engineering Science, 46 (1991) 715-722.

23. T. Canal, N.A. Peppas, Correlation between mesh size and equilibrium degree of swelling of polymeric networks, Journal of Biomedical Materials Research, 23 (1989) 1183-1193.
24. P.J. Flory, N. Rabjohn, M.C. Shaffer, Dependence of elastic properties of vulcanized rubber on the degree of cross linking, Journal of Polymer Science, 4 (1949) 225-245.
25. T. Alfrey, E. Gurnee, W. Lloyd, Diffusion in glassy polymers, Journal of Polymer Science Part C: Polymer Symposia, Wiley Online Library, 1966, pp. 249-261.
26. G.R. Davidson, N.A. Peppas, Solute and penetrant diffusion in swellable polymers: V. Relaxation-controlled transport in P (HEMA-co-MMA) copolymers, Journal of Controlled Release, 3 (1986) 243-258.
27. J. Vrentas, C. Jarzebski, J. Duda, A Deborah number for diffusion in polymer solvent systems, AIChE Journal, 21 (1975) 894-901.
28. J. Vrentas, J. Duda, Diffusion in polymer–solvent systems. III. Construction of Deborah number diagrams, Journal of Polymer Science: Polymer Physics Edition, 15 (1977) 441-453.
29. G.R. Davidson, N.A. Peppas, Solute and penetrant diffusion in swellable polymers: VI. The Deborah and swelling interface numbers as indicators of the order of biomolecular release, Journal of Controlled Release, 3 (1986) 259-271.
30. G. CameraRoda, G.C. Sarti, Mass transport with relaxation in polymers, AIChE Journal, 36 (1990) 851-860.
31. J. Wilmers, S. Bargmann, Simulation of non-classical diffusion in polymers, Heat and Mass Transfer, 50 (2014) 1543-1552.
32. J. Tritt-Goc, J. Kowalczuk, N. Piślewski, MRI study of Fickian, case II and anomalous diffusion of solvents into hydroxypropylmethylcellulose, Applied Magnetic Resonance, 29 (2005) 605-615.
33. J. Tritt-Goc, J. Kowalczuk, N. Pislewski, Hydration of hydroxypropylmethyl cellulose: effects of pH and molecular mass, Acta Physica Polonica-Series A General Physics, 108 (2005) 197-206.
34. D. Caccavo, G. Lamberti, A.A. Barba, S. Abrahmsén-Alami, A. Viridén, A. Larsson, Modeling of extended release matrix tablet performance: water up-take, polymer and drug release, and shape deformation, (in preparation).
35. N.A. Peppas, N.M. Franson, The swelling interface number as a criterion for prediction of diffusional solute release mechanisms in swellable polymers, Journal of Polymer Science: Polymer Physics Edition, 21 (1983) 983-997.
36. G. Grassi, R. Lapasin, M. Grassi, I. Colombo, Understanding Drug Release and Absorption Mechanisms A Physical and Mathematical Approach, 2007.
37. B. Amsden, Solute diffusion within hydrogels. Mechanisms and models, Macromolecules, 31 (1998) 8382-8395.
38. B. Amsden, Solute diffusion in hydrogels: an examination of the retardation effect, Polymer Gels and Networks, 6 (1998) 13-43.
39. L. Masaro, X. Zhu, Physical models of diffusion for polymer solutions, gels and solids, Progress in Polymer Science, 24 (1999) 731-775.
40. R. Cukier, Diffusion of Brownian spheres in semidilute polymer solutions, Macromolecules, 17 (1984) 252-255.
41. R. Phillips, W. Deen, J. Brady, Hindered transport of spherical macromolecules in fibrous membranes and gels, AIChE Journal, 35 (1989) 1761-1769.

42. A. Ogston, B. Preston, J. Wells, On the transport of compact particles through solutions of chain-polymers, in: Proceedings of the Royal Society of London A: Mathematical, Physical and Engineering Sciences, The Royal Society, 1973, pp. 297-316.
43. L. Johansson, C. Elvingson, J.E. Loefroth, Diffusion and interaction in gels and solutions. 3. Theoretical results on the obstruction effect, Macromolecules, 24 (1991) 6024-6029.
44. D.S. Tsai, W. Strieder, Effective conductivities of random fiber beds, Chemical Engineering Communications, 40 (1986) 207-218.
45. L. Johansson, J.E. Löfroth, Diffusion and interaction in gels and solutions. 4. Hard sphere Brownian dynamics simulations, The Journal of Chemical Physics, 98 (1993) 7471-7479.
46. D.S. Clague, R.J. Phillips, Hindered diffusion of spherical macromolecules through dilute fibrous media, Physics of Fluids (1994-present), 8 (1996) 1720-1731.
47. H. Yasuda, A. Peterlin, C.K. Colton, K.A. Smith, E.W. Merrill, Permeability of solutes through hydrated polymer membranes. Part III. Theoretical background for the selectivity of dialysis membranes, Die Makromolekulare Chemie, 126 (1969) 177-186.
48. N.A. Peppas, C.T. Reinhart, Solute diffusion in swollen membranes. Part I. A new theory, Journal of Membrane Science, 15 (1983) 275-287.
49. S.R. Lustig, N.A. Peppas, Solute diffusion in swollen membranes. IX. Scaling laws for solute diffusion in gels, Journal of Applied Polymer Science, 36 (1988) 735-747.
50. W. Hennink, H. Talsma, J. Borchert, S. De Smedt, J. Demeester, Controlled release of proteins from dextran hydrogels, Journal of Controlled Release, 39 (1996) 47-55.
51. H. Fujita, Diffusion in polymer-diluent systems, in: Fortschritte Der Hochpolymeren-Forschung, Springer, Berlin, Heidelberg, 1961, pp. 1-47.
52. R.W. Korsmeyer, S.R. Lustig, N.A. Peppas, Solute and penetrant diffusion in swellable polymers. I. Mathematical modeling, Journal of Polymer Science Part B: Polymer Physics, 24 (1986) 395-408.
53. R.W. Korsmeyer, E. Von Meerwall, N.A. Peppas, Solute and penetrant diffusion in swellable polymers. II. Verification of theoretical models, Journal of Polymer Science Part B: Polymer Physics, 24 (1986) 409-434.
54. N. Graham, M. McNeill, Hydrogels for controlled drug delivery, Biomaterials, 5 (1984) 27-36.
55. S. Chirico, A. Dalmoro, G. Lamberti, G. Russo, G. Titomanlio, Analysis and modeling of swelling and erosion behavior for pure HPMC tablet, Journal of Controlled Release, 122 (2007) 181-188.
56. J. Siepmann, H. Kranz, R. Bodmeier, N. Peppas, HPMC-matrices for controlled drug delivery: a new model combining diffusion, swelling, and dissolution mechanisms and predicting the release kinetics, Pharmaceutical Research, 16 (1999) 1748-1756.
57. R.T. Ju, P.R. Nixon, M.V. Patel, Drug release from hydrophilic matrices. 1. New scaling laws for predicting polymer and drug release based on the polymer disentanglement concentration and the diffusion layer, Journal of Pharmaceutical Sciences, 84 (1995) 1455-1463.
58. R.T. Ju, P.R. Nixon, M.V. Patel, D.M. Tong, Drug release from hydrophilic matrices. 2. A mathematical model based on the polymer disentanglement concentration and the diffusion layer, Journal of Pharmaceutical Sciences, 84 (1995) 1464-1477.
59. R. Bettini, P. Catellani, P. Santi, G. Massimo, N. Peppas, P. Colombo, Translocation of drug particles in HPMC matrix gel layer: effect of drug solubility and influence on release rate, Journal of Controlled Release, 70 (2001) 383-391.

60. P.I. Lee, Kinetics of drug release from hydrogel matrices, Journal of Controlled Release, 2 (1985) 277-288.

61. K. Sung, P.R. Nixon, J.W. Skoug, T.R. Ju, P. Gao, E. Topp, M. Patel, Effect of formulation variables on drug and polymer release from HPMC-based matrix tablets, International Journal of Pharmaceutics, 142 (1996) 53-60.

62. J. Nerurkar, H. Jun, J. Price, M. Park, Controlled-release matrix tablets of ibuprofen using cellulose ethers and carrageenans: effect of formulation factors on dissolution rates, European Journal of Pharmaceutics and Biopharmaceutics, 61 (2005) 56-68.

63. K. Mitchell, J. Ford, D. Armstrong, P. Elliott, J. Hogan, C. Rostron, The influence of the particle size of hydroxypropylmethylcellulose K15M on its hydration and performance in matrix tablets, International Journal of Pharmaceutics, 100 (1993) 175-179.

64. S. Zuleger, B.C. Lippold, Polymer particle erosion controlling drug release. I. Factors influencing drug release and characterization of the release mechanism, International Journal of Pharmaceutics, 217 (2001) 139-152.

65. C. Maderuelo, A. Zarzuelo, J.M. Lanao, Critical factors in the release of drugs from sustained release hydrophilic matrices, Journal of Controlled Release, 154 (2011) 2-19.

66. S. Jamzad, L. Tutunji, R. Fassihi, Analysis of macromolecular changes and drug release from hydrophilic matrix systems, International Journal of Pharmaceutics, 292 (2005) 75-85.

67. S. Jamzad, R. Fassihi, Development of a controlled release low dose class II drug-Glipizide, International Journal of Pharmaceutics, 312 (2006) 24-32.

68. P.L. Mamani, R. Ruiz-Caro, M.D. Veiga, Matrix tablets: the effect of hydroxypropyl methylcellulose/anhydrous dibasic calcium phosphate ratio on the release rate of a water-soluble drug through the gastrointestinal tract I. In vitro tests, AAPS PharmSciTech, 13 (2012) 1073-1083.

69. A.A. Barba, M. d'Amore, S. Cascone, S. Chirico, G. Lamberti, G. Titomanlio, On the behavior of HPMC/theophylline matrices for controlled drug delivery, Journal of Pharmaceutical Sciences, 98 (2009) 4100-4110.

70. U.P. XXIII, The United States Pharmacopoeia Convention Inc, Rockville, 1995, pp 557.

71. M.U. Ghori, G. Ginting, A.M. Smith, B.R. Conway, Simultaneous quantification of drug release and erosion from hypromellose hydrophilic matrices, International Journal of Pharmaceutics, 465 (2014) 405-412.

72. C. Remunan-Lopez, R. Bodmeier, Mechanical, water uptake and permeability properties of crosslinked chitosan glutamate and alginate films, Journal of Controlled Release, 44 (1997) 215-225.

73. P. Gao, R.H. Meury, Swelling of hydroxypropyl methylcellulose matrix tablets. 1. Characterization of swelling using a novel optical imaging method, Journal of Pharmaceutical Sciences, 85 (1996) 725-731.

74. K. Tahara, K. Yamamoto, T. Nishihata, Overall mechanism behind matrix sustained release (SR) tablets prepared with hydroxypropyl methylcellulose 2910, Journal of Controlled Release, 35 (1995) 59-66.

75. A.A. Barba, M. d'Amore, S. Chirico, G. Lamberti, G. Titomanlio, Swelling of cellulose derivative (HPMC) matrix systems for drug delivery, Carbohydrate Polymers, 78 (2009) 469-474.

76. A. Rajabi-Siahboomi, R. Bowtell, P. Mansfield, A. Henderson, M. Davies, C. Melia, Structure and behaviour in hydrophilic matrix sustained release dosage forms: 2. NMR-imaging studies of dimensional changes in the gel layer and core of HPMC tablets undergoing hydration, Journal of Controlled Release, 31 (1994) 121-128.
77. P. Gao, P.E. Fagerness, Diffusion in HPMC gels. I. Determination of drug and water diffusivity by pulsed-field-gradient spin-echo NMR, Pharmaceutical Research, 12 (1995) 955-964.
78. W.E. Baille, C. Malveau, X.X. Zhu, R.H. Marchessault, NMR imaging of high-amylose starch tablets. 1. Swelling and water uptake, Biomacromolecules, 3 (2002) 214-218.
79. S. Abrahmsén-Alami, A. Körner, I. Nilsson, A. Larsson, New release cell for NMR microimaging of tablets: swelling and erosion of poly (ethylene oxide), International Journal of Pharmaceutics, 342 (2007) 105-114.
80. F. Tajarobi, S. Abrahmsén-Alami, A.S. Carlsson, A. Larsson, Simultaneous probing of swelling, erosion and dissolution by NMR-microimaging—effect of solubility of additives on HPMC matrix tablets, European Journal of Pharmaceutical Sciences, 37 (2009) 89-97.
81. A. Viridén, S. Abrahmsén-Alami, B. Wittgren, A. Larsson, Release of theophylline and carbamazepine from matrix tablets–consequences of HPMC chemical heterogeneity, European Journal of Pharmaceutics and Biopharmaceutics, 78 (2011) 470-479.
82. L. Yang, B. Johnson, R. Fassihi, Determination of continuous changes in the gel layer thickness of poly (ethylene oxide) and HPMC tablets undergoing hydration: a texture analysis study, Pharmaceutical Research, 15 (1998) 1902-1906.
83. S. Nazzal, M. Nazzal, Y. El-Malah, A novel texture-probe for the simultaneous and real-time measurement of swelling and erosion rates of matrix tablets, International Journal of Pharmaceutics, 330 (2007) 195-198.
84. H. Li, X. Gu, Correlation between drug dissolution and polymer hydration: a study using texture analysis, International Journal of Pharmaceutics, 342 (2007) 18-25.
85. G. Lamberti, S. Cascone, M.M. Cafaro, G. Titomanlio, M. d'Amore, A.A. Barba, Measurements of water content in hydroxypropyl-methyl-cellulose based hydrogels via texture analysis, Carbohydrate Polymers, 92 (2013) 765-768.
86. S. Cascone, G. Lamberti, G. Titomanlio, M. d'Amore, A.A. Barba, Measurements of non-uniform water content in hydroxypropyl-methyl-cellulose based matrices via texture analysis, Carbohydrate Polymers, 103 (2014) 348-354.
87. P. Colombo, P. Catellani, N. Peppas, L. Maggi, U. Conte, Swelling characteristics of hydrophilic matrices for controlled release new dimensionless number to describe the swelling and release behavior, International Journal of Pharmaceutics, 88 (1992) 99-109.
88. R. Bettini, P. Colombo, G. Massimo, P.L. Catellani, T. Vitali, Swelling and drug release in hydrogel matrices: polymer viscosity and matrix porosity effects, European Journal of Pharmaceutical Sciences, 2 (1994) 213-219.
89. P. Colombo, R. Bettini, N.A. Peppas, Observation of swelling process and diffusion front position during swelling in hydroxypropyl methyl cellulose (HPMC) matrices containing a soluble drug, Journal of Controlled Release, 61 (1999) 83-91.
90. S. Kikuchi, Y. Onuki, H. Kuribayashi, K. Takayama, Relationship between diffusivity of water molecules inside hydrating tablets and their drug release behavior elucidated by magnetic resonance imaging, Chemical and Pharmaceutical Bulletin, 60 (2012) 536-542.

91. K.O. Hewlett, J. L'Hote-Gaston, M. Radler, K.R. Shull, Direct measurement of the time-dependent mechanical response of HPMC and PEO compacts during swelling, International Journal of Pharmaceutics, 434 (2012) 494-501.

92. S. Zuleger, R. Fassihi, B.C. Lippold, Polymer particle erosion controlling drug release. II. Swelling investigations to clarify the release mechanism, International Journal of Pharmaceutics, 247 (2002) 23-37.

93. K. Huanbutta, K. Terada, P. Sriamornsak, J. Nunthanid, Advanced technologies for assessment of polymer swelling and erosion behaviors in pharmaceutical aspect, European Journal of Pharmaceutics and Biopharmaceutics, 83 (2013) 315-321.

94. T. Higuchi, Rate of release of medicaments from ointment bases containing drugs in suspension, Journal of Pharmaceutical Sciences, 50 (1961) 874-875.

95. N.A. Peppas, Analysis of Fickian and non-Fickian drug release from polymers, Pharmaceutica Acta Helvetiae, 60 (1985) 110-111.

96. N.A. Peppas, J.J. Sahlin, A simple equation for the description of solute release. III. Coupling of diffusion and relaxation, International Journal of Pharmaceutics, 57 (1989) 169-172.

97. C.-C. Lin, A.T. Metters, Hydrogels in controlled release formulations: network design and mathematical modeling, Advanced Drug Delivery Reviews, 58 (2006) 1379-1408.

98. J.E. Mark, B. Erman, Rubberlike Elasticity: A Molecular Primer, Cambridge University Press, Cambridge, UK, 2007.

99. G.A. Holzapfel, Nonlinear Solid Mechanics, Wiley, Chichester, 2000.

100. F. Horkay, G. McKenna, Polymer networks and gels, in: J. Mark (Ed.) Physical Properties of Polymers Handbook, Springer, New York, 2007, pp. 497-523.

101. E.C. Achilleos, K.N. Christodoulou, I.G. Kevrekidis, A transport model for swelling of polyelectrolyte gels in simple and complex geometries, Computational and Theoretical Polymer Science, 11 (2001) 63-80.

102. J. Ricka, T. Tanaka, Swelling of ionic gels: quantitative performance of the Donnan theory, Macromolecules, 17 (1984) 2916-2921.

103. P. Chiarelli, D. De Rossi, Polyelectrolyte intelligent gels: design and applications, in: Ionic Interactions in Natural and Synthetic Macromolecules, Wiley, Hoboken, 2012, pp. 581-620.

104. T. Wallmersperger, Modelling and simulation of the chemo-electro-mechanical behaviour, in: G. Gerlach, K.-F. Arndt (Eds.) Hydrogel Sensors and Actuators, Springer, Berlin, Heidelberg, 2010, pp. 137-163.

105. W. Hong, Z. Liu, Z. Suo, Inhomogeneous swelling of a gel in equilibrium with a solvent and mechanical load, International Journal of Solids and Structures, 46 (2009) 3282-3289.

106. J. Siepmann, H. Kranz, R. Bodmeier, N.A. Peppas, HPMC-matrices for controlled drug delivery: a new model combining diffusion, swelling, and dissolution mechanisms and predicting the release kinetics, Pharmaceutical Research, 16 (1999) 1748-1756.

107. S. Kiil, K. Dam-Johansen, Controlled drug delivery from swellable hydroxypropylmethylcellulose matrices: model-based analysis of observed radial front movements, Journal of Controlled Release, 90 (2003) 1-21.

108. A.A. Barba, M. d'Amore, S. Chirico, G. Lamberti, G. Titomanlio, A general code to predict the drug release kinetics from different shaped matrices, European Journal of Pharmaceutical Sciences, 36 (2009) 359-368.

109. T. Coviello, M. Grassi, R. Lapasin, A. Marino, F. Alhaique, Scleroglucan/borax: characterization of a novel hydrogel system suitable for drug delivery, Biomaterials, 24 (2003) 2789-2798.

110. G. Lamberti, I. Galdi, A.A. Barba, Controlled release from hydrogel-based solid matrices. A model accounting for water up-take, swelling and erosion, International Journal of Pharmaceutics, 407 (2011) 78-86.

111. E. Kaunisto, S. Abrahmsen-Alami, P. Borgquist, A. Larsson, B. Nilsson, A. Axelsson, A mechanistic modelling approach to polymer dissolution using magnetic resonance microimaging, Journal of Controlled Release : Official Journal of the Controlled Release Society, 147 (2010) 232-241.

112. E. Kaunisto, F. Tajarobi, S. Abrahmsen-Alami, A. Larsson, B. Nilsson, A. Axelsson, Mechanistic modelling of drug release from a polymer matrix using magnetic resonance microimaging, European Journal of Pharmaceutical Sciences, 48 (2013) 698-708.

113. B.R. Bird, W.E. Stewart, E.N. Lightfoot, Transport Phenomena, Wiley, New York, 2007.

114. D. Caccavo, S. Cascone, G. Lamberti, A.A. Barba, Modeling the drug release from hydrogel-based matrices, Molecular Pharmaceutics, 12 (2015) 474-483.

115. D. Caccavo, S. Cascone, G. Lamberti, A.A. Barba, Controlled drug release from hydrogel-based matrices: experiments and modeling, International Journal of Pharmaceutics, 486 (2015) 144-152.

116. E.C. Achilleos, R.K. Prud'homme, I.G. Kevrekidis, K.N. Christodoulou, K.R. Gee, Quantifying deformation in gel swelling: Experiments and simulations, AIChE Journal, 46 (2000) 2128-2139.

117. W. Hong, X. Zhao, J. Zhou, Z. Suo, A theory of coupled diffusion and large deformation in polymeric gels, Journal of the Mechanics and Physics of Solids, 56 (2008) 1779-1793.

118. W. Hong, X. Zhao, Z. Suo, Large deformation and electrochemistry of polyelectrolyte gels, Journal of the Mechanics and Physics of Solids, 58 (2010) 558-577.

119. A. Lucantonio, P. Nardinocchi, L. Teresi, Transient analysis of swelling-induced large deformations in polymer gels, Journal of the Mechanics and Physics of Solids, 61 (2013) 205-218.

120. S.A. Chester, L. Anand, A coupled theory of fluid permeation and large deformations for elastomeric materials, Journal of the Mechanics and Physics of Solids, 58 (2010) 1879-1906.

121. F.P. Duda, A.C. Souza, E. Fried, A theory for species migration in a finitely strained solid with application to polymer network swelling, Journal of the Mechanics and Physics of Solids, 58 (2010) 515-529.

122. M.K. Kang, R. Huang, A variational approach and finite element implementation for swelling of polymeric hydrogels under geometric constraints, Journal of Applied Mechanics, 77 (2010) 061004.

123. X. Wang, W. Hong, A visco-poroelastic theory for polymeric gels, Proceedings of the Royal Society A: Mathematical, Physical and Engineering Sciences, 468 (2012) 3824-3841.

124. J.C. Kurnia, E. Birgersson, A.S. Mujumdar, Computational study of pH-sensitive hydrogel-based microfluidic flow controllers, Journal of Functional Biomaterials, 2 (2011) 195-212.

125. J.C. Kurnia, E. Birgersson, A.S. Mujumdar, Finite deformation of fast-response thermo-sensitive hydrogels – a computational study, Polymer, 53 (2012) 2500-2508.

126. E. Birgersson, H. Li, S. Wu, Transient analysis of temperature-sensitive neutral hydrogels, Journal of the Mechanics and Physics of Solids, 56 (2008) 444-466.

127. Y. Xu, Y. Jia, Z. Wang, Z. Wang, Mathematical modeling and finite element simulation of slow release of drugs using hydrogels as carriers with various drug concentration distributions, Journal of Pharmaceutical Sciences, 102 (2013) 1532-1543.

128. J.C. Kurnia, Computational Study of Transport Phenomena and Deformation Behavior of Stimuli Sensitive Hydrogels, Department of Mechanical Engineering, National University of Singapore, 2011.

129. H. Li, Smart Hydrogel Modelling, Springer, Heidelberg, New York, 2009.

11 Chapter

ANTIBIOTIC DELIVERY SYSTEMS FOR INTRACELLULAR TARGETING OF BACTERIAL PATHOGENS

1. INTRODUCTION: AN OVERVIEW

Infections caused by intracellular bacterial infections are challenging to manage because standard antimicrobial drugs cannot effectively enter, aggregate, or persist within mammalian cells [1]. The escalating issue of antibiotic resistance further complicates the treatment of diseases induced by these medications.

Considering the substantial financial investment required to introduce a new antibiotic to the market and the restricted lifespan of antibiotics, the development of drug delivery systems that facilitate the targeted delivery of antibiotics within cells, enhance their efficacy in various intracellular environments with differing pH and oxygen levels, and minimize dosage and administration frequency may be a judicious strategy [2]. This strategy will facilitate the revival of obsolete antibiotics compromised by resistance or toxicity, enhance the therapeutic index of last-resort antibiotics, broaden the antimicrobial spectrum of antibiotic scaffolds that have failed due to membrane permeability issues, and consequently diminish the disparity between the rising prevalence of drug-resistant pathogens and the advancement of new antibiotics.

This study aims to delineate the limits of various antibiotic classes in addressing intracellular pathogens and to highlight key research trajectories for the advancement of drug delivery technologies facilitating the intracellular release of antibiotics.

2. MICROBIAL ADAPTABILITY TO AN INTRACELLULAR EXISTENCE

Invasion denotes the capacity of infections to breach epithelial barriers via specific pathways, infiltrate host tissue, and proliferate, resulting in adverse outcomes [3]. Invasive microbes can infiltrate host tissues or activate the endocytic function of the substrate, allowing them to sustain survival within host cells [4].

A multitude of dangerous bacteria can endure within eukaryotic, mostly nonphagocytic cells, such as mucosal and endothelial cells of blood vessels. The intracellular environment provides protection to bacteria, allowing them to proliferate or endure.

Certain pathogenic bacteria are facultative intracellular organisms (e.g., *Mycobacterium* spp., *Listeria monocytogenes*, and *Salmonella* spp.), capable of undergoing an intracellular phase during their infectious cycle without a strict reliance on the cellular environment, whereas others are obligate intracellular parasites (Chlamydia spp. and Rickettsia spp.) that cannot survive in the host's extracellular milieu. They infect endothelial cells, epithelial cells, and monocytes.

Invasive organisms typically attach to host cells via a category of molecules known as invasins, which are proteins with adhesion properties that facilitate bacterial entry into the cells [8]. The processes of adhesion initiate or enhance cellular signals that directly or indirectly enable bacterial penetration [9].

Following bacterial adherence, invasion occurs via two mechanisms: (a) the "zipper" mechanism—where adherent bacteria induce alterations in the cytoskeleton, particularly actin filaments, leading to their embedding, and (b) internalization through a pathway that is independent of the membrane molecules facilitating adherence. The contact between the bacterium and the host cell membrane results in localized intrusion (ruffling), subsequently leading to endocytosis [10].

Professional phagocytes possess membrane receptors for conserved structures of microbial pathogens known as pathogen-associated molecular patterns (PAMP), which are absent in mammalian cells. A diverse array of microbial pathogens is identified by a restricted set of host receptor molecules known as pathogen recognition receptors (PRR), which are categorized into the following groups: The TLR family of receptors (Toll-like receptors) identifies various microbial structures, including glycoproteins, lipoproteins, heat shock proteins, and flagellar proteins. Additionally, lectin-type receptors exhibit specificity for common carbohydrates present on bacterial surfaces: (a) mannose-binding lectin (MBL) receptors, which can also detect other carbohydrates such as N-acetylglucosamine, glucose, and L-fucose; (b) galactose receptors that recognize N-acetyl-galactosamine and galactose; (c) fucose receptors and specific membrane molecules like CD14, which target glycolipids (LPS) and lipoarabinomannans (LAM) from mycobacteria.

The necessity for bacterial adhesion to eukaryotic cells to involve the recognition of specific oligosaccharides or glycoproteins was evidenced by in vitro experimental results, which indicated that oligosaccharides serve as the most effective inhibitors of the interaction between bacteria and the eukaryotic cell surface.

The invasion is an active process, maintained by standard cellular activities, with the host cell cytoskeleton facilitating the invasion and embedding mechanisms.

Pathogenic bacteria, including L. monocytogenes, Shigella spp., and Rickettsia spp., utilize mechanisms that trigger cytoskeletal rearrangements in the host cell, resulting in actin condensation and the formation of a propulsion actin comet behind the bacterial cells to facilitate their cytoplasmic and intercellular movement.

Certain bacterial strains may influence host cell apoptosis throughout the infectious cycle [14]. The pro-apoptotic impact may promote the endocytosis of apoptotic bodies containing bacterial cells by neighboring cells, without triggering an inflammatory response; nevertheless, bacteria could simultaneously disseminate into healthy tissues. Bacteria-induced apoptosis is facilitated by the activation of caspases or Fas/FasL pathways, which are associated with the inactivation of antiapoptotic proteins such as NFkB and MAP kinases. Pseudomonas aeruginosa may induce apoptosis in lung epithelial cells, a mechanism via which bacterial cells are eliminated from the lungs or other diseased organs. Nonetheless, *P. aeruginosa* can infiltrate, endure, and proliferate within host cells, eliciting an antiapoptotic response to preserve its host and shield itself from immune response effectors [15].

Through microscope assessment and viable cell count assays, we have shown that clinical strains of P. aeruginosa can endure and proliferate within nonphagocytic epithelial cells, resulting in alterations to cellular morphology, including cytoplasmic wrinkling and the development of elongated, lamellar pseudopodia. The P. aeruginosa strains were capable of modulating the apoptosis of infected cells by upregulating the proapoptotic genes caspase 3 and Bax, while downregulating the antiapoptotic genes Bcl-2 and Mcl-1 [16].

Targeted adhesion to microfold (M) cells constitutes an effective mode of invasion. Bacteria and viruses utilizing M cell transport channels can infect the gastrointestinal mucosa and potentially spread systemically.

M cells, which encompass the Peyer's patches, delineate the epithelium-associated lymphoid follicles from the intestinal lumen. They possess a thin mucous coating, have small microvilli, and demonstrate heightened activity in pinocytosis relative to columnar epithelial cells. Peyer's patches, composed of aggregated lymphoid follicles, are a principal element of the mucosal immune system, serving a specific purpose: to prevent exogenous antigens from entering the internal environment and to limit the systemic immune system's exposure to molecular antigens or cells that penetrate the internal milieu. Mucosa-associated lymphoid tissue (MALT) must remain unresponsive to the typical mucosal microbiota. MALT functions as a "control zone" within the body, interacting with antigens and regulating the efficacy of the systemic immune response. This elucidates that the oral delivery of an antigen in humans or animals generally elicits a mucosal immune response rather than a systemic immunological response. The mechanism remains unidentified; nonetheless, the mucosal immune system inhibits a significant immunological response following exposure to several intestinal antigens, particularly those of dietary origin. Complex antigens from bacteria or viruses can trigger a multifaceted immune response via the mucosal immune system. MALT functional defects subject the organism and systemic immune system to a chronic state of activation that beyond physiological limits, potentially leading to autoimmune disorders [17].

M cells can internalize soluble luminal material via pinocytosis and convey it to the underlying macrophages. Macrophages process antigens and deliver them to neighboring lymphocytes. They possess a limited number of lysosomes, and the included components are not subjected to degradation. M cells transport macromolecules, particles, and bacteria straight into the cellular milieu of the mucosal lymphoid follicles.

M cells lack receptors for polymeric immunoglobulins, signifying their inability to transport IgA, which facilitates antigen access to the mucosal surface. They are adapted for transepithelial transfer. The basolateral surface of M cells is extensively invaginated, featuring extensions of 10 μm in size that create a substantial intraepithelial "pocket" and extend into the underlying lymphoid tissue, where carried macromolecules and particles are discharged. Situated beneath the epithelium M cells is a dense aggregation of macrophages and dendritic cells in close proximity to CD4 T cells possessing the αβ type receptor and B cells. A limited number of lymphocytes are either memory T cells or uncommitted (naive) cells. The folds of M cells serve as the locus for interaction between T cells and antigen-presenting cells, specifically B cells and macrophages.

Microorganisms penetrate the lymphoid follicle structures via the follicular epithelium. The outcome is advantageous as it triggers a protective immune response against luminal bacteria. M cells are considered an early warning mechanism of the immune system. While M cells have developed as a strategic defensive mechanism, their functional characteristics render them genuine gateways—the Achilles heel of the intestine—allowing dangerous bacteria to penetrate deeper structures.

The bacterial cells engage with M cells, likely through carbohydrates [18]. M cells exhibit a diverse array of glycoconjugates that regulate their ability to internalize microbes [19]. Additionally, macrophages and dendritic cells participate in the incorporation of pathogens conveyed by M cells, as well as in the processing and storage of antigens [20].

Specific pathogenic strains of Escherichia coli that inhabit the intestinal mucosa may selectively cling to epithelial cells and engage with M cells. The attachment to intestinal epithelial cells and M cells causes the degradation of microvilli and M cell folds, as well as the formation of specialized structures known as pedestals, resulting from the restructuring of actin filaments at the adhesion point [21].

Shigella sp., a facultative intracellular pathogen, causes significant damage to the mucosa of the small intestine and colon, resulting in the impairment of epithelial barrier function. Shigella sp. cells attach to the cellular membrane, are engulfed, and subsequently released into the cytoplasm following the degradation of the phagosome membrane, where they proliferate, induce the formation of an actin filament tail, and are expelled into a membrane-derived vacuole, which is later phagocytosed by adjacent cells [22].

In vitro studies with enterocytes indicate that Shigella flexneri does not penetrate the apical surface when the epithelial tight connections remain intact. The invasion might occur solely via the basolateral membrane. In vivo, Shigella initially invades the mucosa via M cells, subsequently penetrating epithelial cells through the basolateral surface. Mucosal ulcerations occur most frequently in the ileum and colon, where lymphoid follicles and M cells are more abundant. We have shown that S. flexneri and S. boydii strains altered the expression of various anti- and pro-inflammatory cytokines in HeLa cells by reducing the production of IL-1β, IL-6, TNF-α, and IL-17 [22, 23].

Research on the interplay between viral and bacterial infections indicates that a host's immunity is temporarily diminished during viral infections, leading to a heightened occurrence of bacterial infections, likely due to an upregulation of epithelial cell receptors for bacterial adhesins. Virus-infected host cells may also undergo alterations in the cytoskeleton [24], potentially leading to an increase or decrease in bacterial invasion capabilities. Consequently, we examined the impact of viral preinfection with vaccinia, measles, echovirus 32, and herpes simplex virus 1 strains on the capacity of an enteroinvasive E. coli strain to colonize HeLa cells. Our findings indicate that viral preinfection of the cellular substrate resulted in a diminished invasive capability, suggesting a heightened prevalence of infections by extracellular pathogenic organisms following viral infections [6].

In the small intestine, Vibrio cholerae produces a set of pilus adhesins that facilitate adhesion to enterocytes. The pili retain the vibrio adherent to the mucosal surface, while the cholera toxin stimulates the secretion of chloride ions from intestinal cells into the lumen. V. cholerae also engages intimately with vast regions of the apical membrane of the M cells. The activating signal prompts actin rearrangement, resulting in the phagocytosis of the bacterial cell, without causing damage to the M cell. In this instance, the presence of bacteria within the M cells does not induce disease; rather, it triggers a protective immune response in the mucosa, facilitated by the secretion of anti-toxin and anti-LPS sIgA, which can inhibit mucosal colonization by V. cholerae and consequently avert diarrheal disease.

The introduction of Salmonella cells triggers the infection of Peyer's patches. S. typhi and S. typhimurium swiftly and selectively attach to M cells and immediately penetrate the epithelial villi. Salmonella sp. cells are encapsulated within a substantial endocytic vacuole through a phagocytosis mechanism triggered by the disassembly of apical microvilli and remodeling of the cytoskeleton.

The experiments involving ligated intestinal loops demonstrated that after 30 minutes of injection, Salmonella sp. cells stimulate an increase in the volume of M cells; a swift incorporation of the bacteria was noted, succeeded by the degeneration of M cells and the infiltration of infectious cells into the mucosal structure.

Yersinia sp. cells infiltrate the intestinal mucosa via M cells, to which they preferentially adhere, becoming entrenched and traversing the cytoplasm through transcytosis.

Several bacterial species can directly penetrate host cells after adhering, by localized enzymatic degradation of the host cell membrane. Rickettsia prowazekii secretes phospholipases that facilitate the targeted and regulated breakdown of the host cell membrane. The pathogen directly infiltrates the cytoplasm via membrane lesions [26].

The majority of bacteria, including numerous dangerous strains, are eradicated upon their phagocytosis by macrophages or neutrophils (PMNN). Certain species have evolved techniques that enable them to survive and proliferate within phagocytes.

S. flexneri, L. monocytogenes, and Rickettsia sp. disrupt the first membrane vacuole, thereby accessing the nutrient-rich cytoplasm. Salmonella spp., Mycobacterium spp., and Legionella spp. can obstruct the union of phagosomes and lysosomes, hence evading phagocytosis.

The virulence factors that confer bacterial resistance to lysosomal enzymes and enhance intracellular survival include cell surface protective structures (capsule and LPS), bacterial enzymes that neutralize toxic free radicals and reactive oxygen species, and proteolytic enzymes that degrade host lysosomal enzymes [13].

3. EFFICACY OF VARIOUS ANTIBIOTIC CLASSES AGAINST INTRACELLULAR INFECTIONS

Antibiotics are low molecular weight substances produced by microbial biosynthetic processes or by chemical synthesis, which can be used in low concentrations to specifically inhibit the proliferation or to kill microorganisms [27]. Because of their high specificity, antibiotics exhibit different efficiencies against various microbial species. Antimicrobial drugs act by different mechanisms, such as inhibition of cell wall synthesis, inhibition of cell membrane functions, inhibition of protein synthesis at different stages (translation or transcription), inhibition of nucleic acid synthesis, and blockage of metabolic pathways by competitive inhibition (Figure 1) [28].

Depending on the number and diversity of affected microbial species, the activity spectrum of the antibiotics can be broad (i.e., the spectrum of tetracycline is represented by Gram-negative bacteria, including *Chlamydia* sp. and *Rickettsia* sp. and Gram-positive species; penicillins are active especially against Gram-positive species, and some Gram-negative bacteria, including *Chlamydia* sp., nitrofurans, rifampin, and sulfonamides are active on a large number of Gram-positive and Gram-negative bacteria species), narrow (novobiocin is active on Gram-positive bacteria, especially staphylococci, but also on Gram-negative species, such as *Haemophilus* sp. and *Pasteurella* sp., glycopeptides and bacitracin are active against Gram-positive bacteria), and limited (nitroimidazoles are active only against anaerobic microorganisms).

Even within the same microbial species, there can be large differences regarding the susceptibility of different strains to a particular antibiotic; thus, antibiotic treatment in the clinical setting requires the isolation of the microbial strain, which is the etiologic agent of a specific infection (especially if it belongs to genera and species with a high ability of acquiring clinical resistance) and determining its antibiotic susceptibility spectrum.

The *in vivo* antimicrobial activity is more complex, involving different host-related factors along with the impact of the antibiotic and the nature of the antimicrobial agent. Thus, in the host, a number of local factors (partial pressure of O_2, pH etc.) could influence the activity of the antibiotic. On the other hand, antibiotics are absorbed within the intestinal tract and distributed unevenly in various tissues and body fluids, and very few reach active concentrations in the central nervous system (CNS) or inside most eukaryotic cells. It is also very difficult to maintain an active concentration of the antibiotic for a prolonged period of time, so the interval between doses should be rigorously respected. Some antibiotics have postantibiotic effects (such as observed in the case of carbapenems activity against the Gram-negative bacilli) and may modulate the inflammatory response by indirectly inducing the chronicity of inflammatory reactions due to the accumulation of bacterial fragments. The combination of two or more antimicrobials is recommended for the treatment of severe and chronic infections to avoid the appearance of resistant mutants (i.e., tuberculosis) and also in mixed infections, for obtaining a synergy of action and a strong bactericidal effect (i.e., beta lactams and aminoglycosides, trimethoprim and sulfamethoxazole, amphotericin and flucytosine, beta-lactamase inhibitors and beta-lactam antibiotics).

Some antibiotic classes, such as macrolides, fluoroquinolones, tetracyclines, and ansamycins, are known to be active against obligate intracellular and facultative intracellular organisms, while others, such as beta-lactams and aminoglycosides, show no or only a poor intracellular activity. However, these antibiotics are active against facultative intracellular organisms, including *Mycobacterium tuberculosis*.

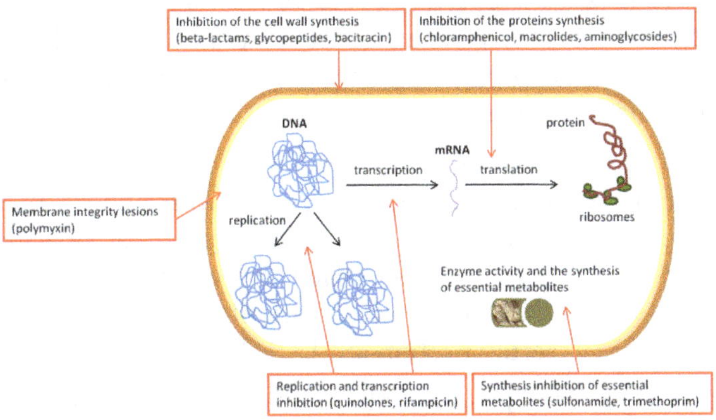

Figure 1. The main mechanisms of action and cellular targets of antibiotics within the bacterial cell.

3.1. Inhibition of Cell Wall Synthesis

Peptidoglycan cell wall is a closed structure, composed by covalently linked units, which allow the sequential addition of new units on the external side of the cytoplasmic membrane, while the old units from the peptidoglycan's structure are shifted outward and released by the action of autolysins.

The synthesis of the peptidoglycan takes place in three stages: (i) low-molecular-weight-soluble precursors (GlcAc UDP and UDP-MurNAc-L-Ala-D-Glu-mezoDap-D-Ala-D-Ala) are synthesized in the cytoplasm; (ii) the nonnucleotide region of the previously synthesized molecular precursor (intermediate *N*-acetyl glucosamine and *N*-acetyl muramic acid-pentapeptide) is attached to a lipid carrier, integrated in the membrane and subsequently modified by adding GlcNAc and pentaglycine, resulting undecaprenol-pyrophosphate MurNac (L-Ala-D-Gln [NH_2 [Gly5] L-Lys-D-Ala-D-Ala]-[beta1-4]-GlcNac), that will be translocated across the plasma membrane and serves as a substrate for a transglycosylation reaction, polymerizing the bacterial glycan chains of the cell wall, to form a repetitive disaccharide $(MurNac\text{-}GlcNAc)_n$; and (iii) the subunits of the peptidoglycan are polymerized by their insertion in the preexisting cell wall, by the reaction of transpeptidation, which takes place at the terminal D-ala-D-ala residues.

The polymerization and cross-linking of the sugar tetrapeptide chains are catalyzed by penicillin-binding protein enzymes (PBP), located in the cytoplasmic membrane and the periplasmic space.

Some antibacterial agents interfere with the early steps of the cell wall synthesis (vancomycin, bacitracin, and cycloserine), while others (β-lactam antibiotics, penicillins, cephalosporins, monobactams, and carbapenems) inhibit the last steps of peptidoglycan synthesis, such as the formation of interpeptidic links, because these antibiotics have structural analogy with terminal D-ala-D-ala dipeptide [29].

Glycopeptides (vancomycin and teicoplanin) inhibit the early stage of the peptidoglycan synthesis by binding to the carboxy-terminal dipeptide D-Ala-D-Ala. It has been revealed that vancomycin shows a slow uptake and modest accumulation into macrophages, especially in the lysosomes compartment (up to eightfold in 24 h) [30, 31], while teicoplanin, a more lipophilic compound, shows a more extensive and faster intracellular accumulation (40- to 60-fold) [32, 33].

A newly investigated glycopeptide antibiotic called oritavancin (LY333328) proved to be avidly accumulated by J774 and THP-1 macrophages and rat fibroblasts and to a lesser extent by LLC-PK1 and Caco-2 cells. The intracellular pharmacokinetic and pharmacodynamic results demonstrated that the level of accumulation reached a plateau (at 370-fold the extracellular concentration) within 24 h, and the effect was partly defeated by a rise in serum protein levels [34].

Bacitracin (a cyclic peptide) prevents the dephosphorylation of the lipid carrier molecule, which transfers a newly synthesized peptidoglycan molecule to the cell membrane during the synthesis of the cell wall. This antibiotic is toxic to kidneys and is not systemically administered but is applied topically to treat skin and mucosa infections.

Cycloserine competitively inhibits the formation of D-ala from L-ala and thus stops the synthesis of the dipeptide D-ala-D-ala. This antibiotic is relatively toxic and is used for the treatment of *M. tuberculosis* infections resistant to other drugs.

Fosfomycin is a pyruvyl-transferase inhibitor, which blocks the synthesis of *N*-acetylmuramic acid.

Cycloserine and fosfomycin act as peptidoglycan precursor analogues. They are very hydrophilic molecules and enter the cytoplasm following the path of transport systems usually utilized for some related metabolites; i.e., fosfomycin is structurally analogous to the phospho-enol-pyruvate and cycloserine is similar to D-alanine.

Beta-lactam antibiotics act as pseudosubstrates and perform the acylation of the active sites of the PBP transpeptidases, which are thus unable to catalyze the polymerization of the peptidoglycan. The acylation reaction of the PBP is very slowly reversible. PBP-deacylated enzymes are unable to catalyze the cross-linking of peptides (Figure

2). Antibiotic-PBP complexes stimulate the release of autolysins, which produce the degradation of the cell wall, leading to osmotic bacterial cell lysis.

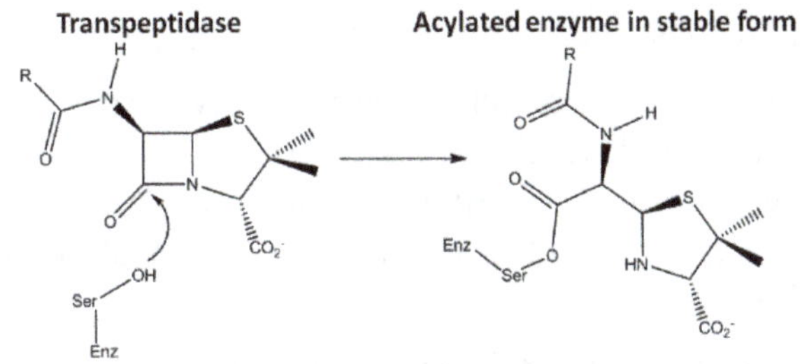

Figure 2. Beta-lactam antibiotics mediate the inactivation of PBP by the acylation reaction.

The inhibitors of beta-lactamase enzymes, such as clavulanic acid, sulbactam, tazobactam, have a high affinity for the respective antibiotic-inactivating enzymes, inducing their acylation and formation of stable, unefficient complexes (Figure 3).

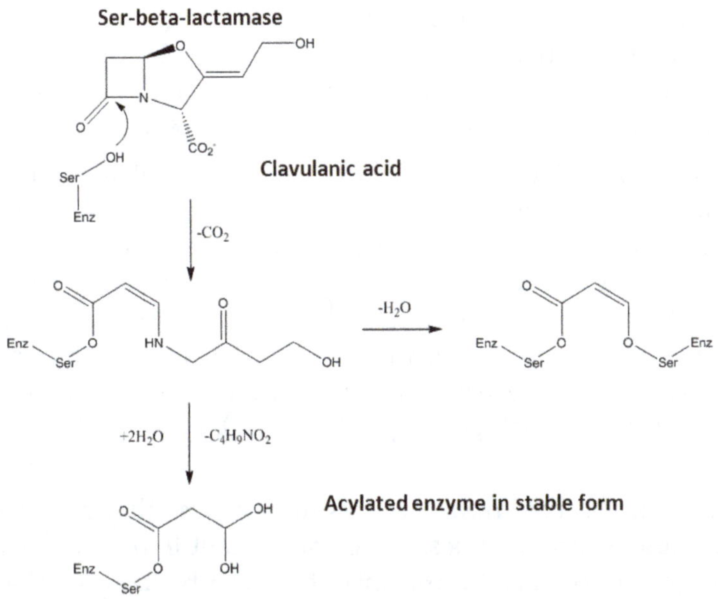

Figure 3. Beta-lactamase enzymes inactivation by acylation in the presence of clavulanic acid.

Penicillin G is the drug of choice for meningococcal and gonococcal intracellular infections. Third-generation cephalosporins (cefotaxime, ceftazidime, ceftriaxone, cefotetan, ceftizoxime, cefoperazone, and cefixime) may cross the blood-brain barrier; therefore, cefotaxime, ceftriaxone, and ceftizoxime are usually intravenously administrated for the treatment of meningitis caused by Gram-negative bacteria. The intracellular concentration of beta-lactams is usually lower than the extracellular amount, as revealed for both phagocytic and nonphagocytic cells [35, 36]. This could be explained by the weak acidic character of these molecules affecting their accumulation in acidic cytosol milieu [37].

3.2. Inhibition of the Cytoplasmic Membrane Function

Cytoplasmic membrane acts as a selective permeability barrier for ions and nutrients and is also the headquartered structural transport system that controls the chemical composition of the cytoplasm. The disruption of structural integrity and/or functional parameters entails the amendment of ion-selective permeability and loss of ionic or macromolecular balance.

Bacteria and fungi have a slightly different cellular membrane as compared with the animal cells, this being injured faster by different therapeutic agents, which enables selective therapy. Biological membranes are comprised of a lipid matrix, wherein the randomly distributed globular proteins penetrate the lipid layer. Cationic, anionic, or neutral detergents may disrupt biological membranes. The effect of polymyxins is similar to the cationic detergents. Their molecule contains hydrophilic and hydrophobic groups. These antibiotics are positively charged at neutral pH and actin similar with the cationic compounds, which are active against the polyanionic outer membrane of Gram-negative bacteria (the load offered by the lipopolysaccharide). Detergents (which are molecules containing lipophilic and hydrophilic group) act by disorganizing the double lipid layer leading to cell disruption.

Polymyxins are polypeptide antibiotics (octapeptides of high molecular weight) with specific chemical and biological properties. There are five known major chemically distinct polymyxins, designated as polymyxin A, B, C, D, and E. All polymyxins are synthesized by *Bacillus polymyxa* and have the same antibacterial spectrum. Polymyxins A and D are nephrotoxic and therefore cannot be used *in vivo*. The most representative are polymyxin B and colistin (or polymyxin E), which are also the less cytotoxic (in concentrations up to 5 μg/ml), being most active against Gram-negative bacteria, such as *Brucella* sp., *Yersinia* sp., *Salmonella* sp., *Shigella* sp.), probably due to their negative lipid charge.

Polymyxins are not absorbed from the intestine, and also they do not accumulate in active concentrations in soft tissues, being not efficient in the treatment of systemic or internal organs infections. In exchange, they can be used for the treatment of superficial, cutaneous, or mucosal infections (wounds, burns, intestinal tract mucosa, and pleural cavity infections), as well as for the prophylaxis of transplant or digestive tract surgery. Polymyxins are used with great effectiveness in the treatment of meningeal, lung, and urinary tract infections. They are often associated with other antibiotics to extend the antimicrobial activity spectrum.

The fixation of the antibiotics within the membrane structure depends on the concentration of divalent environmental cations: their deficiency or excess inhibits the action of polymyxins. Also, the LPS composition, bacterial membrane phospholipids, and proteins influence the sensitivity or resistance of various bacterial species to the action of polymyxins.

Polymyxin and other polycationic molecules bind to the lipid A of LPS in a stoichiometric ratio and are inserted into the membrane structure. Such a molecular patchwork disorganizes the lipid layers so that the cell membrane does not function normally as effective osmotic barrier. Due to structural deterioration of external and internal membranes, osmotic balance is disrupted by the loss of K^+ ions. The permeability changes are associated with the loss of soluble cell constituents and viability. The mechanism is the same as that proposed for hemolysis by the action of ionic detergents. The hemolytic effect occurs due to the disruption of cholesterol–phospholipid–lipoprotein complex from the erythrocyte membrane. Other agents acting on the cytoplasmic membrane are amphotericin B, imidazoles, and triazoles.

3.3. Inhibition of the Protein Synthesis

Several classes of antibiotics are active specifically on the 70S ribosomes, thus blocking protein synthesis at different levels [38].

Aminoglycosides are low molecular weight cationic molecules, but very hydrophilic, which accumulate in the cell only through an energy-dependent transport process. Their accumulation in the bacterial cell occurs through two phases: Phase I is slow and depends on the transmembrane gradient of the electrical potential and thus the oxidative respiratory sinergon, and phase II is quick and translates into an important intracellular accumulation. Intracellular concentrations are approximately 100 times higher than those from the external environment. Slow accumulation causes a bacteriostatic antibiotic, while rapid accumulation produces bactericidal effects. The accumulation rate is conditioned by the size of the electric component ($\Delta\psi$) and the proton-motive force. This explains why microorganisms with transportation systems deficiencies, such as anaerobes, are intrinsically resistant to aminoglycosides. For the same reason, enterococci and other facultative anaerobes are resistant to low concentrations of aminoglycosides [39].

An important role in the intracellular accumulation of aminoglycosides is attributed to the periplasmic proteins whose synthesis is induced by the antibiotic.

Aminoglycosides induce the pleiotropism phenomenon (i.e., simultaneous changes in the expression of many genes) and also produce mRNA reading errors.

Aminoglycosides are rapidly acting antibiotics with broad spectrum of action being active against strict and facultative Gram-positive and negative aerobic bacteria.

Aminoglycosides could slowly accumulate through endocytosis in the lysosomes of the eukaryotic cells to an apparent cellular-to-extracellular ratio of 2 to 4, excepting some tissues like kidney proximal tubular cells, exhibiting binding sites such as megalin and acidic phospholipids where the accumulation is faster [40–43].

Spectinomycin is an aminocyclitol antibiotic related to the aminoglycosides, manifesting bacteriostatic action, usually used for the treatment of gonorrhea produced by penicillin-resistant *Neisseria gonorrhoeae* strains.

The encapsulation of aminoglycosides in liposomes could increase the therapeutic index of the drug by reducing the level of drug delivered at the sites where the antibiotic is toxic to the therapeutic amounts necessary for the treatment of infection. This procedure also increases the aminoglycosides efficiency against intracellular bacteria.

Tetracyclines represent a family of antibiotics inhibitory for the protein synthesis through a mechanism of blocking the attachment of aminoacyl-tRNA complex to the ribosome acceptor site (site A) [44]. These antibiotics have a broad spectrum bacteriostatic effect, being active against Gram-positive Gram-negative bacteria and protozoa, but they also kill normal gut microbiota and produce gastrointestinal disorders.

Tetracyclines have the ability to accumulate in eukaryotic cells, including neutrophils [45].

Tetracyclines are strong chelating agents, their pharmacological properties being influenced by the presence of metal ions. Each of the rings of the tetracycline core can contain only linear carbon atoms in order to keep the antibiotic activity.

Atypical tetracyclines and some of their analogues disrupt the cytoplasmic membrane structure and manifest a bactericidal effect, which contrasts with the bacteriostatic effect of tetracyclines, reversibly inhibiting protein synthesis. Atypical effects of membrane disruption are likely a consequence of the lipophilic nature of the molecule. Because of many side effects derived from their nonspecific interaction with prokaryotic and eukaryotic cell membranes, atypical tetracyclines present no current therapeutic interest.

The use of this antibiotic during pregnancy or in the first 5 years of life results in the deformation of the fetus skull bones and permanent teeth staining due to their ability to bind Ca^{2+}.

In the 80s, before the emergence of resistant strains of *N. gonorrhoeae*, tetracycline was used to treat sexually transmitted infections and is currently used in the treatment of non gonococcal urethritis and chlamydial infections

Tetracycline resistance is widespread in Gram-positive cocci and is present also in *Mycoplasma* sp.

Although the main action of tetracycline is antibacterial, this antibiotic is also active against protozoan parasites, inhibiting *Giardia lamblia, Trichomonas vaginalis, Entamoeba histolytica*, and *Plasmodium falciparum*. The effectiveness of tetracycline derivatives to parasitic protozoa is correlated with the degree of penetration into the cell. The most effective are lipophilic compounds that cross quickly the cytoplasmic membrane (such as the tiotetracycline derivative).

Glicil-tetracyclines are represented by tigecycline, used to treat skin and abdominal infections. The structural feature of tigecycline is the substitution in the position 9 of the tetracycline with a glycine residue. These are broad-spectrum antibiotics against *N. gonorrhoeae, Legionella pneumophila*, and also for fast growing non tubercular mycobacteria.

They are active agents to be used for the prophylaxis of malaria and strains of *P. falciparum* resistant to specific chemotherapeutic agents.

Macrolides, lincosamides, and streptogramins (MLS) have a different chemical structure, but they act in a similar manner on a variety of intracellular bacteria (e.g., Gram-positive, Gram-negative cocci, *Chlamydia* spp., *Mycoplasma* spp., and *Legionella* spp.).

MLSs prevent bacterial ribosomes to translate the RNA in two different ways, either by the inhibition of translocation of peptidyl-tRNA from the acceptor site (A) and the peptidyl donor site (P) or by inhibiting the initial steps of the assembly of the 50S ribosomal subunit.

Macrolides have a marked intracellular accumulation in almost all cells, explained by their weak basic character favoring the accumulation in the acidic cytosol compartment, particularly in the lysosomal apparatus, with a rate depending on the derivative structure, lower for erythromycin and higher for those carrying two basic functions [46, 47].

Regarding their structure, macrolides are characterized by a multiunitar lactone ring with 12, 14, 15, or 16 carbon atoms, with few double bonds, which contain attached 1–3 glucidic residues by glycosidic linkages.

Macrolides are active against Gram-positive and Gram-negative bacteria (*Mycobacterium* spp., *Treponema pallidum*, *Mycoplasma pneumoniae*, *Chlamydia* sp., *Rickettsia* sp.).

Novel molecules, such as azithromycin and clarithromycin, have a superior antibacterial activity as compared with erythromycin because they have higher coefficients of intracellular penetration and are more stable, being more easily absorbed and manifesting lower incidence gastrointestinal side effects. Azithromycin is active against *Mycoplasma* spp. and *Chlamydia* spp. Clarithromycin has significant antibacterial activity *in vitro* against mycobacteria.

Streptogramins are represented by two synergistic components (A and B). Similar with macrolides and lincosamides, the A and B compounds of the streptogramin set at the ribosomal subunit 50S, 23S, and to rRNA.

Lincomycin and clindamycin are macrolides, but many of their biological properties are similar to erythromycin. They consist of an amino acid linked to an amino-sugar. Ketolides (telithromycin) are new chemical entities, characterized by the replacement of L-cladinose in the erythronolide A ring, with a 3-keto function and the C11–C12 carbamate [48]. ABT 773 represents the latest generation of drugs, characterized by 3-keto group that substitutes the sugar rest of the 3-cladinose from erythromycin and clarithromycin [49].

Oxazolidinones (eperezolid and linezolid) represent a unique class of synthetic antimicrobial agents with a unique mechanism of action, which eliminates the risk of extending existing resistance to the available antimicrobial agents. The oxazolidinones are inhibitors of ribosomal protein synthesis in bacteria, preventing the formation of the 70S initiation complex comprising fMet RNA, mRNA, and the two ribosomal subunits.

Linezolid has a good *in vitro* activity against *N. gonorrhoeae, N. meningitidis*, and *M. tuberculosis*.

There are few studies showing the capacity of oxazolidinones (i.e., linezolid) to preferentially and rapidly accumulate intracellularly (in concentrations 1.2 times higher than the extracellular ones within 20 min), both in human phagocytic (PMNs) and in nonphagocytic (McCoy) cells. However, the efflux of the antibiotic is also very rapid, the great amount of the intracellular antibiotic being released in less than 2 min [50].

Sulfonamides are synthetic chemotherapeutic agents, very similar to sulfanilamide (para-amino-benzenesulfonamide). The bacteriostatic action of this antibiotic is due to the interference with the folic acid synthesis pathway.

The best known sulfonamides are sulfadiazine and sulfamethoxazole (cotrimoxazole). As sulfonamides, para-aminosalicylic acid (APAS) and dapsone obtained by chemical synthesis are competitive inhibitors for the para-aminobenzoic acid metabolism and inhibits the synthesis of folic acid, being active against *M. tuberculosis* and *Mycobacterium leprae*.

The family of the diaminopyrimidine derivatives includes trimethoprim and tetroxoprim.

Trimethoprim is an analog of dihydrofolic acid, which competitively inhibits dihydrofolate reductase, an enzyme that converts dihydrofolate to the active cofactor—tetrahydrofolic acid [51].

The blockage of the same biosynthetic pathways sequence under the action of sulfonamides and trimethoprim provides a high degree of synergistic activity against a broad spectrum of microorganisms.

3.4. Chemotherapeutic Agents Acting by Inhibiting DNA Replication and Transcription

Quinolones (also known as 4-quinolones) are the first antimicrobials produced synthetically and form a family of compounds that resemble the core quinolinic existence.

Along with the β-lactam antibiotics and macrolide antibiotics, quinolones represent one of the three major families of antimicrobial agents used in human therapy [52]. Nalidixic acid is an intermediate for the synthesis of quinolones. Subsequently, quinolones have diversified by introducing a fluorine (F) in position 6 and position 7 of a heterocyclic ring (piperazine, pyrrolidine etc.), which generated fluoroquinolones.

Fluoroquinolones (norfloxacin, pefloxacin, ofloxacin, ciprofloxacin etc.) have a broad spectrum of activity against intracellular bacteria, including *Chlamydia* sp., *Rickettsia* sp. and mycobacteria. These molecules penetrate the bacterial cell by passive diffusion and act on specific targets represented by topoisomerases: DNA gyrase (topoisomerase

II) and topoisomerase IV, probably inducing lethal effects such as bacterial DNA damage.

Rifampicin B is naturally synthesized, but in the recent years, the semisynthetic derivatives of rifampicin are the most extensively used. Rifampicin belongs to a group consisting of an aromatic chromophore, which is included in the aliphatic chain. It is associated with the B subunit of DNA-dependent RNA polymerase, thus blocking transcription and RNA synthesis initiation. The antibiotic is widely used in the combinatory therapy of tuberculosis.

It was demonstrated that quinone and hydroquinone forms of rifampin can accumulate in PMNs from normal and chronic granulomatous disease individuals and be active against intracellular staphylococci invading the chronic granulomatous disease PMN [53].

3.5. Other Synthetic Chemotherapeutic Agents

Nicotinic acid hydrazide (isoniazid, INH), introduced in the clinic before 1950, together with rifampin, forms the basis of antituberculosis chemotherapy. Isoniazid is a nicotinamide derivative. The mechanism of action is not known, but it influences the synthesis of lipids, nucleic acids and mycolic acid from *M. tuberculosis*.

It is assumed that isoniazid is active by competing with pyridoxine (vitamin B6) necessary for the growth of *M. tuberculosis* cells or by inhibiting mycolic acid synthesis. It is bactericidal to the growing cells and has a bacteriostatic action against the cells that do not replicate. Together with PASA and dapsone, isoniazid is used to treat infections with *Mycobacterium* sp.

Ethambutol, pyrazinamide, and ethionamide block the enzymatic reactions in the bacterial cell because they are similar but not identical to bacterial vitamins.

Ethambutol inhibits arabinosyl chloride-transferase enzyme involved in the biosynthesis of arabinogalactan and lipoarabinomannan. Other effects attributed to metabolic inhibition action of ethambutol are RNA and phospholipids synthesis, inhibiting the transfer of mycolic acids linked to arabinogalactans of the murine cell wall and also inhibiting the synthesis of spermidine at early stage conversion of glucose into monosaccharides used for the synthesis of parietal polysaccharides and peptidoglycan. It is a very specific and effective drug used in association with isoniazid for tuberculosis treatment. It has a good bacteriostatic effect [54].

Pyrazinamide is a synthetic derivative of nicotinamide, which is metabolized to the pyrazino acid, antibacterial active intermediary.

Ethionamide, a derivative of the isonicotinic acid, is active against *M. tuberculosis* and other mycobacteria, acting through inhibition of mycolic acid synthesis.

Despite the massive amount of literature on the intracellular activity of antibiotics and on its relation to cellular accumulation and disposition, the relationship between drug concentration (or dosing), time of exposure (or other pertinent pharmacokinetic parameters), and chemotherapeutic response (in terms of quantitative measurement of the variation in the bacterial population) is incompletely elucidated [55]. Clinical studies, in this context, are particularly difficult due to the complex extracellular and intracellular pharmacokinetic variables, microbial and host-response variables, and simultaneous presence of extracellular and intracellular foci of infection. Some classes of antibiotics, such as ansamycins, macrolides, tetracyclines, and fluoroquinolones, are generally considered as being active against intracellular pathogens, being already clinically used for the treatment of bacterial infections with obligate and facultative intracellular bacteria. Conversely, there is a consensus over the fact that beta-lactams and aminoglycosides show no or only a poor intracellular activity. However, beta-lactams could exhibit a time-dependent activity against intracellular bacteria when administered in prolonged treatments at the maximal dose to compensate for the lack of accumulation, whereas aminoglycosides, which are concentration-dependent, could be active a high concentrations [56]. For macrolides, activity is clearly observed against phagosomal organisms (phagosomes are neutral or only slightly acidic) at a sufficiently high concentration to cope with the loss of activity caused by low pH or binding to cell constituents. Although some organisms, like *Chlamydia* sp. and *Legionella* sp., are quite sensitive, this may not be the case for others, such as *Staphylococcus aureus*.

The balance between influx and efflux, metabolism, and binding properties determines the intracellular concentration of free active drug; bacterial responsiveness, physico-chemical conditions prevailing at the site of infection, and degree of cooperation (or hindrance) with the host defenses are affecting the intracellular activity of antibiotics.

4. ANTIBIOTICS CARRIERS FOR THE INTRACELLULAR DELIVERY

Intracellular bacterial pathogens are hard to treat because of the inability of conventional antimicrobial agents belonging to widely used classes to penetrate the lipidic membrane. They accumulate in different compartments of the cells and face the limiting conditions of the phagocytic cells, such as the lysosomal acidic pH and inactivating enzymes, low oxygen pressure, etc. [57, 58], requiring the development of efficient delivery systems that could release the antimicrobial agent intracellularly in active concentrations, thus increasing its effectiveness while decreasing the required therapeutic doses, its systemic toxicity, and the probability of selecting resistance [59–61].

Different improved drug carriers have been developed for treating intracellular pathogens, including antibiotics loaded into liposomes and other lipid formulations, microspheres, polymeric carriers, fullerenes, dendrimers and nanoplexes [1, 61–63].

The advantages of using drug delivery systems are represented by the tunable surface/size/shape/functionalization properties, depending on the structure of the transported drug; evasion of the immune system; use of the same carrier to transport more than one drugs; improvement of the biodisponibility, biodistribution, and pharmacokinetics of the drugs; availability of drug carriers for different administration routes; and low probability of selecting resistance [64, 65].

This section will focus on drug delivery systems oriented toward treatment of intracellular infections.

4.1. Polymeric Drug Carriers

Polymeric (both natural and synthetic) biodegradable and/or biocompatible matrixes, such as poly (ε-caprolactone) (PCL), poly(lactic acid) (PLA), poly(lactic-co-glycolic acid) (PLGA), poly(γ-glutamic acid) (PGA), poly(L-lysine) alginate, gelatin, collagen, cellulose, albumin, fibrin, dextran, pectin, chitosan, agar, agarose, and carrageenans, could be used to embed/encapsulate/adsorb/conjugate a certain drug in order to protect it against enzymatic and hydrolytic degradation [66–79] to control the rate of drug release with an optimal maintenance of the biologically active drug level within therapeutic window [80, 81], to prevent toxicity, to target drugs to the site of action, and to improve absorption, bioavailability, and therapeutic efficacy [82, 83].

The polymeric carrier systems could be classified in four different categories: diffusion controlled (the drug is released by diffusion), chemically controlled (the drug molecules are linked to a polymeric backbone often by means of a spacer molecule, being released inside the host tissue by hydrolysis or by the enzymatic cleavage of the linkage between the polymer carrier and the drug, by polymer biodegradation or by bioerosion), solvent activated (controlled by swelling or osmosis allowing the drug inside the system to diffuse outward), and magnetically controlled (the polymer carrier is combined with magnetic microparticles of iron, cobalt, and nickel, which could be oriented inside the body by an externally applied magnetic field) [67, 84–87].

Responsive or smart polymers respond and modulate their properties in accordance with different external parameters (e.g., UV/visible light, electric charges, electromagnetic radiation, temperature, pH, ionic strength, ionic or metallic interactions), leading to degradation, drug release, dissolution/precipitation, swelling/collapsing, and formation of micelles and vesicles [88, 89].

Particulated micro- and nanospheres and capsules prepared from natural polymers have been synthesized by emulsion polymerization, solvent evaporation, ionic gelation, self-assembly, nanoprecipitation, and supercritical fluid technology for drug delivery [90–92].

While microparticles are likely to remain in time at the injection place and can be engulfed only by phagocytes, the smaller nanoparticles can diffuse from the injection place and cross biological barriers, including the cellular membrane of different cell types [93, 94].

Nanoparticle-based drug delivery systems were applied in the treatment of different infectious diseases with intracellular pathogens, such as acquired immune deficiency syndrome (AIDS), malaria, and tuberculosis [95, 96]. Polymeric nanoparticles represent also a promising solution for the local delivery of therapeutics to the central nervous system through the blood–brain barrier [96, 97].

The polymeric micelles consisting of a hydrophilic shell and a drug-containing core were used to incorporate extremely hydrophobic drugs, to assure prolonged drug circulation time, drug stability, and escape from the reticuloendothelial system due to their nanometer size [98]. Nanoparticles formulated using biodegradable polymers have been also shown to enhance the delivery of antibiotics intracellularly and to improve their effectiveness as revealed by the reduced microbial burden.

In comparison with other delivery systems, natural polymers are generally safer and more stable, easier to obtain, and offer better control over agent release [82, 99].

Dextran, a biodegradable, biocompatible, nonimmunogenic, and nonantigenic polymer of bacterial origin, composed essentially of α-1,6-linked D-glucopyranose units [100], proved to improve the activity of polar molecules such as penicillins, aminoglycosides, rifampicines, and quinolones and to efficiently challenge the drug delivery into the infected cells in an active form, leaving the host cells intact [101]. Dextran microspheres could act as macromolecular carriers for the small molecules antibiotics and induce endocytosis of the drug by the target cell *via* a specific receptor, followed by the subcellular distribution of the drug to sites where the microbial cells are localized [102].

Chitosan-dextran sulfate (CD) nanocapsules were assessed for their efficiency in delivering ciprofloxacin or ceftriaxone drugs against *Salmonella* using a murine salmonellosis model. CD nanocapsules proved to efficiently target and kill the intracellular pathogen at a significantly lower dose, as compared to the free antibiotic, assuring also a more increased retention time of ciprofloxacin in the blood and organs [103].

Cyclodextrin, a cyclic oligosaccharide consisting of six to eight glucopyranose units joined by α-(1 →→ 4) glucosidic linkages, exhibits an internal lipophilic cavity, which can be complexed with hydrophobic agents [104], improving drug solubility, stability, and bioavailability [105, 106].

Hyaluronic acid, a linear anionic polysaccharide of animal or microbial origin, belonging to the glycosaminoglycans family, consisting of alternating units of *N*-acetyl-D-glucosamine and glucuronic acid, is a promising delivery vehicle for antibiotics [107].

Alginate nanoparticles increased the activity of rifampicin, isoniazid, pyrazinamide, and ethambutol against *M. turberculosis* by assuring a higher drug payload and therapeutic efficacy as well as an improved pharmacokinetic [96].

Some pathogens can survive for a prolonged period of time in the first-line anti-infective defense cells represented by polymorphonuclear leukocytes (PMNs). The amorphous chitin nanoparticles with a size of 350 ± 50 nm in diameter proved to achieve a sustained release of rifampin till 72 h and significantly enhanced the drug accumulation into the intracellular compartments of PMNs [108].

Synthetic polymers are preferentially used for the development of drug delivery systems due to their excellent and tailor-made properties (biocompatibility; water compatibility; lack of immunogenicity; optimal degradation time coinciding with their function; appropriate mechanical properties in terms of toughness, flexibility, and swelling; generation of nontoxic degradation products that can be easily resorbed or excreted; flexibility for chemical modification to get increased biocompatibility and to enlarge the variety of the loaded agent; they do not need to be removed from the body being able to be degraded and excreted or resorbed; the existence of FDA and European Medicine Agency approval for drug delivery systems for parenteral administration; and protection of the loaded agent from degradation, assuring its sustained and targeted release) [99, 109–114].

Amoxicillin-loaded PLGA microspheres successfully eliminated *L. monocytogenes* from vital organs (kidney, spleen, and brain) and also increased the survival rate of treated animals in comparison with the free antibiotic, suggesting the targeted delivery of the antibiotic to the infected macrophages, as well as its sustained release over an prolonged period of time [115].

The PLGA nanoparticles proved to be efficient in encapsulating and releasing the rifampicin drug, showing an initial burst followed by the sustained release of this primary tuberculostatic agent [116, 117]. Also, rifampicin-loaded polybutylcyanoacrylate nanoparticles potentiated the *in vitro* and *in vivo* activity of rifampin and ciprofloxacin against *Mycobacterium avium* due to an effective delivery of drugs to macrophages [118, 119].

Gentamicin-loaded PLGA nanoparticles have been obtained for the treatment of brucellosis, proving to achieve high intracellular bactericidal activity of the antibiotic [120].

The PLGA microparticles proved efficient for the delivery of the antibacterial phosphorylcholine and of the dietary antigen beta lactoglobulin in a mouse model, inducing protective mucosal immunity against intestinal infection by *S. typhimurium* [121].

PLGA nanoparticles have been shown to efficiently accumulate in inclusions in both acutely and persistently infected *Chlamydia*-infected cells, while the encapsulation of rifampin and azithromycin antibiotics in PLGA nanoparticles enhanced the effectiveness of the antibiotics in reducing microbial burden. The combination of rifampin and azithromycin was more effective than the individual drugs [122].

Gentamicin was ion-paired with the anionic AOT surfactant to obtain a hydrophobic complex (GEN-AOT) that was formulated as a particulated material either by the precipitation method or by encapsulation into PLGA nanoparticles. The *in vitro* studies against the intracellular bacteria *Brucella melitensis* demonstrated that the bactericidal activity of gentamicin was unmodified, proving their use for the treatment of infections caused by intracellular bacteria [123].

Rapamycin-loaded PLGA microparticles effectively released the active drug inside dendritic cells, under intra-phagosomal (pH 5) and extracellular (pH 7.4) conditions [124].

Amoxicillin-bearing human serum albumin and, more evident, amoxicillin-dopped PLGA microparticles proved to be efficient in combating *L. monocytogenes* infection in a mouse experimental model, as revealed by the decreased bacterial burden in various organs and reduced viable counts, the results clearly demonstrating that the respective microparticles successfully target the infected macrophages [106].

Poly(isohexylcyanoacrylate) (PIHCA) nanospheres improved the activity of ampicillin against *S. typhimurium* and *L. monocytogenes,* but the particles themselves exhibited also antimicrobial activity [125, 126].

Ampicillin-encapsulated poly(isohexylcyanoacrylate) nanoparticles prove to be more efficient than the free antibiotic against *L. monocytogenes* infecting mouse peritoneal macrophage, as revealed by the more drastic decrease of viable cell counts. However, the nanoparticles acted on the intracellular bacteria after a lag period of 6–9 h, probably due to a required period for the degradation of the polymer [127].

Poly-lactide-co-glycolide (PLG) nanoparticles enhanced the bioavailability and pharmacodynamic properties of rifampicin, isoniazid, pyrazinamide, and ethambutol against *M. turberculosis* [128].

Amphiphilic, cationic polymers with an amino moiety, a low molecular weight, and short alkyl chains designed to mimic the host secreted microbicidal peptides are considered promising candidates for potent and highly selective antimicrobial agents (acting on microbial walls or mitochondrial activity) with decreased risk to select resistance [129, 130].

The polyketal nanoparticles formulated from the hydrophobic polymer poly(1,4-phenyleneacetone dimethylene ketal) (PPADK) improved the activity of superoxide-dismutase to scavenge reactive oxygen species produced by macrophages [131, 132].

Poly-butyl cyanoacryle proved to increase the efficiency of the moxifloxacin fluoroquinolone against *M. tuberculosis* infecting the THP-1 cells [133].

Polyalkycyanoacrylate nanoparticles proved to improve the activity of ciprofloxacin and colistin against *S. typhimurium* at the early stages of the infection in mice and/or *in vitro* models. Ciprofloxacin-loaded nanoparticles induced a significant decrease of bacterial counts in the liver whatever the stage of infection and the form used. However, none of the treatments were able to sterilize the spleen or the liver. In the *in vitro* study, colistin was only active against bacteria recovered during the early phase of infection, whereas ciprofloxacin exerted its activity at all times postinfection [134].

Amphiphilic block copolymers could self-assemble, resulting in vesicles called polymersomes [135]. Polymersomes of (poly[2-[methacryloyloxy]ethyl phosphorylcholine] [PMPC]–poly[2-[diisopropylamino]ethyl methacrylate] [PDPA] block copolymers) proved to successfully deliver metronidazole and doxycycline in *Porphyromonas gingivalis*-infected oral keratinocytes significantly increasing their activity [136].

4.2. Liposomes

Liposomes are small spherical, uni- or multilamellar vesicles in which the central aqueous cavities are surrounded by amphipatic molecules, being thus able to entrap both hydrophilic and hydrophobic drugs [137]. After intravenous injections, liposomes are taken up by macrophages in the liver and in the spleen, representing thus a promising option for fighting infections due to facultative intracellular bacteria, parasites, or viruses [138].

The incorporation of different tuberculostatic agents in liposomes (such as ciprofloxacin) has shown good antibacterial efficacy both in both macrophage cell lines and in animal tuberculosis models [139, 140].

Streptomycin inclusion in phosphatidyl glycerol, phosphatidyl choline, and cholesterol-containing liposomes showed an increased antimicrobial activity against *Mycobacterium avium* [141].

The encapsulation of antibiotics in liposomes could represent a viable solution for the drug penetration into the systemic circulation through the alveolar-capillary barrier, followed by its accumulation in different organ tissues or for the direct administration to the lung [142].

Phosphatidylcholine, cholesterol, dicetylphosphate, *O*-steroyl amylopectin, and monosialogangliosides/distearylphosphatidylethanolamine-poly (ethylene glycol) 2000 liposomes have been shown to act as a promising targeted delivery systems for isoniazid and rifampicin to the lung in mice experimental model [143].

The liposomal encapsulation of membrane-impermeative antibiotics, like gentamicin is among the most used approaches to achieve intracellular antibiotic delivery and therefore increase the drug's therapeutic activity against intracellular pathogens.

Gentamicin, encapsulated in plurilamellar liposomal vesicles, proved to be active against intracellular *Brucella abortus* infecting murine monocytes [144].

Gentamicin entrapped within stable multilamellar liposomes was used to treat mice orally infected with *Salmonella dublin* and proved to achieve high and persistent (up to 10 days) concentrations of gentamicin in the spleen, while bacterial counts in the lymph nodes decreased. Also, gentamicin entrapped in liposomes was less toxic in mice than its free form [145]. Ciprofloxacin encapsulation in dipalmitoylphosphatidylcholine, dipalmitoylphosphatidylglycerol, and cholesterol containing liposomes also proved increased anti-*Salmonella dublin* activity demonstrated by the decreased mortality of animals and good distribution of liposomes to all areas of infection [145].

The encapsulation of ampicillin in liposomes reduced the *L. monocytogenes* viable counts in mice peritoneal macrophages [146]. The DOPE (dioleoylphosphatidylethanolamine) liposomes, sensitive to pH proved to be efficient in the ampicillin uptake by the macrophages infected with *L. monocytogenes*, correlated with an increase in the microbicidal activity. The efficiency of this drug delivery system was also proven in an *in vivo* mouse infection model, as revealed by the decrease of viable cell counts in the liver and spleen [147].

Liposomes, as well as nanoparticles coated with a lipid bilayer have been used to encapsulate drugs for the passive transport through the blood–brain barrier due to the enhanced lipophilic transport of drugs to the target tissues [148–150].

Streptomycin and doxycycline were entrapped into macromolecular nanoplexes with anionic homo- and block copolymers enabling the simultaneous binding of both antibiotics into the nanoplexes, which significantly reduced the *B. melitensis* load in the spleens and livers of the infected mice [151].

It was demonstrated that gentamicin can be easily introduced into membrane vesicles of Gram-negative pathogens that naturally bleb off the bacterium throughout its growth cycle and delivered directly not only to other Gram-positive and Gram-negative pathogens but also to mammalian cells [152].

4.3. Niosomes

Niosomes or nonionic surfactant vesicles are microscopic, spherical, uni- or multilamellar, and polyhedral vesicles of 10–1000 nm formed by self-assembly of a mixture of cholesterol and a single alkyl chain nonionic and nontoxic surfactant with subsequent hydration [153]. Niosomes can be used for the delivery of hydrophilic, lipophilic, and amphiphilic drugs, irrespective of their degree of solubility [153]. Niosomes improve the activity of isoniazid and rifampicin against *M. tuberculosis* infecting the J774 macrophage cell line [154, 155].

4.4. Solid Lipid Nanoparticles (SLN)

Solid lipid nanoparticles (SLN) (50 nm–1 nm) are colloidal carriers for lipophilic and hydrophilic drugs, containing natural lipids dispersed in water or in the aqueous surfactant solution [156].

Mannose-conjugated SLNs were successfully used to selectively deliver rifabutin, isoniazid, and pyrazinamide to alveolar and lymphatic tissues [157]. Stearic acid SLN improved the activity of rifampicin, isoniazid, and pyrazinamide against *M. tuberculosis* by increasing the residence time and the drug bioavailability while decreasing the administration frequency [158].

Nanosuspensions could be used for nebulization procedures for delivering drugs poorly soluble in the lung secretions [159], as already proved by the antitubercular drugs (rifampicin, isoniazid, and pyrazinamide) incorporated into various formulations of solid lipid particles ranging from 1.1 to 2.1 μm and nebulized to guinea pigs [160].

4.5. Fullerenes

Fullerenes are a new form of carbon, with hollow sphere, ellipsoid, or tube size. The cationic fullerene derivatives bearing a substituted-quinazolin-4(3H)-one moiety as a side arm were reported to have a very good inhibitory potential on *M. tuberculosis* [161].

4.6. Dendrimers

Mannosylated dendrimers proved to be an efficient drug delivery system for rifampicin in a rat alveolar macrophages, the sustained release taking place in a pH-dependent manner [162].

The mannosylated fifth-generation poly(propyleneimine) dendrimer nanocarriers proved to be very efficient for the intracellular uptake of lamivudine, a nucleoside/nucleotide reverse transcriptase inhibitor, and the reduction of the HIV-1 viral load in the infected MT2 cells [163].

Pegylated lysine-based copolymeric dendrimer improved the proved anti-*P. falciparum* of artemether drug, as revealed by the increased drug stability, enhanced solubility, and prolonged drug circulation half-life [164].

A fourth-generation hydroxyl-terminated poly(amidoamine) (PAMAM) dendrimer was used as the intracellular vehicle of azithromycin for the treatment of chlamydial inclusions, proving to be more efficient than the free drug with a sustained effect lasting for 24–48 h post-infection [165].

4.7. Zeolites

Zeolites are crystalline materials with frameworks comprising Si, Al, and O [166]. The zeolites possess nanochannels and cages of regular dimensions [167]. The nanochannels (pores) of zeolites are open allowing the diffusion of therapeutic agents from the exterior to the interior of the zeolites. These networks exhibit a large specific surface area and a good stability in different environments [167].

Mesoporous silica nanoparticles proved to increase the efficiency of the rifampin and isoniazid against *M. tuberculosis* infecting the THP-1 cells [168].

The capability of porous sol-gel processed silica as a carrier for gentamicin has been demonstrated, showing a significantly higher rate of bacterial clearance from organs than did the free drug [169].

4.8. Erythrocytes

Erythrocytes possess significant potential to serve as an effective therapeutic against intracellular infections. Amikacin encapsulation in human erythrocytes exhibited a gradual and sustained release from the carrier over 48 hours, indicating the possible application of erythrocytes as a slow-release method for antibiotics.

5. CONCISE SUMMARY

Recent years have witnessed significant advancements in the enhancement of medication delivery systems for combating intracellular bacterial infections. The proposed solutions resulted in diminished toxicity, higher bioavailability, and extended, sustained release, which correlated with a lower frequency of dosage and improved antimicrobial efficacy. The design of an optimum drug carrier for the intracellular release of various antibiotics must depend on the understanding of the intracellular kinetics, including accumulation, degradation, and dispersion throughout distinct intracellular compartments and activities of the respective medicines.

Promising outcomes have been achieved through the utilization of natural or synthetic polymers, liposomes, and other lipid formulation carriers, whose efficacy has been validated by in vitro and in vivo studies, along with clinical trials. Consequently, these approaches may serve as effective strategies for combating severe microbial infections caused by facultative or obligate intracellular microorganisms, as well as viral infections.

REFERENCES

1. Salouti M, Ahangari A. Nanoparticle Based Drug Delivery Systems for Treatment of Infectious Diseases. 2014. 2014-07-25.
2. Antibiotic Resistance: Implications for Global Health and Novel Intervention Strategies: Workshop Summary. Washington, DC: The National Academies Press. 2010. 496 p.
3. Todar K. Web Review of Todar's Online Textbook of Bacteriology. http://wwwtextbookofbacteriologynet/Rickettsiahtml. 2009.
4. Wilson JW, Schurr MJ, LeBlanc CL, Ramamurthy R, Buchanan KL, Nickerson CA. Mechanisms of bacterial pathogenicity. Postgraduate Medical Journal. 2002 April 1, 2002;78(918):216–24.
5. Chifiriuc MC, Lixandru M, Iordache C, Bleotu C, Larion C, Olguta D, et al. Internalization of Staphylococcus aureus and Pseudomonas aeruginosa bacterial cells by non-phagocytic, epithelial human cells. Romanian Biotechnological Letters. 2008;13(2).
6. Bleotu C, Chifiriuc MC, Dracea, O., Iordache C, Delcaru C, Lazar V. In vitro modulation of adherence and invasion ability of enteroinvasive Escherichia Coli by different viruses. International Journal of Applied Biology and Pharmaceutical Technology. 2010:1359–63.
7. Chifiriuc MC, Mihaescu G, Lazar V. Medical Microbiology and Virology. University of Bucharest Publishing House. 2011;ISBN 978-973-737-985-6579.61.
8. Mihaescu G, Chifiriuc C, Ditu L. General microbiology University of Bucharest Publishing House. 2007;ISBN-9789737372689:552.
9. Chifiriuc MC, Bleotu C, Pelinescu DR, Lazar V, Ditu LM, Vassu T, et al. Patterns of colonization and immune response elicited from interactions between enteropathogenic bacteria, epithelial cells and probiotic fractions. International Journal of Medicine and Biomedical Research. 2010;1(4):47–57.
10. Madigan M, Martinko J, J. P. Brock's Biology of Microorganisms. 8th edition. New Jersey: Prentice Hall. 1997.
11. Nizet V, Esko JD. Bacterial and Viral Infections. Essentials of Glycobiology. CSH Press. 2009.
12. Galan JE, Wolf-Watz H. Protein delivery into eukaryotic cells by type III secretion machines. Nature. 2006;444:567–73.
13. Chifiriuc MC, Bloetu C, Sokolov D, Mihaescu GLV. Host immune response to Chlamydia infection. In: Mares M, editor. The Book Chlamydia. Intech Open Access. 2011;ISBN 978-953-51-0470-4.
14. Weinrauch Y, Zychlinsky A. The induction of apoptosis by bacterial pathogens. Annual Review of Microbiology. 1999;53(1):155–87. PubMed PMID: 10547689.

15. Grassme H, Kirschnek S, Riethmueller J, Riehle A, von Kurthy G, Lang F, et al. CD95/CD95 ligand interactions on epithelial cells in host defense to Pseudomonas aeruginosa. Science. 2000 Oct 20;290(5491):527–30. PubMed PMID: 11039936. Epub 2000/10/20. eng.

16. Iordache C, Bleotu C, Holban A, Lixandru M, Cotar A, Lazar V, et al. Differential effects on caspase mediated apoptosis of hela cells induced by different Pseudomonas aeruginosa culture fractions. International Journal of Applied Biology and Pharmaceutical Technology. 2011;2(1):132–8.

17. Mihaescu G, Chifiriuc C, Ditu LM. Imunobiology. University of Bucharest Publication House. 2009;ISBN 978-973-737-734-0:572.

18. Reid CW, Fulton KM, Twine SM. Never take candy from a stranger: the role of the bacterial glycome in host-pathogen interactions. Future Microbiology. 2010 Feb;5(2):267–88. PubMed PMID: 20143949. Epub 2010/02/11. eng.

19. Vimr ER, Kalivoda KA, Deszo EL, Steenbergen SM. Diversity of microbial sialic acid metabolism. Microbiology and Molecular Biology Reviews. 2004;68(1):132–53. PubMed PMID: PMC362108.

20. Lazar V, Balotescu C, Cernat R, Bulai D, Stewart-Tull D. Imunobiologie. Ed Univ din Bucuresti. 2005;ISBN-973-73-7124-0:250.

21. Yatsuyanagi J, Saito S, Sato H, Miyajima Y, Amano K-I, Enomoto K. Characterization of enteropathogenic and enteroaggregative Escherichia coli isolated from diarrheal outbreaks. Journal of Clinical Microbiology. 2002 07/09/received 09/03/revised 10/21/accepted;40(1):294-7. PubMed PMID: PMC120118.

22. Chifiriuc MC, Bleotu C, Marutescu L, Cristea D, Lazar V. The modulation of HeLa cells secretory patterns by invasive Shigella spp. and enteroinvasive E. coli bacterial cells and their soluble components. Roumanian Archives of Microbiology and Immunology. 2010 Jul–Sep;69(3):139–44. PubMed PMID: 21434590. Epub 2011/03/26. eng.

23. Cristea D, Ceciu S, Chitoiu DT, Bleotu C, Lazar V, Chifiriuc MC. Comparative study of pathogenicity tests for Shigella spp. and enteroinvasive Escherichia coli strains. Roumanian Archives of Microbiology and Immunology. 2009 Jan–Mar;68(1):44–9. PubMed PMID: 19507627. Epub 2009/06/11. eng.

24. de la Torre JC, Borrow P. Chapter 22 Virus-induced alterations in cells. Principles of Medical Biology1998. p. 365–79.

25. Israil AM, Balotescu C, Alexandru A, Cojocaru R, Bucurenci N, Chicu V, et al. Characterization of V. cholerae strain isolated in the Republic of Moldavia between 1995–1999. Roumanian Biotechnological Letters. 2005;10(6):2441–57.

26. Mihaescu G, Chifiriuc (Balotescu) MC. Toxins and other potentially toxic substances. Romanian Academy Publishing House. 2005;ISBN 973-27-1136-1:364.

27. Mihaescu G, Chifiriuc MC, L.M. D. Antibiotics and antimicrobial chemotherapeutic substances. Romanian Academy Publishing House. 2008;ISBN 978-973-27-1573-4.:358.

28. Brooks GF, Caroll KC, Butel JS, S.A. M. Jawetz, Melnick, & Adelberg's Medical Microbiology, 24th Edition. wwwaccessmedicinecom. 2007.

29. Collier L, Balows A, Sussman M. Topley and Wilson's Microbiology and Microbial Infections, Vol. I, II. 1998.

30. Beauchamp D, Gourde P, Simard M, Bergeron MG. Subcellular localization of tobramycin and vancomycin given alone and in combination in proximal tubular cells, determined by immunogold labeling. Antimicrobial Agents and Chemotherapy. 1992;36(10):2204–10. PubMed PMID: PMC245477.

31. Van Bambeke F, Snoeck A, Chanteux H, Mingeot-Leclercq M, Tulkens P. Is LY333328 glycopeptide a new cell-associated antibiotic? Comparative studies with vancomycin and azithromycin in a model of J774 mouse macrophages. 11th European Congress of Clinical Microbiology and Infectious Diseases Istanbul, Turkey, April 1–4, 2001. 2001.
32. Pascual A, Tsukayama D, Kovarik J, Gekker G, Peterson P. Uptake and activity of rifapentine in human peritoneal macrophages and polymorphonuclear leukocytes. Antimicrobial Agents and Chemotherapy. 1987 Apr;6(2):152–7. PubMed PMID: 2954817. Epub 1987/04/01. eng.
33. Maderazo EG, Breaux SP, Woronick CL, Quintiliani R, Nightingale CH. High teicoplanin uptake by human neutrophils. Chemotherapy. 1988;34(3):248–55. PubMed PMID: 2970950. Epub 1988/01/01. eng.
34. Van Bambeke F, Carryn S, Seral C, Chanteux H, Tyteca D, Mingeot-Leclercq MP, et al. Cellular pharmacokinetics and pharmacodynamics of the glycopeptide antibiotic oritavancin (LY333328) in a model of J774 mouse macrophages. Antimicrobial Agents and Chemotherapy. 2004 Aug;48(8):2853–60. PubMed PMID: 15273091. PubMed Central PMCID: PMC478544. Epub 2004/07/27. eng.
35. Jacobs RF, Thompson JW, Kiel DP, Johnson D. Cellular uptake and cell-associated activity of third generation cephalosporins. Pediatric Research. 1986 Sep;20(9):909–12. PubMed PMID: 3489219. Epub 1986/09/01. eng.
36. Carryn S, Van Bambeke F, Mingeot-Leclercq MP, Tulkens PM. Comparative intracellular (THP-1 macrophage) and extracellular activities of beta-lactams, azithromycin, gentamicin, and fluoroquinolones against Listeria monocytogenes at clinically relevant concentrations. Antimicrobial Agents and Chemotherapy. 2002 Jul;46(7):2095–103. PubMed PMID: 12069960. PubMed Central PMCID: PMC127291. Epub 2002/06/19. eng.
37. Wilkinson G. Pharmacokinetics: the dynamics of drugs absorption, distribution and elimination. In: Hardman JG, Limbird LL, editors. Goodman & Gilman's the Pharmacological Basis of Therapeutics. New York: McGraw Hill Medical Publishing Division. 2001:3–30.
38. Mingeot-Leclercq MP, Glupczynski Y, Tulkens PM. Aminoglycosides: activity and resistance. Antimicrobial Agents and Chemotherapy. 1999 Apr;43(4):727–37. PubMed PMID: 10103173. PubMed Central PMCID: PMC89199. Epub 1999/04/02. eng.
39. Vakulenko SB, Mobashery S. Versatility of aminoglycosides and prospects for their future. Clinical Microbiology Reviews. 2003;16(3):430–50. PubMed PMID: PMC164221.
40. 40.Tulkens P, Trouet A. The uptake and intracellular accumulation of aminoglycoside antibiotics in lysosomes of cultured rat fibroblasts. Biochemical Pharmacology. 1978 Feb 15;27(4):415–24. PubMed PMID: 24449. Epub 1978/02/15. eng.
41. Just M, Erdmann G, Habermann E. The renal handling of polybasic drugs. 1. Gentamicin and aprotinin in intact animals. Naunyn-Schmiedeberg's Archives of Pharmacology. 1977 Oct;300(1):57–66. PubMed PMID: 304182. Epub 1977/10/25. eng.
42. Nagai J, Tanaka H, Nakanishi N, Murakami T, Takano M. Role of megalin in renal handling of aminoglycosides. American Journal of Physiology. Renal Physiology. 2001 Aug;281(2):F337–44. PubMed PMID: 11457726. Epub 2001/07/18. eng.
43. Sastrasinh M, Knauss TC, Weinberg JM, Humes HD. Identification of the aminoglycoside binding site in rat renal brush border membranes. Journal of Pharmacology and Experimental Therapeutics. 1982 Aug;222(2):350–8. PubMed PMID: 7097555. Epub 1982/08/01. eng.

44. Chopra I, Roberts M. Tetracycline antibiotics: mode of action, applications, molecular biology, and epidemiology of bacterial resistance. Microbiology and Molecular Biology Reviews. 2001 Jun;65(2):232–60; second page, table of contents. PubMed PMID: 11381101. PubMed Central PMCID: PMC99026. Epub 2001/05/31. eng.

45. Coates TD, Torres M, Harman J, Williams V. Localization of chlorotetracycline fluorescence in human polymorphonuclear neutrophils. Blood. 1987 Apr;69(4):1146–52. PubMed PMID: 3828534. Epub 1987/04/01. eng.

46. Carlier MB, Garcia-Luque I, Montenez JP, Tulkens PM, Piret J. Accumulation, release and subcellular localization of azithromycin in phagocytic and non-phagocytic cells in culture. International Journal of Tissue Reactions. 1994;16(5–6):211–20. PubMed PMID: 7558665. Epub 1994/01/01. eng.

47. Van Bambeke F, Gerbaux C, Michot JM, d'Yvoire MB, Montenez JP, Tulkens PM. Lysosomal alterations induced in cultured rat fibroblasts by long-term exposure to low concentrations of azithromycin. Journal of Antimicrobial Chemotherapy. 1998 Dec;42(6):761–7. PubMed PMID: 10052900. Epub 1999/03/03. eng.

48. Ackermann G, Tang YJ, Kueper R, Heisig P, Rodloff AC, Silva J, Jr., et al. Resistance to moxifloxacin in toxigenic Clostridium difficile isolates is associated with mutations in gyrA. Antimicrobial Agents and Chemotherapy. 2001 Aug;45(8):2348–53. PubMed PMID: 11451695. PubMed Central PMCID: PMC90652. Epub 2001/07/14. eng.

49. Vester B, Douthwaite S. Macrolide resistance conferred by base substitutions in 23S rRNA. Antimicrobial Agents and Chemotherapy. 2001;45(1):1–12. PubMed PMID: PMC90232.

50. Pascual A, Ballesta S, Garcia I, Perea EJ. Uptake and intracellular activity of linezolid in human phagocytes and nonphagocytic cells. Antimicrobial Agents and Chemotherapy. 2002 Dec;46(12):4013–5. PubMed PMID: 12435714. PubMed Central PMCID: PMC132792. Epub 2002/11/19. eng.

51. Wistreich AG. Microbiology Laboratory Fundamentals and Applications (Hardcover). 1996.

52. Wolfson JS, Hooper DC. Fluoroquinolone antimicrobial agents. Clinical Microbiology Reviews. 1989;2(4):378–424. PubMed PMID: PMC358131.

53. Hoger PH, Vosbeck K, Seger R, Hitzig WH. Uptake, intracellular activity, and influence of rifampin on normal function of polymorphonuclear leukocytes. Antimicrobial Agents and Chemotherapy. 1985 Nov;28(5):667–74. PubMed PMID: 3004324. PubMed Central PMCID: PMC176354. Epub 1985/11/01. eng.

54. Musser JM. Antimicrobial agent resistance in mycobacteria: molecular genetic insights. Clinical Microbiology Reviews. 1995 Oct;8(4):496–514. PubMed PMID: 8665467. PubMed Central PMCID: PMC172873. Epub 1995/10/01. eng.

55. Carryn S, Chanteux H, Seral C, Mingeot-Leclercq MP, Van Bambeke F, Tulkens PM. Intracellular pharmacodynamics of antibiotics. Infectious Disease Clinics of North America. 2003 Sep;17(3):615–34. PubMed PMID: 14711080. Epub 2004/01/09. eng.

56. Dulhunty JM, Roberts JA, Davis JS, Webb SA, Bellomo R, Gomersall C, et al. Continuous infusion of beta-lactam antibiotics in severe sepsis: a multicenter double-blind, randomized controlled trial. Clinical Infectious Diseases. 2013 Jan;56(2):236–44. PubMed PMID: 23074313. Epub 2012/10/18. eng.

57. Seral C, Van Bambeke F, Tulkens PM. Quantitative analysis of gentamicin, azithromycin, telithromycin, ciprofloxacin, moxifloxacin, and oritavancin (LY333328) activities against intracellular Staphylococcus aureus in mouse J774 macrophages. Antimicrobial Agents

and Chemotherapy. 2003 Jul;47(7):2283–92. PubMed PMID: 12821480. PubMed Central PMCID: PMC161849. Epub 2003/06/25. eng.

58. Abed N, Couvreur P. Nanocarriers for antibiotics: a promising solution to treat intracellular bacterial infections. International Journal of Antimicrobial Agents. 2014 Jun;43(6):485–96. PubMed PMID: 24721232. Epub 2014/04/12. eng.

59. Singh R, Smitha MS, Singh SP. The role of nanotechnology in combating multi-drug resistant bacteria. Journal of Nanoscience and Nanotechnology. 2014 Jul;14(7):4745–56. PubMed PMID: 24757944. Epub 2014/04/25. eng.

60. Pelgrift RY, Friedman AJ. Nanotechnology as a therapeutic tool to combat microbial resistance. Advanced Drug Delivery Reviews. 2013 Nov;65(13–14):1803–15. PubMed PMID: 23892192. Epub 2013/07/31. eng.

61. Zhang L, Pornpattananangku D, Hu CM, Huang CM. Development of nanoparticles for antimicrobial drug delivery. Current Medicinal Chemistry. 2010;17(6):585–94. PubMed PMID: 20015030. Epub 2009/12/18. eng.

62. Pinto-Alphandary H, Andremont A, Couvreur P. Targeted delivery of antibiotics using liposomes and nanoparticles: research and applications. International Journal of Antimicrobial Agents. 2000 Jan;13(3):155–68. PubMed PMID: 10724019. Epub 2000/03/21. eng.

63. Briones E, Colino CI, Lanao JM. Delivery systems to increase the selectivity of antibiotics in phagocytic cells. Journal of Controlled Release. 2008 Feb 11;125(3):210–27. PubMed PMID: 18077047. Epub 2007/12/14. eng.

64. Huh AJ, Kwon YJ. "Nanoantibiotics": a new paradigm for treating infectious diseases using nanomaterials in the antibiotics resistant era. Journal of Controlled Release. 2011 Dec 10;156(2):128–45. PubMed PMID: 21763369. Epub 2011/07/19. eng.

65. Rawat M, Singh D, Saraf S, Saraf S. Nanocarriers: promising vehicle for bioactive drugs. Biological and Pharmaceutical Bulletin. 2006 Sep;29(9):1790–8. PubMed PMID: 16946487. Epub 2006/09/02. eng.

66. Mahapatro A, Singh DK. Biodegradable nanoparticles are excellent vehicle for site directed in-vivo delivery of drugs and vaccines. Journal of Nanobiotechnology. 2011;9:55. PubMed PMID: 22123084. PubMed Central PMCID: PMC3238292. Epub 2011/11/30. eng.

67. Kumari A, Yadav SK, Yadav SC. Biodegradable polymeric nanoparticles based drug delivery systems. Colloids and Surfaces B: Biointerfaces. 2010 1/1/;75(1):1–18.

68. 68.Maham A, Tang Z, Wu H, Wang J, Lin Y. Protein-based nanomedicine platforms for drug delivery. Small (Weinheim an der Bergstrasse, Germany). 2009 Aug 3;5(15):1706–21. PubMed PMID: 19572330. Epub 2009/07/03. eng.

69. Kanokpanont S, Damrongsakkul S, Ratanavaraporn J, Aramwit P. An innovative bi-layered wound dressing made of silk and gelatin for accelerated wound healing. International Journal of Pharmaceutics. 2012 Oct 15;436(1–2):141–53. PubMed PMID: 22771972. Epub 2012/07/10. eng.

70. Kuehn C, Graf K, Mashaqi B, Pichlmaier M, Heuer W, Hilfiker A, et al. Prevention of early vascular graft infection using regional antibiotic release. Journal of Surgical Research. 2010 Nov;164(1):e185–91. PubMed PMID: 20828762. Epub 2010/09/11. eng.

71. Hou T, Xu J, Li Q, Feng J, Zen L. In vitro evaluation of a fibrin gel antibiotic delivery system containing mesenchymal stem cells and vancomycin alginate beads for treating bone infections and facilitating bone formation. Tissue Engineering Part A. 2008 Jul;14(7):1173–82. PubMed PMID: 18593356. Epub 2008/07/03. eng.

72. Portilla-Arias JA, Camargo B, Garcia-Alvarez M, de Ilarduya AM, Munoz-Guerra S. Nanoparticles made of microbial poly(gamma-glutamate)s for encapsulation and delivery of drugs and proteins. Journal of Biomaterials Science, Polymer Edition. 2009;20(7–8):1065–79. PubMed PMID: 19454169. Epub 2009/05/21. eng.

73. Okamoto S, Matsuura M, Akagi T, Akashi M, Tanimoto T, Ishikawa T, et al. Poly(gamma-glutamic acid) nano-particles combined with mucosal influenza virus hemagglutinin vaccine protects against influenza virus infection in mice. Vaccine. 2009 Sep 25;27(42):5896–905. PubMed PMID: 19647814. Epub 2009/08/04. eng.

74. Matsuo K, Ishii Y, Matsuo K, Yoshinaga T, Akashi M, Mukai Y, et al. The utility of poly(gamma-glutamic acid) nanoparticles as antigen delivery carriers in dendritic cell-based cancer immunotherapy. Biological and Pharmaceutical Bulletin. 2010;33(12):2003–7. PubMed PMID: 21139241. Epub 2010/12/09. eng.

75. Takehara M, Hibino A, Saimura M, Hirohara H. High-yield production of short chain length poly(epsilon-L-lysine) consisting of 5–20 residues by Streptomyces aureofaciens, and its antimicrobial activity. Biotechnology Letters. 2010 Sep;32(9):1299–303. PubMed PMID: 20464451. Epub 2010/05/14. eng.

76. Couffin-Hoarau AC, Aubertin AM, Boustta M, Schmidt S, Fehrentz JA, Martinez J, et al. Peptide-poly(L-lysine citramide) conjugates and their in vitro anti-HIV behavior. Biomacromolecules. 2009 Apr 13;10(4):865–76. PubMed PMID: 19296658. Epub 2009/03/20. eng.

77. Ravi Kumar MNV. A review of chitin and chitosan applications. Reactive and Functional Polymers. 2000 11//;46(1):1–27.

78. Hench LL. Biomaterials: a forecast for the future. Biomaterials. 1998 Aug;19(16):1419–23. PubMed PMID: 9794512. Epub 1998/10/30. eng.

79. Khoushab F, Yamabhai M. Chitin Research Revisited. Marine Drugs. 2010 06/28 05/02/received 05/24/revised 05/08/accepted;8(7):1988–2012. PubMed PMID: PMC2920538.

80. Jain KK. Drug delivery systems—an overview. Methods in Molecular Biology (Clifton, NJ). 2008;437:1–50. PubMed PMID: 18369961. Epub 2008/03/29. eng.

81. Bajpai AK, Shukla SK, Bhanu S, Kankane S. Responsive polymers in controlled drug delivery. Progress in Polymer Science. 2008 11//;33(11):1088–118.

82. Chifiriuc MC, Grumezescu AM, Grumezescu V, Bezirtzoglou E, Lazar V, Bolocan A. Biomedical applications of natural polymers for drug delivery. Current Organic Chemistry. 2014;18(2):152–64.

83. Tiwari G, Tiwari R, Sriwastawa B, Bhati L, Pandey S, Pandey P, et al. Drug delivery systems: an updated review. International Journal of Pharmaceutical Investigation. 2012 Jan;2(1):2–11. PubMed PMID: 23071954. PubMed Central PMCID: PMC3465154. Epub 2012/10/17. eng.

84. Schmaljohann D. Thermo- and pH-responsive polymers in drug delivery. Advanced Drug Delivery Reviews. 2006 Dec 30;58(15):1655–70. PubMed PMID: 17125884. Epub 2006/11/28. eng.

85. von Burkersroda F, Schedl L, Gopferich A. Why degradable polymers undergo surface erosion or bulk erosion. Biomaterials. 2002 Nov;23(21):4221–31. PubMed PMID: 12194525. Epub 2002/08/27. eng.

86. Keraliya RA, Patel C, Patel P, Keraliya V, Soni TG, Patel RC, et al. Osmotic Drug Delivery System as a Part of Modified Release Dosage Form. ISRN Pharmaceutics. 2012 07/17 03/09/received 05/08/accepted;2012:528079. PubMed PMID: PMC3407637.

87. Urbina MC, Zinoveva S, Miller T, Sabliov CM, Monroe WT, Kumar CSSR. Investigation of magnetic nanoparticle-polymer composites for multiple-controlled drug delivery. Journal of Physical Chemistry C. 2008 2008/07/01;112(30):11102–8.

88. Mano JF. Stimuli-responsive polymeric systems for biomedical applications. Advanced Engineering Materials. 2008;10(6):515–27.

89. Qiu J, Charleux B, Matyjaszewski K. Controlled/living radical polymerization in aqueous media: homogeneous and heterogeneous systems. Progress in Polymer Science. 2001 12//;26(10):2083–134.

90. Kingsley JD, Dou H, Morehead J, Rabinow B, Gendelman HE, Destache CJ. Nanotechnology: a focus on nanoparticles as a drug delivery system. Journal of Neuroimmune Pharmacology. 2006 Sep;1(3):340–50. PubMed PMID: 18040810. Epub 2007/11/28. eng.

91. Pinto Reis C, Neufeld RJ, Ribeiro AJ, Veiga F. Nanoencapsulation I. Methods for preparation of drug-loaded polymeric nanoparticles. Nanomedicine: Nanotechnology, Biology, and Medicine. 2006 Mar;2(1):8–21. PubMed PMID: 17292111. Epub 2007/02/13. eng.

92. Lee LY, Wang CH, Smith KA. Supercritical antisolvent production of biodegradable micro- and nanoparticles for controlled delivery of paclitaxel. Journal of Controlled Release. 2008 Jan 22;125(2):96–106. PubMed PMID: 18054107. Epub 2007/12/07. eng.

93. Thiele L, Diederichs JE, Reszka R, Merkle HP, Walter E. Competitive adsorption of serum proteins at microparticles affects phagocytosis by dendritic cells. Biomaterials. 2003 Apr;24(8):1409–18. PubMed PMID: 12527282. Epub 2003/01/16. eng.

94. Ravi Kumar MN. Nano and microparticles as controlled drug delivery devices. Journal of Pharmacy and Pharmaceutical Sciences. 2000 May–Aug;3(2):234–58. PubMed PMID: 10994037. Epub 2000/09/20. eng.

95. Date AA, Joshi MD, Patravale VB. Parasitic diseases: liposomes and polymeric nanoparticles versus lipid nanoparticles. Advanced Drug Delivery Reviews. 2007 Jul 10;59(6):505–21. PubMed PMID: 17574295. Epub 2007/06/19. eng.

96. Ahmad Z, Pandey R, Sharma S, Khuller GK. Alginate nanoparticles as antituberculosis drug carriers: formulation development, pharmacokinetics and therapeutic potential. Indian Journal of Chest Diseases and Allied Sciences. 2006 Jul–Sep;48(3):171–6. PubMed PMID: 18610673. Epub 2008/07/10. eng.

97. Nagpal K, Singh SK, Mishra DN. Chitosan nanoparticles: a promising system in novel drug delivery. Chemical and Pharmaceutical Bulletin. 2010 Nov;58(11):1423–30. PubMed PMID: 21048331. Epub 2010/11/05. eng.

98. Huh KM, Lee SC, Cho YW, Lee J, Jeong JH, Park K. Hydrotropic polymer micelle system for delivery of paclitaxel. Journal of Controlled Release. 2005 Jan 3;101(1–3):59–68. PubMed PMID: 15588894. Epub 2004/12/14. eng.

99. Bertesteanu S, Chifiriuc MC, Grumezescu AM, Printza AG, Marie-Paule T, Grumezescu V, et al. Biomedical applications of synthetic, biodegradable polymers for the development of anti-infective strategies. Current Medicinal Chemistry. 2014;21(29):3383–90. PubMed PMID: 24606501. Epub 2014/03/13. eng.

100. Hornig S, Bunjes H, Heinze T. Preparation and characterization of nanoparticles based on dextran-drug conjugates. Journal of Colloid and Interface Science. 2009 Oct 1;338(1):56–62. PubMed PMID: 19635622. Epub 2009/07/29. eng.

101. 101.Roseeuw E, Coessens V, Balazuc A-M, Lagranderie M, Chavarot P, Pessina A, et al. Synthesis, degradation, and antimicrobial properties of targeted macromolecular prodrugs of norfloxacin. Antimicrobial Agents and Chemotherapy. 2003 12/13/received 04/14/revised 08/11/accepted;47(11):3435–41. PubMed PMID: PMC253810.

102. Jiang D, Salem AK. Optimized dextran-polyethylenimine conjugates are efficient non-viral vectors with reduced cytotoxicity when used in serum containing environments. International Journal of Pharmaceutics. 2012 May 1;427(1):71–9. PubMed PMID: 22037445. PubMed Central PMCID: PMC3295901. Epub 2011/11/01. eng.

103. Gnanadhas DP, Ben Thomas M, Elango M, Raichur AM, Chakravortty D. Chitosan-dextran sulphate nanocapsule drug delivery system as an effective therapeutic against intraphagosomal pathogen Salmonella. Journal of Antimicrobial Chemotherapy. 2013 Nov;68(11):2576–86. PubMed PMID: 23798672. Epub 2013/06/27. eng.

104. De Paula EE, De Sousa FB, Da Silva JC, Fernandes FR, Melo MN, Frezard F, et al. Insights into the multi-equilibrium, superstructure system based on beta-cyclodextrin and a highly water soluble guest. International Journal of Pharmaceutics. 2012 Dec 15;439(1–2):207–15. PubMed PMID: 23022296. Epub 2012/10/02. eng.

105. Jain A, Gupta Y, Jain SK. Perspectives of biodegradable natural polysaccharides for site-specific drug delivery to the colon. Journal of pharmacy & pharmaceutical sciences: a publication of the Canadian Society for Pharmaceutical Sciences, Societe Canadienne des Sciences Pharmaceutiques. 2007;10(1):86–128. PubMed PMID: 17498397. Epub 2007/05/15. eng.

106. Farazuddin M, Chauhan A, Khan RM, Owais M. Amoxicillin-bearing microparticles: potential in the treatment of Listeria monocytogenes infection in Swiss albino mice. Bioscience Reports. 2011 Aug;31(4):265–72. PubMed PMID: 20687896. Epub 2010/08/07. eng.

107. Heijink A, Yaszemski MJ, Patel R, Rouse MS, Lewallen DG, Hanssen AD. Local antibiotic delivery with OsteoSet, DBX, and Collagraft. Clinical Orthopaedics and Related Research. 2006 Oct;451:29–33. PubMed PMID: 16906070. Epub 2006/08/15. eng.

108. Smitha KT, Nisha N, Maya S, Biswas R, Jayakumar R. Delivery of rifampicin-chitin nanoparticles into the intracellular compartment of polymorphonuclear leukocytes. International Journal of Biological Macromolecules. 2015 Mar;74:36–43. PubMed PMID: 25475841. Epub 2014/12/06. eng.

109. Puoci F, Cirillo G, Curcio M, Parisi OI, Iemma F, Picci N. Molecularly imprinted polymers in drug delivery: state of art and future perspectives. Expert Opinion on Drug Delivery. 2011 Oct;8(10):1379–93. PubMed PMID: 21933031. Epub 2011/09/22. eng.

110. Sah H, Thoma LA, Desu HR, Sah E, Wood GC. Concepts and practices used to develop functional PLGA-based nanoparticulate systems. International Journal of Nanomedicine. 2013;8:747–65. PubMed PMID: 23459088. PubMed Central PMCID: PMC3582541. Epub 2013/03/06. eng.

111. Kaditi E, Mountrichas G, Pispas S, Demetzos C. Block copolymers for drug delivery nano systems (DDnSs). Current Medicinal Chemistry. 2012;19(29):5088–100. PubMed PMID: 22963634. Epub 2012/09/12. eng.

112. Kluin OS, van der Mei HC, Busscher HJ, Neut D. Biodegradable vs non-biodegradable antibiotic delivery devices in the treatment of osteomyelitis. Expert Opinion on Drug Delivery. 2013 Mar;10(3):341–51. PubMed PMID: 23289645. Epub 2013/01/08. eng.

113. Ulery BD, Nair LS, Laurencin CT. Biomedical applications of biodegradable polymers. Journal of Polymer Science Part B: Polymer Physics. 2011;49(12):832–64.

114. Danhier F, Ansorena E, Silva JM, Coco R, Le Breton A, Preat V. PLGA-based nanoparticles: an overview of biomedical applications. Journal of Controlled Release. 2012 Jul 20;161(2):505–22. PubMed PMID: 22353619. Epub 2012/02/23. eng.

115. Farazuddin M, Alam M, Khan AA, Khan N, Parvez S, Dutt GU, et al. Efficacy of amoxicillin bearing microsphere formulation in treatment of Listeria monocytogenes infection in Swiss albino mice. Journal of Drug Targeting. 2010 Jan;18(1):45–52. PubMed PMID: 19624287. Epub 2009/07/25. eng.

116. Malathi S, Balasubramanian S. Synthesis of biodegradable polymeric nanoparticles and their controlled drug delivery for tuberculosis. Journal of Biomedical Nanotechnology. 2011 Feb;7(1):150–1. PubMed PMID: 21485846. Epub 2011/04/14. eng.

117. Pandey R, Sharma A, Zahoor A, Sharma S, Khuller GK, Prasad B. Poly (DL-lactide-co-glycolide) nanoparticle-based inhalable sustained drug delivery system for experimental tuberculosis. Journal of Antimicrobial Chemotherapy. 2003 Dec;52(6):981–6. PubMed PMID: 14613962. Epub 2003/11/14. eng.

118. Skidan IN, Gel'perina SE, Severin SE, Guliaev AE. [Enhanced activity of rifampicin loaded with polybutyl cyanoacrylate nanoparticles in relation to intracellularly localized bacteria]. Antibiotiki i Khimioterapiia = Antibiotics and Chemoterapy [sic]/Ministerstvo Meditsinskoi i Mikrobiologicheskoi Promyshlennosti SSSR. 2003;48(1):23–6. PubMed PMID: 12741319. Epub 2003/05/14. Povyshenie aktivnosti rifampitsina, assotsiirovannogo s nanochastitsami iz polibutiltsianoakrilata, v otnoshenii bakterii, lokalizovannykh vnutri kletok. rus.

119. Fawaz F, Bonini F, Maugein J, Lagueny AM. Ciprofloxacin-loaded polyisobutylcyanoacrylate nanoparticles: pharmacokinetics and in vitro antimicrobial activity. International Journal of Pharmaceutics. 1998 6/15/;168(2):255–9.

120. Lecaroz C, Gamazo C, Renedo MJ, Blanco-Prieto MJ. Biodegradable micro- and nanoparticles as long-term delivery vehicles for gentamicin. Journal of Microencapsulation. 2006 Nov;23(7):782–92. PubMed PMID: 17123922. Epub 2006/11/25. eng.

121. Fattal E, Pecquet S, Couvreur P, Andremont A. Biodegradable microparticles for the mucosal delivery of antibacterial and dietary antigens. International Journal of Pharmaceutics. 2002 Aug 21;242(1–2):15–24. PubMed PMID: 12176221. Epub 2002/08/15. eng.

122. Toti US, Guru BR, Hali M, McPharlin CM, Wykes SM, Panyam J, et al. Targeted delivery of antibiotics to intracellular chlamydial infections using PLGA nanoparticles. Biomaterials. 2011 Sep;32(27):6606–13. PubMed PMID: 21652065. PubMed Central PMCID: PMC3133877. Epub 2011/06/10. eng.

123. Imbuluzqueta E, Elizondo E, Gamazo C, Moreno-Calvo E, Veciana J, Ventosa N, et al. Novel bioactive hydrophobic gentamicin carriers for the treatment of intracellular bacterial infections. Acta Biomaterialia. 2011 Apr;7(4):1599–608. PubMed PMID: 21115143. Epub 2010/12/01. eng.

124. Jhunjhunwala S, Raimondi G, Thomson AW, Little SR. Delivery of rapamycin to dendritic cells using degradable microparticles. Journal of Controlled Release. 2009 Feb 10;133(3):191–7. PubMed PMID: 19000726. PubMed Central PMCID: PMC2925512. Epub 2008/11/13. eng.

125. Gaspar R, Preat V, Opperdoes FR, Roland M. Macrophage activation by polymeric nanoparticles of polyalkylcyanoacrylates: activity against intracellular Leishmania donovani associated with hydrogen peroxide production. Pharmaceutical Research. 1992 Jun;9(6):782–7. PubMed PMID: 1409361. Epub 1992/06/01. eng.

126. Fattal E, Youssef M, Couvreur P, Andremont A. Treatment of experimental salmonellosis in mice with ampicillin-bound nanoparticles. Antimicrobial Agents and Chemotherapy. 1989;33(9):1540–3. PubMed PMID: PMC172698.

127. Forestier F, Gerrier P, Chaumard C, Quero AM, Couvreur P, Labarre C. Effect of nanoparticle-bound ampicillin on the survival of Listeria monocytogenes in mouse peritoneal macrophages. Journal of Antimicrobial Chemotherapy. 1992 Aug;30(2):173–9. PubMed PMID: 1399927. Epub 1992/08/01. eng.

128. Pandey R, Khuller GK. Oral nanoparticle-based antituberculosis drug delivery to the brain in an experimental model. Journal of Antimicrobial Chemotherapy. 2006 Jun;57(6):1146–52. PubMed PMID: 16597631. Epub 2006/04/07. eng.

129. Kuroda K, Caputo GA. Antimicrobial polymers as synthetic mimics of host-defense peptides. Nanomedicine and Nanobiotechnology. 2013 Jan–Feb;5(1):49–66. PubMed PMID: 23076870. Epub 2012/10/19. eng.

130. Palermo EF, Kuroda K. Structural determinants of antimicrobial activity in polymers which mimic host defense peptides. Applied Microbiology and Biotechnology. 2010 Aug;87(5):1605–15. PubMed PMID: 20563718. Epub 2010/06/22. eng.

131. Lee S, Yang SC, Heffernan MJ, Taylor WR, Murthy N. Polyketal microparticles: a new delivery vehicle for superoxide dismutase. Bioconjugate Chemistry. 2007 Jan–Feb;18(1):4–7. PubMed PMID: 17226951. Epub 2007/01/18. eng.

132. Seshadri G, Sy JC, Brown M, Dikalov S, Yang SC, Murthy N, et al. The delivery of superoxide dismutase encapsulated in polyketal microparticles to rat myocardium and protection from myocardial ischemia-reperfusion injury. Biomaterials. 2010 Feb;31(6):1372–9. PubMed PMID: 19889454. PubMed Central PMCID: PMC2813932. Epub 2009/11/06. eng.

133. Kalluru R, Fenaroli F, Westmoreland D, Ulanova L, Maleki A, Roos N, et al. Poly(lactide-co-glycolide)-rifampicin nanoparticles efficiently clear Mycobacterium bovis BCG infection in macrophages and remain membrane-bound in phago-lysosomes. Journal of Cell Science. 2013 Jul 15;126(Pt 14):3043–54. PubMed PMID: 23687375. Epub 2013/05/21. eng.

134. Page-Clisson ME, Pinto-Alphandary H, Chachaty E, Couvreur P, Andremont A. Drug targeting by polyalkylcyanoacrylate nanoparticles is not efficient against persistent Salmonella. Pharmaceutical Research. 1998 Apr;15(4):544–9. PubMed PMID: 9587949. Epub 1998/05/20. eng.

135. Discher BM, Won YY, Ege DS, Lee JC, Bates FS, Discher DE, et al. Polymersomes: tough vesicles made from diblock copolymers. Science. 1999 May 14;284(5417):1143–6. PubMed PMID: 10325219. Epub 1999/05/15. eng.

136. Wayakanon K, Thornhill MH, Douglas CW, Lewis AL, Warren NJ, Pinnock A, et al. Polymersome-mediated intracellular delivery of antibiotics to treat Porphyromonas gingivalis-infected oral epithelial cells. FASEB Journal. 2013 Nov;27(11):4455–65. PubMed PMID: 23921377. Epub 2013/08/08. eng.

137. Coune A. Liposomes as drug delivery system in the treatment of infectious diseases. Potential applications and clinical experience. Infection. 1988 May–Jun;16(3):141–7. PubMed PMID: 3042625. Epub 1988/05/01. eng.

138. Kelly C, Jefferies C, Cryan S-A. Targeted liposomal drug delivery to monocytes and macrophages. Journal of Drug Delivery. 2011;2011:11.

139. Khuller GK, Kapur M, Sharma S. Liposome technology for drug delivery against mycobacterial infections. Current Pharmaceutical Design. 2004;10(26):3263–74. PubMed PMID: 15544514. Epub 2004/11/17. eng.

140. Yanagihara K. Design of anti-bacterial drug and anti-mycobacterial drug for drug delivery system. Current Pharmaceutical Design. 2002;8(6):475–82. PubMed PMID: 12069384. Epub 2002/06/19. eng.

141. Gangadharam PR, Ashtekar DA, Ghori N, Goldstein JA, Debs RJ, Duzgunes N. Chemotherapeutic potential of free and liposome encapsulated streptomycin against experimental Mycobacterium avium complex infections in beige mice. Journal of Antimicrobial Chemotherapy. 1991 Sep;28(3):425–35. PubMed PMID: 1960123. Epub 1991/09/01. eng.

142. Patton JS, Fishburn CS, Weers JG. The lungs as a portal of entry for systemic drug delivery. Proceedings of the American Thoracic Society. 2004;1(4):338–44. PubMed PMID: 16113455. Epub 2005/08/23. eng.

143. Deol P, Khuller GK. Lung specific stealth liposomes: stability, biodistribution and toxicity of liposomal antitubercular drugs in mice. Biochimica et Biophysica Acta. 1997 Mar 15;1334(2–3):161–72. PubMed PMID: 9101710. Epub 1997/03/15. eng.

144. Vitas AI, Díaz R, Gamazo C. Effect of composition and method of preparation of liposomes on their stability and interaction with murine monocytes infected with Brucella abortus. Antimicrobial Agents and Chemotherapy. 1996;40(1):146–51. PubMed PMID: PMC163073.

145. Fierer J, Hatlen L, Lin JP, Estrella D, Mihalko P, Yau-Young A. Successful treatment using gentamicin liposomes of Salmonella dublin infections in mice. Antimicrobial Agents and Chemotherapy. 1990 Feb;34(2):343–8. PubMed PMID: 2327780. PubMed Central PMCID: PMC171584. Epub 1990/02/01. eng.

146. Bakker-Woudenberg IA, Lokerse AF, Roerdink FH. Effect of lipid composition on activity of liposome-entrapped ampicillin against intracellular Listeria monocytogenes. Antimicrobial Agents and Chemotherapy. 1988;32(10):1560–4. PubMed PMID: PMC175919.

147. Lutwyche P, Cordeiro C, Wiseman DJ, St-Louis M, Uh M, Hope MJ, et al. Intracellular delivery and antibacterial activity of gentamicin encapsulated in pH-sensitive liposomes. Antimicrobial Agents and Chemotherapy. 1998 Oct;42(10):2511–20. PubMed PMID: 9756749. PubMed Central PMCID: PMC105873. Epub 1998/10/03. eng.

148. Lockman PR, Mumper RJ, Khan MA, Allen DD. Nanoparticle technology for drug delivery across the blood–brain barrier. Drug Development and Industrial Pharmacy. 2002 Jan;28(1):1–13. PubMed PMID: 11858519. Epub 2002/02/23. eng.

149. Roney C, Kulkarni P, Arora V, Antich P, Bonte F, Wu A, et al. Targeted nanoparticles for drug delivery through the blood–brain barrier for Alzheimer's disease. Journal of Controlled Release. 2005 Nov 28;108(2–3):193–214. PubMed PMID: 16246446. Epub 2005/10/26. eng.

150. Kreuter J. Nanoparticulate systems for brain delivery of drugs. Advanced Drug Delivery Reviews. 2001 Mar 23;47(1):65–81. PubMed PMID: 11251246. Epub 2001/03/17. eng.

151. Seleem MN, Jain N, Pothayee N, Ranjan A, Riffle JS, Sriranganathan N. Targeting Brucella melitensis with polymeric nanoparticles containing streptomycin and doxycycline. FEMS Microbiology Letters. 2009 May;294(1):24–31. PubMed PMID: 19493005. Epub 2009/06/06. eng.

152. Kadurugamuwa JL, Beveridge TJ. Delivery of the non-membrane-permeative antibiotic gentamicin into mammalian cells by using Shigella flexneri membrane vesicles. Antimicrobial Agents and Chemotherapy. 1998 Jun;42(6):1476–83. PubMed PMID: 9624497. PubMed Central PMCID: PMC105625. Epub 1998/06/13. eng.

153. Kamboj S, Saini V, Maggon N, Bala S, Jhawat V. Vesicular drug delivery systems: a novel approach for drug targeting. International Journal of Drug Delivery. 2013;5(2):10. Epub 2013-09-17.

154. Singh G, Dwivedi H, Saraf S, Saraf S. Niosomal delivery of isoniazid: development and characterization. Tropical Journal of Pharmaceutical Research. 2011;10(2):203–10.

155. Jain C, Vyas S, VK. D. Niosomal system for delivery of rifampicin to lymphatics. Indian Journal of Pharmaceutical Sciences. 2006;68(5):575–8.

156. Mukherjee S, Ray S, Thakur RS. Solid lipid nanoparticles: a modern formulation approach in drug delivery system. Indian Journal of Pharmaceutical Sciences. 2009 Jul;71(4):349–58. PubMed PMID: 20502539. PubMed Central PMCID: PMC2865805. Epub 2010/05/27. eng.

157. Nimje N, Agarwal A, Saraogi GK, Lariya N, Rai G, Agrawal H, et al. Mannosylated nanoparticulate carriers of rifabutin for alveolar targeting. Journal of Drug Targeting. 2009 Dec;17(10):777–87. PubMed PMID: 19938949. Epub 2009/11/27. eng.

158. Pandey R, Khuller GK. Solid lipid particle-based inhalable sustained drug delivery system against experimental tuberculosis. Tuberculosis (Edinburgh, Scotland). 2005 Jul;85(4):227–34. PubMed PMID: 15922668. Epub 2005/06/01. eng.

159. Muller RH, Jacobs C. Buparvaquone mucoadhesive nanosuspension: preparation, optimisation and long-term stability. International Journal of Pharmaceutics. 2002 Apr 26;237(1–2):151–61. PubMed PMID: 11955813. Epub 2002/04/17. eng.

160. Aggarwal P, Hall JB, McLeland CB, Dobrovolskaia MA, McNeil SE. Nanoparticle interaction with plasma proteins as it relates to particle biodistribution, biocompatibility and therapeutic efficacy. Advanced Drug Delivery Reviews. 2009 Jun 21;61(6):428–37. PubMed PMID: 19376175. PubMed Central PMCID: PMC3683962. Epub 2009/04/21. eng.

161. Patel MB, Harikrishnan U, Valand NN, Modi NR, Menon SK. Novel cationic quinazolin-4(3H)-one conjugated fullerene nanoparticles as antimycobacterial and antimicrobial agents. Archiv der Pharmazie. 2013 Mar;346(3):210–20. PubMed PMID: 23359525. Epub 2013/01/30. eng.

162. Kumar PV, Asthana A, Dutta T, Jain NK. Intracellular macrophage uptake of rifampicin loaded mannosylated dendrimers. Journal of Drug Targeting. 2006 Sep;14(8):546–56. PubMed PMID: 17050121. Epub 2006/10/20. eng.

163. Dutta T, Jain NK. Targeting potential and anti-HIV activity of lamivudine loaded mannosylated poly (propyleneimine) dendrimer. Biochimica et Biophysica Acta. 2007 Apr;1770(4):681–6. PubMed PMID: 17276009. Epub 2007/02/06. eng.

164. Bhadra D, Bhadra S, Jain NK. Pegylated lysine based copolymeric dendritic micelles for solubilization and delivery of artemether. Journal of Pharmacy and Pharmaceutical Sciences. 2005;8(3):467–82. PubMed PMID: 16401394. Epub 2006/01/13. eng.

165. Mishra MK, Kotta K, Hali M, Wykes S, Gerard HC, Hudson AP, et al. PAMAM dendrimer-azithromycin conjugate nanodevices for the treatment of Chlamydia trachomatis infections. Nanomedicine: Nanotechnology, Biology, and Medicine. 2011 Dec;7(6):935–44. PubMed PMID: 21658474. Epub 2011/06/11. eng.

166. Corma A, Garcia H. Supramolecular host–guest systems in zeolites prepared by ship-in-a-bottle synthesis. European Journal of Inorganic Chemistry. 2004;2004(6):1143–64.

167. Vilaça N, Amorim R, Machado AF, Parpot P, Pereira MFR, Sardo M, et al. Potentiation of 5-fluorouracil encapsulated in zeolites as drug delivery systems for in vitro models of colorectal carcinoma. Colloids and Surfaces B: Biointerfaces. 2013 12/1/;112(0):237–44.

168. Clemens DL, Lee BY, Xue M, Thomas CR, Meng H, Ferris D, et al. Targeted intracellular delivery of antituberculosis drugs to Mycobacterium tuberculosis-infected macrophages via functionalized mesoporous silica nanoparticles. Antimicrobial Agents and

Chemotherapy. 2012 May;56(5):2535–45. PubMed PMID: 22354311. PubMed Central PMCID: PMC3346638. Epub 2012/02/23. eng.

169. Seleem MN, Munusamy P, Ranjan A, Alqublan H, Pickrell G, Sriranganathan N. Silica-antibiotic hybrid nanoparticles for targeting intracellular pathogens. Antimicrobial Agents and Chemotherapy. 2009 08/10 06/17/received 07/12/revised 08/03/accepted;53(10):4270–4. PubMed PMID: PMC2764215.

170. Gutierrez Millan C, Bax BE, Castaneda AZ, Marinero ML, Lanao JM. In vitro studies of amikacin-loaded human carrier erythrocytes. Translational Research. 2008 Aug;152(2):59–66. PubMed PMID: 18674740. Epub 2008/08/05. eng.

12 Chapter

INTEGRITY OF DRUG-ELUTING DEPOT STENT FOR INTELLIGENT DRUG DELIVERY

1. INTRODUCTION: AN OVERVIEW

Percutaneous coronary intervention (PCI), commonly referred to as angioplasty, is the prevailing technique for treating coronary artery disease. A metallic stent is a tiny, coiled wire-mesh tube that can be inserted into an artery and extended via a catheter during angioplasty to alleviate arterial constriction. Intimal cells may multiply following arterial injury during stenting, frequently resulting in in-stent restenosis. Restenosis, the re-narrowing of the artery following intervention, is the most prevalent complication after angioplasty treatments in the initial period.

Over the past decade, stent technology has progressed from metallic stents to drug-eluting stents (DES). A drug-eluting stent comprises a metallic stent framework coated with an anti-proliferative agent (e.g., Sirolimus or Everolimus) that is recognized for its ability to inhibit the restenosis process. The medication is generally combined with a polymer ingredient (either durable or biodegradable) to accurately regulate its release rate and timing to the arterial wall. The implementation of drug-eluting stents has significantly reduced restenosis rates from 20-30% for metallic stents to single digits, resulting in global acceptance of this innovative healthcare treatment. The advent of drug-eluting stents has diminished the prevalence of restenosis in the management of coronary artery disorders. Consequently, the drug-eluting stent has established itself as the gold standard for percutaneous coronary intervention treatments.

Despite the significant effectiveness of drug-eluting stents in reducing restenosis, stenting technology persists in its evolution in pursuit of superior solutions. The biodegradable vascular scaffold (BVS) represents the forthcoming frontier. Biodegradable stents remain in the blood vessel for a finite duration, provide mechanical support, and subsequently decompose into non-toxic chemicals. The prospective benefits of the stent's dissolution at the treated location encompass less late stent thrombosis, enhanced capacity for further interventions at the same site, and immunity from restenosis caused by fractures. The biodegradable stents composed of poly lactic acid (PLA) have excellent physical features, including high strength and processability; they will decompose into natural components in an appropriate disposal environment [6-8]. BVS possesses the capability to function as localized drug delivery systems. Consequently, it is feasible to engineer a BVS that not only provides structural support to the vessel wall but also incorporates a pharmacological strategy for the prevention of thrombus formation and intimal proliferation [9-11].

In recent years, a new concept in smart drug delivery has emerged: the depot stent, a metallic stent laser-drilled with micro-sized holes, referred to as "reservoirs," which can be filled with one or multiple medications, perhaps in varying quantities or formulas. The drug-polymer combination can be adjusted between reservoirs, facilitating a great degree of flexibility in the regulated release of various medications. For instance, on the outside of the reservoirs adjacent to the arterial wall, agents that restrict neointimal proliferation might be administered, whilst on the interior of the reservoirs near the bloodstream, platelet inhibitors can be utilized to avert stent thrombosis (Figure 1). Furthermore, this stent concept is anticipated to be particularly effective in instances such as the renal indication for the simultaneous treatment of renal artery stenosis (RAS) and its related kidney diseases, given that RAS is typically associated with progressive hypertension, renal insufficiency, or kidney failure in a reciprocal manner. For instance, agents that inhibit neointimal proliferation may be administered on the external surfaces of the reservoirs adjacent to the arterial wall, while agents for renal disorders can be encapsulated within the reservoirs and transported via the bloodstream to the distal kidney for targeted therapy. This proposed solution may simultaneously address two issues. Figure 2 illustrates that several drug kinds may be administered independently at each step following intervention.

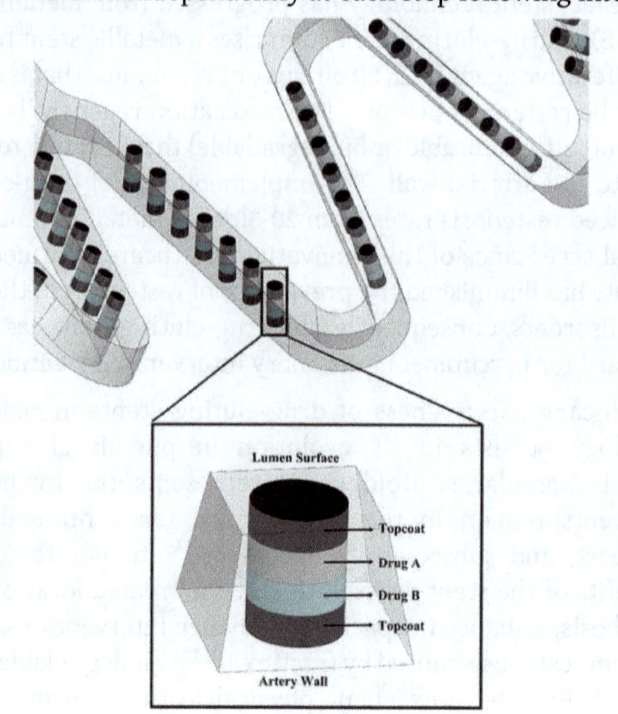

Figure 1. Depot stent concept with different types of drugs and release rates administered independently of opposite sides of the stent.

The depot stent possesses additional benefits. In contrast to drug-eluting stents, the depot stent does not require a surface coating. Consequently, it lacks surface coating layers, so minimizing direct contact between the arterial wall and the polymer component. This interaction is thought to elevate the possible risk of chronic inflammation or delayed stent thrombosis. Another benefit is the reduction of the overall stent profile resulting from the lack of surface coating layers. A reduced stent profile facilitates access to narrower lesion locations and enhances deliverability for clinicians. Despite these potential benefits, the formation of reservoirs on the stent struts inherently diminishes the structural integrity of the stent, undermining its mechanical properties, specifically its capacity to endure diverse loading scenarios, such as crimping onto a balloon catheter during production, stent expansion upon deployment, radial resistance against inward collapse of blood vessels, and long-term fatigue resistance to systolic and diastolic pressure fluctuations. The aim of this paper is to examine the effect of micro-sized reservoirs on the overall mechanical integrity of the depot stent.

Computational modeling has become an effective instrument for optimizing stent designs and can be utilized alongside bench testing to enhance clinical efficacy of stents [14-18]. These computational methods could yield significant insights into stent design strategies, thereby mitigating the risks of vascular damage and restenosis. It provides comprehensive information in a highly controlled environment, enabling the evaluation of multiple design iterations before expensive prototyping. Consequently, this work involved the development of computational models to evaluate essential clinical characteristics of the depot stent by finite element analysis (FEA). In light of these findings, we propose an ideal depot stent design to enhance medication capacity without substantially compromising its mechanical integrity.

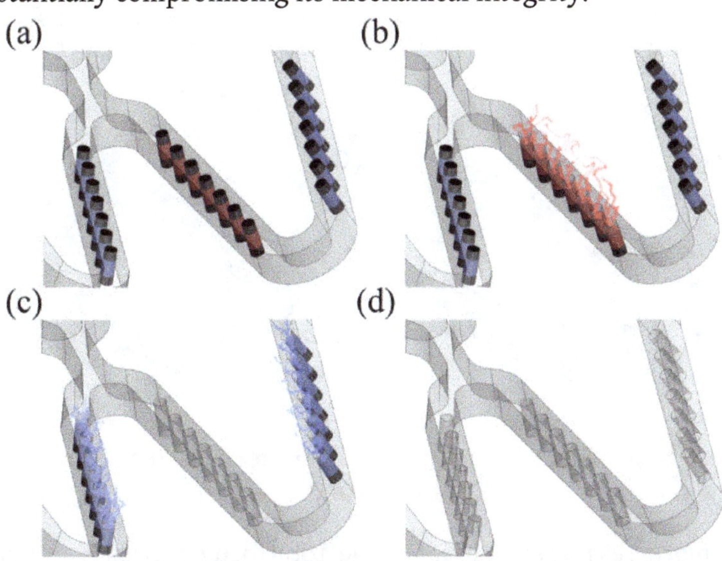

Figure 2. Schematic of sequential release of multiple drugs for each period after intervention.

2. DEPOT STENT CONFIGURATION

An L-605 cobalt–chromium balloon-expandable stent was used as the "standard" stent for baseline in this study. Micro-sized drug reservoirs were created on this standard stent struts in order to investigate their effects on the stent mechanical integrity. The stent was designed to form a series of nested rings interconnected with bridging connectors (CO). The design parameters such as crown radius (CR) and strut dimension were tailored to optimize the overall stent performance.

The standard stent, which has exactly the same geometry as the investigated depot stents but without drug reservoirs, was first evaluated to establish the baseline information. The FEA simulation was then conducted to investigate the effects of reservoir location on the mechanical integrity of the depot stent. Five equally spaced circular (cylindrical if considering depth) reservoirs were created on three major locations of the depot stent, namely, connectors, bar arms (BA), and crowns (Figure 3). The diameter of each circular reservoir was 50% of the strut width, whereas the reservoir depth was varied for evaluation. The spacing between two adjacent reservoirs was 0.15 mm, as defined by the length between two reservoir centers along the strut centerline. The choice of the reservoir number and size was based on the condition that the total reservoir capacity of the drug–polymer mix inside the reservoirs of the depot stent was able to fully replace the total volume of surface coating layers on a typical drug-eluting stent with an average coating thickness of 5μm [4].

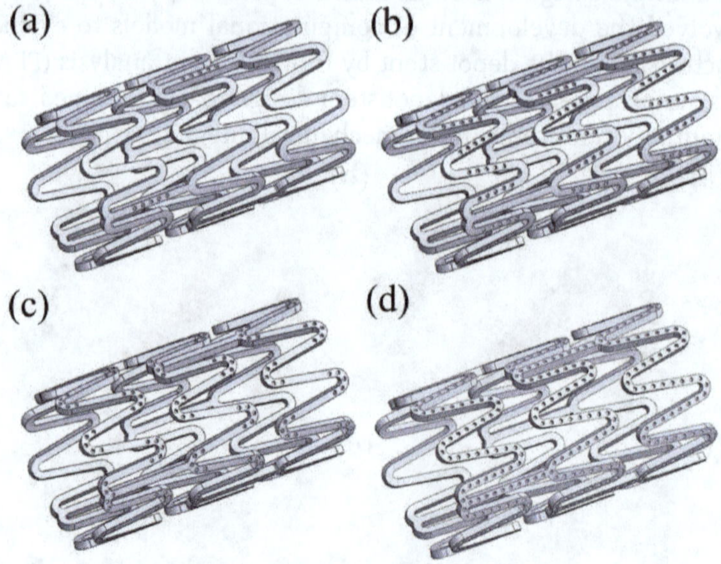

Figure 3. Depot stent with reservoirs on (a) connectors, (b) bar arms, (c) crowns, and (d) entire stent surfaces.

Since adding more reservoirs increases the total drug capacity, investigation was also carried out on the depot stent with reservoirs uniformly spread on the entire stent to understand whether the mechanical integrity of such a depot stent is further compromised or not (Figure 3(d)). In this special case, the entire stent was covered by reservoirs with the same circular diameter and depth aforementioned. Another method of increasing the total drug capacity is by drilling through-holes instead of blind-holes into the stent struts. Therefore, FEA simulation was also conducted to investigate the effects of reservoir depth on the mechanical integrity. Further studies were conducted on the depot stent to investigate whether the reservoir shape, size, and number affect the stent mechanical integrity or not.

3. DEVELOPMENT OF COMPUTATIONAL MODELS

3.1. Stent Mechanical Integrity Assessment

On 18 April 2010, the US Food and Drug Administration (FDA) released an official document titled "Non-Clinical Engineering Tests and Recommended Labeling for Intravascular Stents and Associated Delivery Systems" to provide guidance for the medical device industry. This paper enumerates various clinically significant functional features that the FDA considers when evaluating future stent submissions, in addition to standard dimensions tests such as dimensional verification, % surface area, foreshortening, and recoil. The essential therapeutic properties of the balloon-expandable stent encompass radial strength, stress-strain characteristics, and fatigue resistance. Each of these qualities can function as a signal about different facets of stent integrity. This study employed three primary clinical parameters to evaluate the mechanical integrity of the depot stent.

3.1.1. Radial Strength (RS)

One of the most important functions of the stent is to create a scaffolding structure in the artery and exert radial force against the artery wall to prevent its reclosure. Radial strength represents the ability of a stent to resist radial collapse under external pressure loadings exerted by the artery wall. It is defined as the maximum pressure at which the stent experiences irreversible deformation.

3.1.2. Equivalent plastic strain (PEEQ)

Since the in vivo deployment of a balloon-expandable stent involves large plastic deformation, the equivalent plastic stresses and strains have to be calculated throughout the stent. This stress analysis provides a risk assessment of acute device failure. The stress or strain contour plots provide the overall distribution of plastic stresses or strains and identify the most fracture-prone locations of a stent. Stent fracture may cause loss of the radial strength or perforation of the blood vessel by the fractured stent struts.

3.1.3. Fatigue Safety Factor (FSF)

Stent fracture due to long-term pulsatile fatigue loading may result in loss of the radial strength, thrombus formation, focal restenosis, or perforation of the blood vessel by the fractured stent struts. FDA recommends using a Goodman life analysis to determine the fatigue resistance of a stent to clinically relevant pressure loadings up to 4×108 cycles. The Goodman life analysis, combined with the stress analysis aforementioned and accelerated fatigue bench testing, provides a comprehensive risk assessment of long-term stent durability. The resulting fatigue safety factor shows how safe a stent is from fatigue failure based on the Goodman life analysis.

3.2. Finite Element Analysis

3.2.1. Finite Element Model

A stent placed in the vascular system experiences multiple loading conditions that may ultimately jeopardize its mechanical integrity during its operational lifespan. This work created finite element models to assess the mechanical integrity and fatigue resistance of a stent under various loading circumstances associated with its fabrication and deployment in accordance with existing practices. The complete stress–strain history of the stent during each loading phase was analyzed to account for the influence of accumulated residual stress–strains throughout the procedures. It encompasses manufacture (attached to a balloon catheter), in vivo deployment (expanded within an artery), and the associated recoil and pulsatile loading under systolic and diastolic pressures. The FEA simulation ascertains the distribution of stress and strain, the fatigue safety factor, and the radial strength through the subsequent steps:

Step 1. Crimping a stent from 2.54 mm to 2 mm OD (crimp).

Step 2. Removing outer constraint to allow stent recoil after crimping (crimp-recoil).

Step 3. Expanding a stent to 6.0 mm ID (expansion).

Step 4. Removing inner constraint to allow stent recoil after expansion (expansion-recoil).

Step 5. Applying 180/80 mmHg systolic/diastolic pressures for stent fatigue assessment (or applying external pressure for radial strength assessment).

It should be noted that step 5 can be used to calculate either the fatigue safety factor or radial strength of a stent.

3.2.2. Stent Geometry and Meshing

The ABAQUS/standard finite element solver (Dassault Systemes Simulia Corp., Providence, RI, USA) was employed to conduct the stent finite element analysis. To conserve computational time, three typical rings were modeled instead of the full stent, due to the stent's repetitive patterns in both axial and circumferential directions (Figure 3). To replicate the manufacturing (crimping onto a balloon catheter) and in-vivo deployment (expansion within an artery) processes, two hard cylinders with diameters of 2.54 mm and 1.12 mm were integrated into the stent model, with one cylinder positioned inside the stent and the other outside. Gervaso et al. and De Beule et al. established that employing the displacement-control expansion of a rigid cylinder to simulate balloon expansion can yield reliable and precise data concerning stent morphology, stress-strain characteristics, and other relevant parameters upon achieving the stent's nominal diameter [19, 20]. Consequently, the displacement-control simplification was employed in this investigation, as it is less computationally intensive than simulations utilizing balloon-driven expansion. Our objective is to evaluate the influence of drug reservoirs on the "standard" stent in a comparative manner, so the displacement-control expansion effectively fulfills this aim.The stent model was meshed with the eight-node linear brick element in incompatible mode (C3D8I) with the element size of one-sixth of the strut width and one-third of strut thickness. This specific mesh size was chosen after a mesh sensitivity study to ensure that stress–strain variation on the stent was adequately captured. The inside and outside rigid cylinders were meshed with the four-node quadrilateral surface element (SFM3D4).

3.2.3. Material properties and boundary conditions

The material properties of L-605 cobalt–chromium alloy along with the ABAQUS von Mises plasticity model with isotropic hardening for large deformation analysis were used. Its Young's modulus, Poisson ratio, yield stress, ultimate stress, ultimate strain, and fatigue endurance limit are 203 GPa, 0.3, 590 MPa, 1689 MPa, 60%, and 483 MPa, respectively.

A frictionless contact was used to prevent penetration between two surfaces of the model during crimping and expansion, with the following contact pairs implemented:

1. The first contact pair was defined as the surface contact between the inner surface of the outer rigid cylinder and the outer surface of the stent.
2. The second contact pair was defined as the surface contact between the outer surface of the inner rigid cylinder and the inner surface of the stent.
3. The third contact pair was defined as the side contact between any two stent struts during crimping.

3.2.4. Stent stress–strain analysis

In step 1, stress–strain analysis was conducted to simulate the crimping of a stent onto a balloon catheter. The outer rigid cylinder was compressed in the radial direction with the displacement control, forcing the stent to collapse inward. In step 2, stent recoil after crimping due to elastic strain energy was modeled by removing the outer rigid cylinder to allow for the stent recovery. In step 3, to simulate the in-vivo deployment, the inner rigid cylinder was expanded in the radial direction with the displacement control to simulate the stent deployment to the target size. In the final step, stent recoil after expansion due to elastic strain energy was modeled by removing the inner rigid cylinder to allow for the stent recovery. Figure 4 demonstrates the configuration of the stent and rigid cylinders at each step of the modeling scheme.

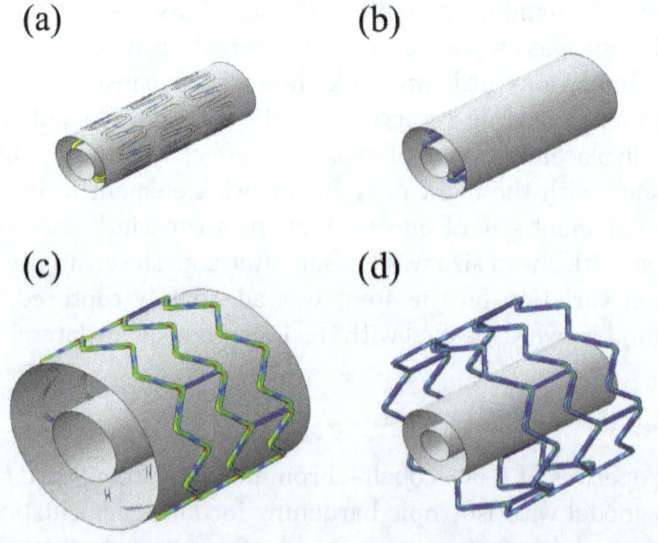

Figure 4. Configuration of the stent/cylindrical surfaces at each stage of the loading scheme: (a) crimp, (b) crimp-recoil, (c) expansion, and (d) expansion-recoil.

3.2.5. Stent Goodman life analysis

Following the previous four steps, systolic/diastolic arterial blood pressures of 180/80 mmHg were applied to simulate the pulsatile fatigue loading. In order to account for the external loading exerted by the arterial wall, an arterial pressure loading corresponding to the interaction between the stent and the artery was also imposed on the stent. The Goodman life analysis was performed using the multi-axial stress state experienced during the pulsatile fatigue loading to determine the fatigue resistance of a stent after implant [14]. It states that fatigue failure will occur if the stress state satisfies the following relationship:

$$\left(\frac{\sigma_a}{\sigma_e}\right)+\left(\frac{\sigma_m}{\sigma_u}\right)\geq 1 \tag{1}$$

where σ_a is the stress amplitude applied to the stent, σ_e is the modified material endurance limit for nonzero mean stress, σ_m is the mean stress applied to the stent, and σ_u is the material ultimate strength.

The Goodman diagram is a plot of the normalized stress amplitude σ_a/σ_e (on the y-axis) versus the normalized mean stress σ_m/σ_u (on the x-axis). The equation $(\sigma_a/\sigma_e)+(\sigma_m/\sigma_u)=1$ represents the failure line on the Goodman diagram for nonzero mean stress with the modified endurance limit defined as:

$$\sigma_e=\sigma_{e0}\left(1-\frac{\sigma_m}{\sigma_u}\right) \tag{2}$$

where σ_{e0} is the material endurance limit for zero mean stress. The fatigue safety factor (FSF) is defined as the ratio of the modified endurance limit divided by the stress amplitude. An FSF smaller than 1.0 indicates the fatigue failure:

$$FSF = \frac{\sigma_e}{\sigma_a} \tag{3}$$

4. DEPOT STENT MANUFACTURING

4.1. Laser Cutting by Integrated Laser Module

When making a stent, a design drawing is first sketched on the 2D plane, wrapped around a target cylinder, and coded into the 3D cylindrical coordinate using the CAD/CAM software. The coded stent geometry is then input into the laser cutting machine and the design pattern is cut onto a seamless hypotube of 1–2 mm. During the laser cutting process, the hypotube was rotated and translated in the axial direction by the motor stage while the laser source remained stationary.

In this study, a laser module consisting of a 100W Yb-doped pulsed fiber laser (Rofin-Baasel Taiwan Ltd.), a linear X-Y motor stage (Aerotech, Inc.), and a Z-direction server motor was assembled and integrated (Figure 5). The precision motor stage provides linear motion and rotation of the hypotube, whereas the Z-direction server motor controls the distance between the laser source and hypotube surface for the optimal focal position (Figure 6). The X-Y motor stage accuracy is ±2 μm and ±25 arc-second in the axial and circumstantial direction, respectively; on the other hand, the linear encoder resolution for the Z-direction server motor is up to 0.5 μm. Position synchronized output (PSO), a control algorithm that greatly enhances the efficiency and quality of the laser cutting, was used to coordinate the linear X-Y motor stage with the timing of laser firing. It can minimize the heat-affected zone (HAZ) during the laser cutting process. A3200 controller (Aerotech, Inc.) allows us to perform up to 32 axes of synchronized motion control and therefore could accomplish very sophisticated laser cutting patterns effortlessly.

The principles of laser cutting and drilling are based on fusion cutting, which involves a melting mechanism where the heated materials transformed into a molten state are expelled from the cut kerf by a high pressure assisted gas such as nitrogen or argon. Laser cutting quality is typically controlled by several input laser parameters such as focal position, average laser power, pulse repetition rate, assisted gas pressure, etc. An appropriate position of the laser focal spot significantly improves the cutting outcome. The focal position of our laser module was assessed by measuring the kerf width on the hypotube while adjusting the distance between the laser source and hypotube surface. The smallest kerf width can be achieved by precisely focusing the laser sweet spot on the hypotube surface. A proper selection of laser power is crucial to the outcome as well, as excessive laser power results in a wider kerf and a thicker recast layer. On the other hand, insufficient laser power produces dross due to incomplete melting [21, 22]. Pulse repetition rate is another important laser parameter related to surface roughness and material removal. A higher pulse repetition rate corresponds to a better cutting surface and more effective material removal. Inert gas is a favorable assisted gas since it can avoid oxidation of the materials. High pressure inert gas was used during the cutting process to enhance drag forces and achieve high cutting quality [23].

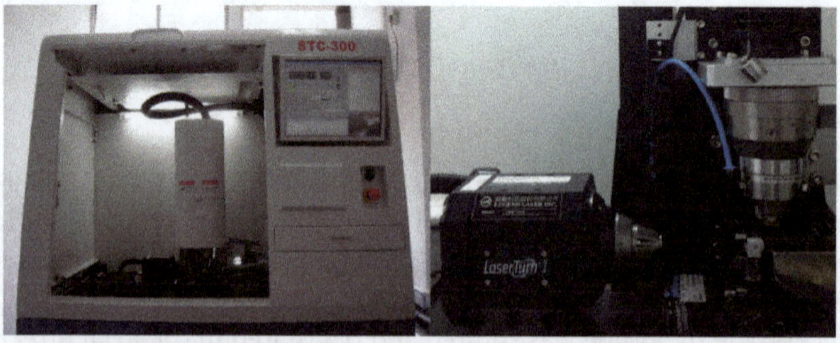

Figure 5. Integrated laser module with a magnified view of the linear X-Y motor stage and laser source in the right window.

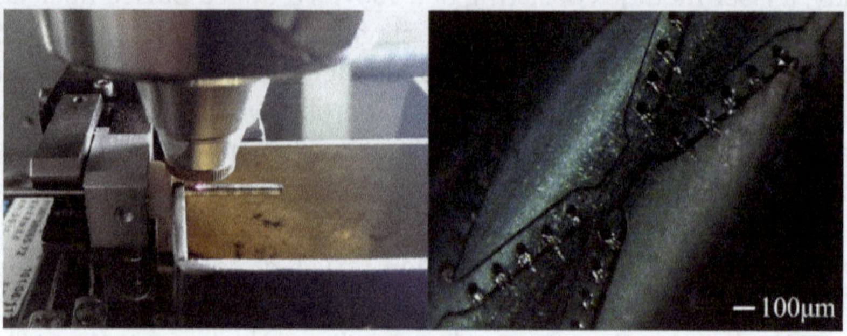

Figure 6. Stent design pattern cut onto a seamless hypotube by laser.

4.2. Surface Finishing by Electro-Polishing

The laser cutting process inevitably generates dross, heat-affected zone, and other defects at stent surface. To achieve high quality of mirror-like surface, electro-polishing was performed on laser-cut depot stent prototypes. A 100 ml glass beaker was used as a bath. The experiment setup used for electro-polishing is illustrated in Figure 7. The stent was used as an anode, whereas the cathode was made of a thin lead sheet. The electrolyte consisted of 60 wt% phosphoric acid (H_3PO_4), 20 wt% sulfuric acid (H_2SO_4), and 20 wt% distilled water. Electro-polishing process was performed with continuous stirring of electrolyte to prevent oxygen bubbles from adhering to stent surface. Furthermore, several important polishing parameters including bath temperature, current, and time were determined through experiments to find the optimal conditions for electro-polishing of depot stents. The stents were then cleaned ultrasonically using distilled water for 5 minutes and were dried by air blowing as the final step.

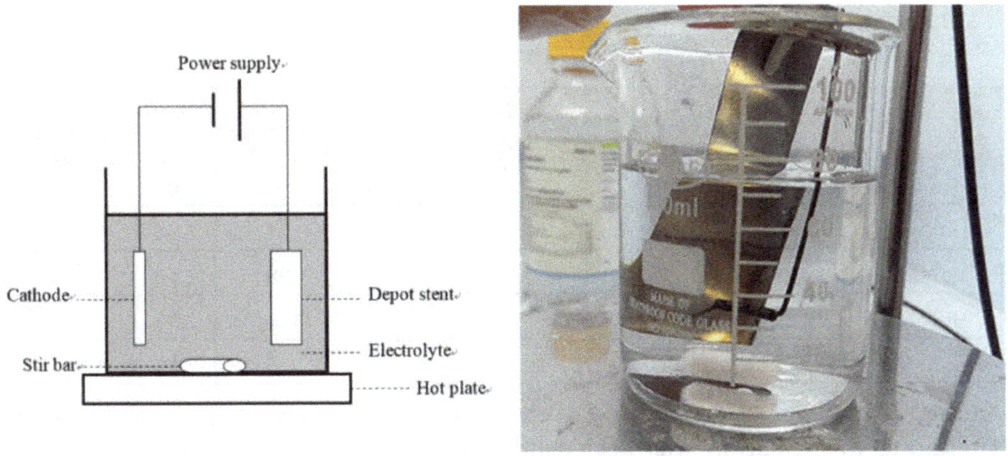

Figure 7. Experimental setup for electro-polishing of depot stent prototypes.

5. RESULTS AND DISCUSSION

5.1. Effects of Reservoir Location on Stent Mechanical Integrity

The "standard" stent was first evaluated to establish the baseline information for this study. The FEA simulation was then conducted to investigate the impact of reservoir location on the mechanical integrity of the depot stent (e.g., equivalent plastic strain, radial strength, and fatigue safety factor). Five equally spaced circular (cylindrical if considering depth) and blind-hole reservoirs were cut on three major locations of the depot stent, namely, connectors, bar arms, and crowns (Figure 3).

From Table 1, it is clear that the creation of blind-hole reservoirs on either bar arms or connectors resulted in little or no change in equivalent plastic strain and radial strength. However, the degradation in the fatigue safety factor was the most significant among major clinical attributes investigated, with a 16–18% reduction compared to the "standard" stent. This indicates that the depot stent with reservoirs on the bar arms or connectors is resistant to vessel collapse or acute stent fracture but susceptible to long-term stent fatigue failure. In other words, the depot stent is more sensitive to dynamic loading than static loading.

However, the depot stent with blind-hole reservoirs on the crowns led to noticeable changes in equivalent plastic strain (+12%) and radial strength (-8%). Its fatigue safety factor declined further from the standard case of 3.05 to 2.33, a significant 24% reduction. By comparing these three reservoir locations, it is clear that cutting reservoirs on the stent crowns has the most significant impact among the three major locations investigated. This is not surprising considering the standard case that the maximum von Mises stress and maximum equivalent plastic strain always occur on the inner surface of the curved crowns, whereas the connectors and the bar arms are mostly under elastic deformation.

Table 1. Effects of reservoir location on stent mechanical integrity (blind-hole reservoirs).

Model	RS (N/mm)	Variation (%)	PEEQ (%Strain)	Variation (%)	FSF	Variation (%)
Standard	3.78	-	40.5	-	3.05	-
Hole- CO	3.77	-0.26	40.2	-0.74	2.56	-16.07
Hole- BA	3.66	-3.17	39.7	-1.98	2.49	-18.36
Hole- CR	3.49	-7.67	45.2	11.6	2.33	-23.61
Hole- All	3.45	-8.73	45.1	11.36	2.17	-28.85

Adding the number of reservoirs increases the total drug capacity of the depot stent. Therefore, investigation was also conducted for reservoirs evenly spread on the entire stent to understand whether the mechanical integrity of such a stent is further compromised or not (Figure 3(d)). Simulation results show that this specific depot stent followed a similar trend to the previous case (blind-hole reservoirs on the crowns only). Their equivalent plastic strain and radial strength were almost identical, whereas the fatigue safety factor continued to decline further, with a 29% reduction compared to the "standard" stent. This again demonstrates that the mechanical integrity of the depot stent is mainly dominated by the reservoirs located on the stent crowns.

5.2. Effects of Reservoirs Depth on Stent Mechanical Integrity

Another method of increasing the total drug capacity is to cut through-holes instead of blind-holes into the stent struts. The through-hole reservoir design also allows different types of drugs with different release rates to be administered independently on opposite sides of the stent. Since this dual-side drug delivery concept is quite interesting, simulation was then carried out to investigate the effects of reservoir depth on the mechanical integrity of the depot stent. The depth of the reservoirs was increased from 50% to 75% and 100% of the strut thickness, with the last case equivalent to the through-hole scenario.

Table 2 summarizes the effects of reservoir depth on the key stent attributes for the case of depot reservoirs evenly spread on the entire stent. Figures 8 and 9 show the contour plot comparisons of the equivalent plastic strain developed during different stages of the loading process (crimping and expansion, respectively) between the standard case and the depot stent with through-hole reservoirs on the entire stent. It shows again that the maximum equivalent plastic strain occurred on the inner surface of the most critical region of the stent, the curved crowns. The maximum equivalent plastic strain was increased by 16%, and its strain distribution, as indicated by the colors, changed significantly due to the appearance of the through-hole reservoirs on the stent crowns. It was more evenly spread along the crown arc for the standard case but became non-uniform when the maximum stress–strain occurred at the 6 o'clock location of each reservoir.

Table 2. Effects of reservoir location on stent mechanical integrity (blind-hole reservoirs).

Model	RS (N/mm)	Variation (%)	PEEQ (%Strain)	Variation (%)	FSF	Variation (%)
Standard	3.78	-	40.5	-	3.05	-
Hole- All (50%)	3.45	-8.73	45.1	11.36	2.17	-28.85
Hole- All (75%)	3.33	-11.9	46.8	15.56	2.06	-32.46
Hole- All (100%)	3.08	-18.52	46.8	15.56	2.02	-33.77

Figure 10 shows the radial strength comparison between the "standard" stent and the depot stent with through-hole reservoirs on the entire stent. The radial strength dropped by 19% in this case, and its peak value shifted toward the right by 0.1 mm when compared to the "standard" stent. This suggests that the through-hole depot stent is not as strong as its standard counterpart and could be collapsed by the arterial pressure at an earlier stage. Figure 11 shows the Goodman diagram comparison of the pulsatile fatigue loading between the "standard" stent and the depot stent with through-hole reservoirs on the entire stent. Simulation data of the "standard" stent were far below the Goodman diagram failure line, indicating that the "standard" stent is able to pass the fatigue life of 4 x 10^8 cycles with ease under pulsatile fatigue loading. Comparing Figure 11 (top) with Figure 11 (bottom), wherein the same stent but with through-hole reservoirs was evaluated for pulsatile fatigue loading, shows that the simulation data of the depot stent migrated toward the Goodman diagram failure line, indicating a significant drop of 34% in FSF and thus much lower fatigue resistance to systolic/diastolic blood pressures in this specific case.

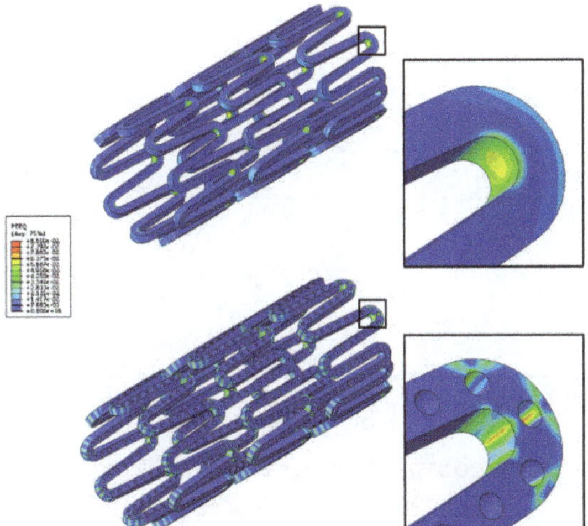

Figure 8. Contour plot of the PEEQ of the standard stent (top) and the depot stent with through-hole reservoirs (bottom) at crimping with a magnified view of the stent crown in the right window.

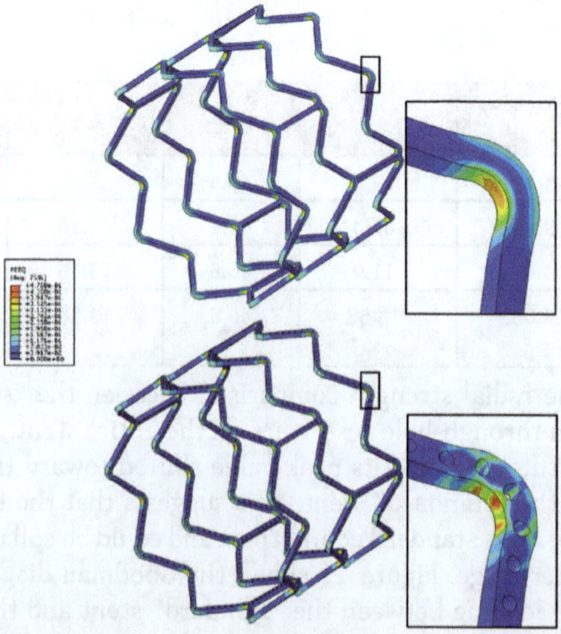

Figure 9. Contour plot of the PEEQ of the standard stent (top) and the depot stent with through-hole reservoirs (bottom) at expansion with a magnified view of the stent crown in the right window.

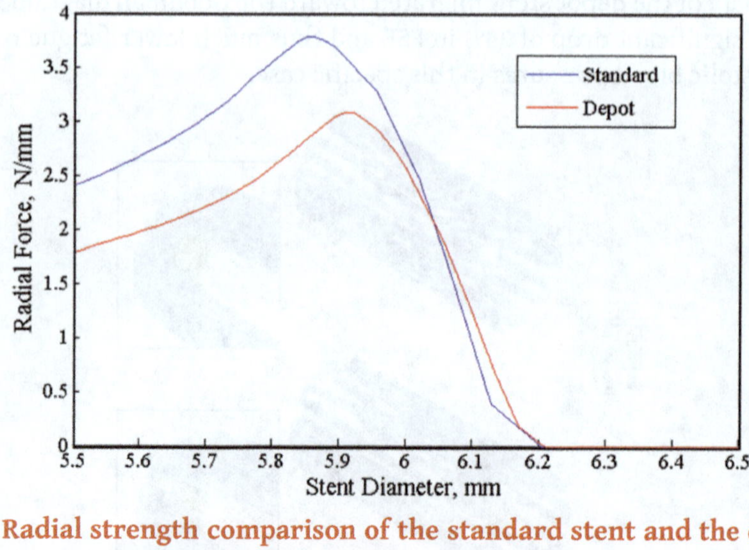

Figure 10. Radial strength comparison of the standard stent and the depot stent with through-hole reservoirs.

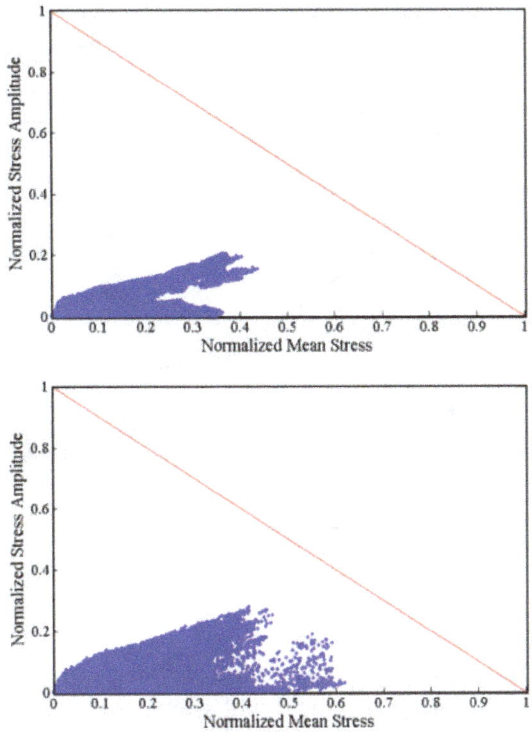

Figure 11. Goodman diagram comparison of the standard stent (top) and the depot stent with through-hole reservoirs (bottom).

Figure 12 shows the effects of reservoir depth on the key stent attributes of the depot stent with the reservoir depth ranging from 50%, 75% to 100% of the strut thickness on the entire stent. It is shown that the radial strength decayed almost linearly with the reservoir depth. The loss in radial strength reached the maximum, a 19% reduction compared to the standard case, when the reservoirs were completely cut through. The equivalent plastic strain rose moderately with the reservoir depth but eventually reached a plateau for an approximately 15–20% gain. The fatigue safety factor remained the most critical factor among these key stent attributes. According to the chart, it fell significantly right from the beginning, even with shallow blind holes, but eventually reached a plateau and settled with an approximately 30–35% loss when compared to the standard case. Since the major stent clinical attributes suffered significant losses, it is not a good idea to pursue this specific design with through-hole reservoirs spread all over the entire stent. Given the fact that the crown is a critical region in a stent, we propose that an optimal depot stent should have through-hole reservoirs on the stent bar arms and/or connectors for the maximum drug capacity without compromising its mechanical integrity significantly. It should be noted that although the depot stent has the wonderful feature of precise and programmable drug release control, it was found that its fatigue safety factor could be compromised to certain degrees for all various forms of the depot stent.

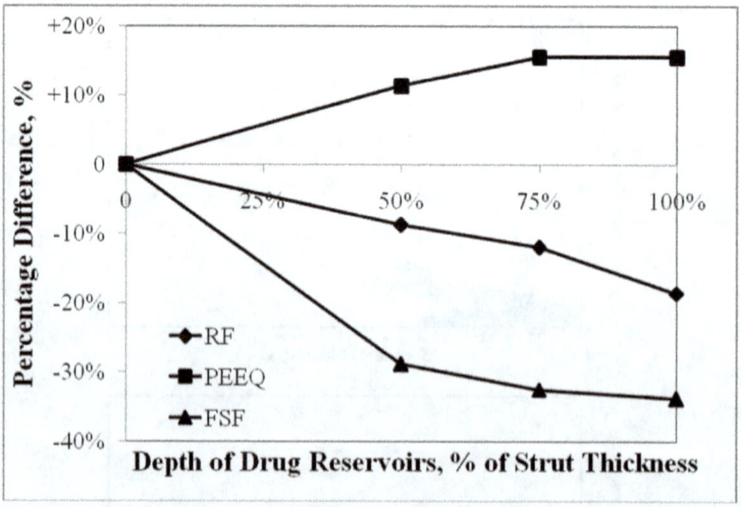

Figure 12. Variation of key clinically relevant functional attributes versus drug reservoir depth.

5.3. Depot Stent Drug Capacity

A typical DES (3-ring model) with a 5 μm coating thickness carries a total drug-polymer volume of 0.0535 mm^3 (Table 3). For the depot stent, our chosen reservoir size is 50% of the strut width and 100% completely through the strut thickness. Such a design is able to carry approximately 0.0004 mm^3 of drug-polymer mix per reservoir. Therefore, by creating 135 through-hole reservoirs on the 3-ring depot stent model, its total reservoir capacity is enough to fully replace the surface coating layers of 0.0535 mm^3 on a typical drug-eluting stent. This helps to completely eliminate the surface coating layers and thus reduce the overall stent profile.

The density and size of the reservoirs could be changed to increase the total drug capacity of the depot stent. For example, the total volume of the drug-polymer mix can be quadrupled to 0.221 mm^3 when the through-hole reservoirs are evenly distributed on the entire stent, as shown in Figure 3(d). Our proposed depot stent in the next section, same stent as the one in Figure 3(d) without reservoirs on the crowns, also triples the total volume to 0.149 mm^3.

Table 3. Estimated drug capacity of a depot stent (3-ring model).

Model	Number of reservoirs	Drug-polymer compound carried (mm^3)
5-μm thickness coating on stent surface	-	0.0535
Through-hole reservoir (per reservoir)	-	0.0004
Through-hole reservoirs on CO	30	0.012

Model	Number of reservoirs	Drug-polymer compound carried (mm^3)
Through-hole reservoirs on BA	270	0.108
Through-hole reservoirs on CR	270	0.108
Through-hole reservoirs on entire stent	552	0.221
Proposed depot stent	372	0.149

5.4. Proposed Depot Stent and Its Variants

5.4.1. Proposed Depot Stent

An optimal depot stent is proposed, featuring reservoirs uniformly distributed across the entire stent, excluding the crown region, to enhance total drug capacity while minimally affecting mechanical integrity (Figure 13). The depot stent comprises eight reservoirs on the connectors and six reservoirs on the bar arms, with an inter-reservoir spacing of approximately 0.15 mm. Simulation results regarding the variations of key clinical attributes are presented in Table 4, alongside comparative data on other stents. Figure 14 presents a comparison of contour plots illustrating the equivalent plastic strain generated during the expansion stage for the standard case, the depot stent featuring through-hole reservoirs throughout the entire stent, and the proposed depot stent. The proposed depot stent demonstrated a 9% reduction in maximum equivalent plastic strain, with a more uniform strain distribution compared to the standard case. This was due to the development of through-hole reservoirs on the bar arms, which effectively redirected the stress-strains from the crown reservoirs and redistributed them along the crown arcs. The radial strength decreased by 10%. The fatigue safety factor decreased by 13% relative to the standard case, while the identical stent featuring through-hole reservoirs throughout exhibited a significant reduction of 34%. The notable increase in fatigue safety factor resulted partly from the elimination of through-hole reservoirs on the crowns and partly from the aforementioned stress–strain redistribution.

In conclusion, the total drug capacity of the proposed depot stent may be increased threefold, with minimal compromise in key clinical attributes: radial strength and fatigue safety factor were diminished by only 10% and 13%, respectively. This depot stent has the potential to carry a greater quantity of drugs and facilitate more precise delivery compared to contemporary drug-eluting stents, thus creating numerous new treatment possibilities for conditions such as renal disease and targeted cancer therapy.

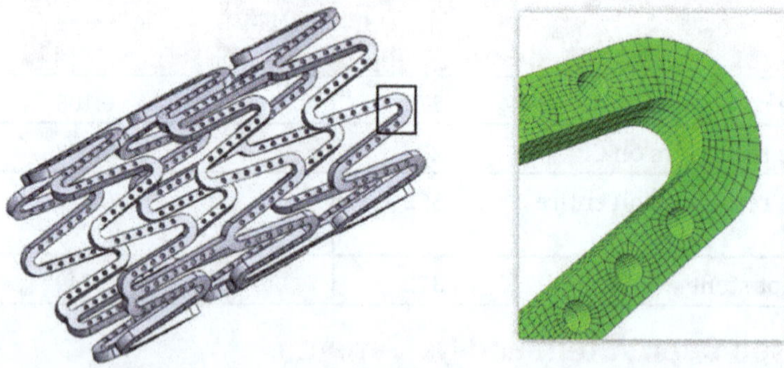

Figure 13. Proposed depot stent with a magnified view of the stent mesh in the right window.

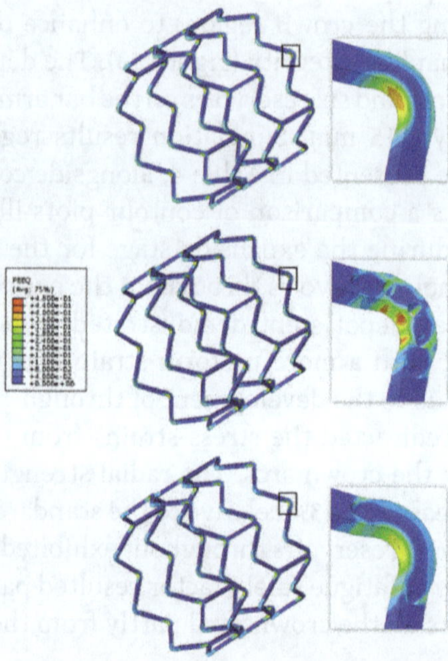

Figure 14. Contour plot of the equivalent plastic strain of the standard stent (top), the depot stent with reservoirs on the entire stent (middle), and the proposed depot stent (bottom) at expansion with a magnified view of the stent crown in the right window.

5.4.2. Effects of Reservoir Shape

Besides the circular (cylindrical if considering depth) reservoirs aforementioned, other reservoir shapes were also investigated, for example, hexagonal and square reservoirs (Figure 15). The length on each side of the hexagonal and square reservoirs (0.0349 mm and 0.0563 mm, respectively) was determined in a way that each reservoir capacity was identical to that of a circular reservoir. The location of the reservoir center remained unchanged.

Table 4 lists the mechanical integrity of the depot stent as a function of the reservoir shape. Simulation results show that the changes in the reservoir shape caused little differences in equivalent plastic strain and radial strength, with approximately 10% across-the-board reductions when compared to the "standard" stent. In terms of the fatigue safety factor, the hexagonal reservoir had a slight 5% advantage over the circular and square reservoirs. This could be attributed to the stress re-distribution within the stent and the hexagonal reservoir makes a bigger impact than reservoirs with other shapes.

(a)

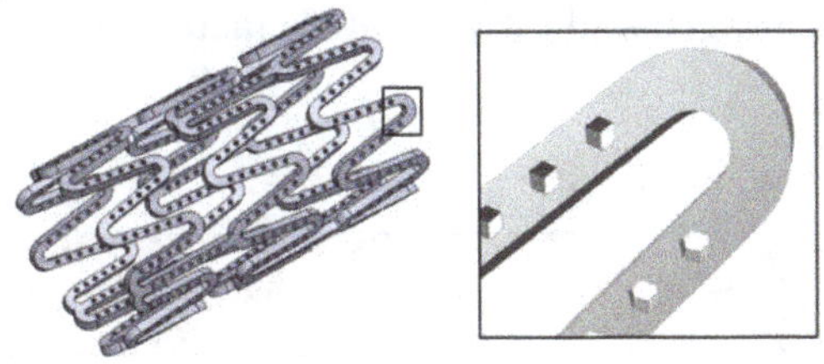

(b)

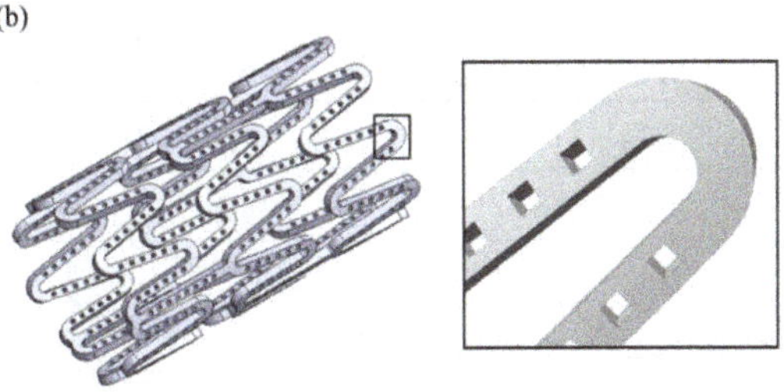

Figure 15. Depot stent with (a) hexagonal and (b) square reservoirs.

Table 4. Effects of reservoir shape on stent mechanical integrity.

Model	RS (N/mm)	Variation (%)	PEEQ (%Strain)	Variation (%)	FSF	Variation (%)
Standard	3.78	-	40.5	-	3.05	-
Proposed depot stent	3.41	-9.79	36.7	-9.38	2.66	-12.79
Hexagonal reservoir	3.43	-9.26	36.4	-10.12	2.80	-8.20
Square reservoir	3.38	-10.58	36.1	-10.86	2.65	-13.11

5.4.3. Effects of reservoir size and number

Effects of the reservoir size and number of the depot stent were also investigated (Figure 16). The total drug loading capacity on each bar arm/connector was intended to maintain the same, whereas the size and number of the reservoirs were adjusted accordingly. Stent variation #1 had smaller but more reservoirs, with 8 reservoirs on the bar arms and 10 reservoirs on the connectors; on the other hand, stent variation #2 had larger but fewer reservoirs, with four reservoirs on the bar arms and six reservoirs on the connectors. In all cases, the total length between the farther edges of two end reservoirs remained unchanged.

Table 5 lists the mechanical integrity of the depot stent as a function of the reservoir size and number. Simulation results show that, for the same drug loading capacity, stent variation #2 with larger and fewer reservoirs yielded lower radial strength, but smaller equivalent plastic strain and thus higher fatigue safety factor. In addition, the fatigue safety factor seems to be more sensitive than the equivalent plastic strain and radial strength in this case. Its value increased from 2.36 to 2.88, a 17% jump from stent variation #1 to #2, which is consistent with the earlier observation. Therefore, stent variation #2 of larger and fewer reservoirs is a better candidate for drug delivery; its total drug capacity could be tripled with marginal trade-off in its major clinical attributes: the radial strength and fatigue safety factor were reduced by only 11% and 6%, respectively.

Table 5. Effects of reservoir size and number on stent mechanical integrity.

Model	RS (N/mm)	Variation (%)	PEEQ (%Strain)	Variation (%)	FSF	Variation (%)
Standard	3.78	-	40.5	-	3.05	-
Proposed depot stent	3.41	-9.79	36.7	-9.38	2.66	-12.79
Variation #1	3.48	-7.94	37.6	-7.16	2.36	-22.62
Variation #2	3.38	-10.58	34.8	-14.70	2.88	-5.57

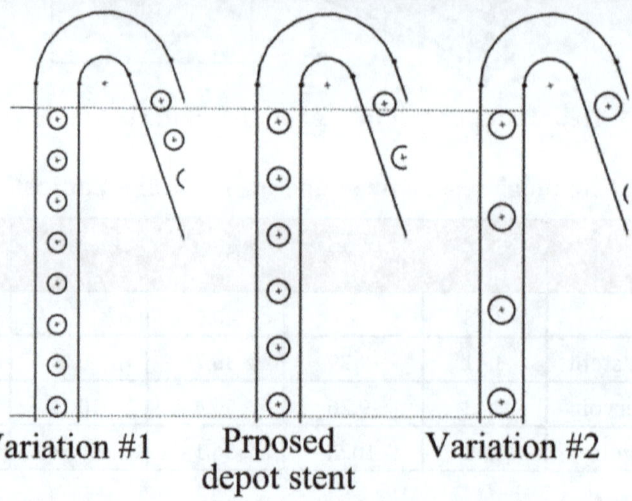

Figure 16. Proposed depot stent and its variation #1 and #2.

5.5. Depot Stent Prototyping

In this study, the input laser parameters used for cutting stents are listed as follows: average power 37.5 W, pulse repetition rate 80 KHz, cutting speed 5 mm/s, and Argon pressure 12 bar. Optical microscopy was used to measure the kerf width and observe the surface conditions of each stent.

Figure 17 shows the relationship of the average kerf width vs. the distance between the laser source and hypotube surface. The kerf width had the minimum value of 23.2 μm at the distance of 0.37 mm. When the distance was between 0.27 mm and 0.51 mm, the laser beam was able to penetrate through the hypotube, resulting in successful cutting within a focal-depth range of 0.24 mm. Figure 6 is the depot stent design pattern cut onto a seamless hypotube by laser prior to material removal and electro-polishing.

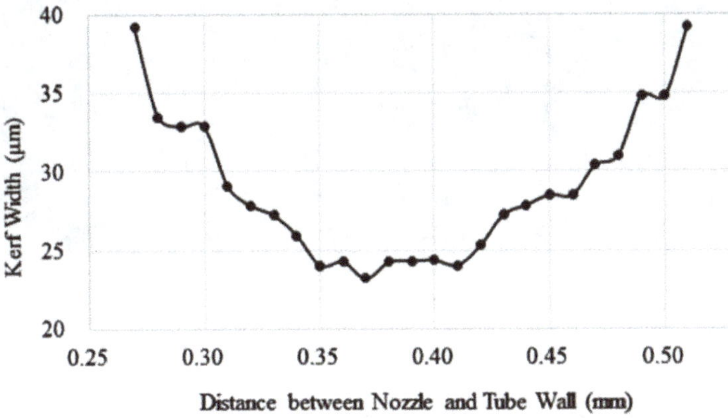

Figure 17. Average kerf width vs. distance between laser source and hypotube surface.

The polishing parameters for the surface finishing of depot stent prototypes are detailed in Table 6. Figure 18 illustrates the depot stent prototype prior to and subsequent to electro-polishing. These stents attained a superior mirror-like surface finish post-polishing. Figure 19 illustrates the prototype of our suggested depot stent, measuring 2 mm in diameter and 22 mm in length, to demonstrate our design concept.

Table 6. Electro-polishing conditions for surface finishing of depot stents.

Stirring speed (RPM)	Current (A)	Time (sec)	Temperature (Co)
500–550	0.242	105–135	50–55

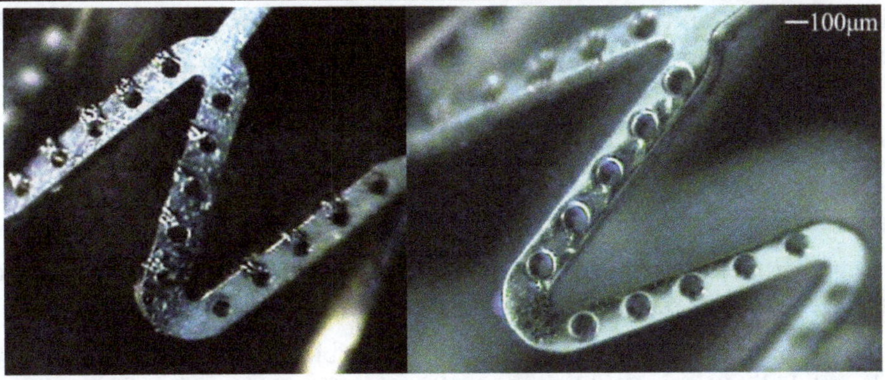

Figure 18. Surface conditions of manufactured depot stents before (left) and after (right) electro-polishing.

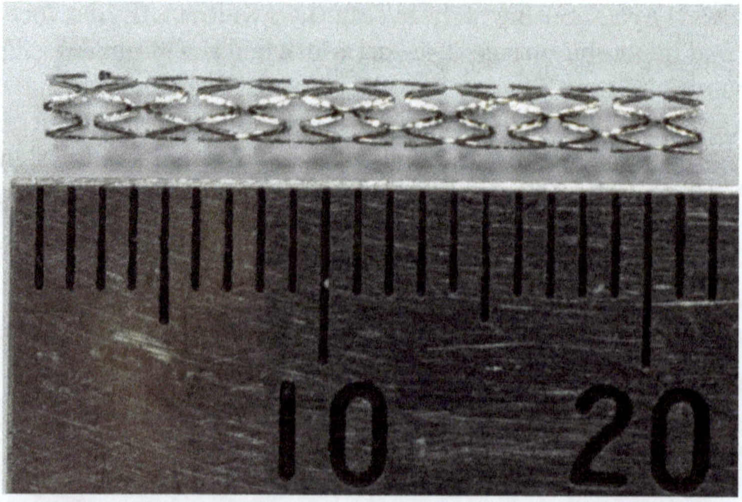

Figure 19. Prototype of our proposed depot stent.

6. CONCISE SUMMARY

The depot stent including micro-sized drug reservoirs represents an innovative approach to intelligent drug delivery, offering significant potential for the precise release of various drugs with programmable spatial and temporal control. Nonetheless, the formation of drug reservoirs on the stent struts inherently diminishes the stent's scaffolding strength and undermines its mechanical integrity. The influence of these drug reservoirs on key clinical characteristics of the depot stent was methodically examined. This investigation yielded several conclusions:

The reservoirs on either bar arms or connectors had little effects in equivalent plastic strain and radial strength when compared to the "standard" drug-eluting stent. However, the fatigue safety factor was reduced more significantly, suggesting that the depot stent is resistant to acute stent fracture or vessel collapse but susceptible to long-term stent fatigue failure.

Creating reservoirs on the crown region of the depot stent has the most significant impact among all major locations.

The degradation in mechanical integrity is more sensitive to reservoir location than reservoir depth.

The hexagonal reservoirs resulted in a marginal increase in fatigue resistance when compared to the circular and square reservoirs.

For the same drug loading capacity, larger and fewer reservoirs resulted in a noticeable increase in the fatigue resistance over smaller and more reservoirs.

Our proposed depot stent was proven to be a feasible design. Its total drug capacity could be tripled with acceptable/marginal trade-off in major clinical attributes: the radial strength and the fatigue safety factor of our proposed depot stent were reduced by only 10% and 13%, respectively.

A prototype of our proposed depot stent (2 mm diameter and 22 mm long) was manufactured for the feasibility demonstration of our design concept.

This study may provide a framework for future depot stent designs to optimize the balance between stent mechanical integrity and intelligent drug administration.

REFERENCES

1. M. R. Bell, P. B. Berger, J. F. Bresnahan, G. S. Reeder, K. R. Bailey, and D. Holmes, "Initial and long-term outcome of 354 patients after coronary balloon angioplasty of total coronary artery occlusions," Circulation, vol. 85, pp. 1003-1011, 1992.
2. C. Landau, R. A. Lange, and L. D. Hillis, "Percutaneous transluminal coronary angioplasty," New England Journal of Medicine, vol. 330, pp. 981-993, 1994.
3. B. L. Van der Hoeven, N. M. Pires, H. M. Warda, P. V. Oemrawsingh, B. J. van Vlijmen, P. H. Quax, et al., "Drug-eluting stents: results, promises and problems," International Journal of Cardiology, vol. 99, pp. 9-17, 2005.
4. M.-C. Morice, P. W. Serruys, J. E. Sousa, J. Fajadet, E. Ban Hayashi, M. Perin, et al., "A randomized comparison of a sirolimus-eluting stent with a standard stent for coronary revascularization," New England Journal of Medicine, vol. 346, pp. 1773-1780, 2002.
5. J. W. Moses, M. B. Leon, J. J. Popma, P. J. Fitzgerald, D. R. Holmes, C. O'Shaughnessy, et al., "Sirolimus-eluting stents versus standard stents in patients with stenosis in a native coronary artery," New England Journal of Medicine, vol. 349, pp. 1315-1323, 2003.
6. A. Colombo and E. Karvouni, "Biodegradable stents "fulfilling the mission and stepping away"," Circulation, vol. 102, pp. 371-373, 2000.
7. H. R. Kricheldorf, I. KreiserSaunders, C. Jürgens, and D. Wolter, "Polylactidessynthesis, characterization and medical application," Macromolecular Symposia, pp. 85-102, 1996.
8. J. A. Ormiston and P. W. Serruys, "Bioabsorbable coronary stents," Circulation: Cardiovascular Interventions, vol. 2, pp. 255-260, 2009.
9. T. Tsuji, H. Tamai, K. Igaki, E. Kyo, K. Kosuga, T. Hata, et al., "Biodegradable stents as a platform to drug loading," International Journal of Cardiovascular Interventions, vol. 5, pp. 13-16, 2003.
10. R. Waksman, "Biodegradable stents: they do their job and disappear," The Journal of Invasive Cardiology, vol. 18, pp. 70-74, 2006.
11. R. Blindt, K. Hoffmeister, H. Bienert, G. Bartsch, H. Thissen, D. Klee, et al., "Development of a new biodegradable intravascular polymer stent with simultaneous incorporation of bioactive substances," The International Journal of Artificial Organs, vol. 22, pp. 843-853, 1999.
12. P. W. Serruys, G. Sianos, A. Abizaid, J. Aoki, P. den Heijer, H. Bonnier, et al., "The effect of variable dose and release kinetics on neointimal hyperplasia using a novel paclitaxel-eluting stent platform: the Paclitaxel In-Stent Controlled Elution Study (PISCES)," Journal of the American College of Cardiology, vol. 46, pp. 253-260, 2005.
13. A. Finkelstein, D. McClean, S. Kar, K. Takizawa, K. Varghese, N. Baek, et al., "Local drug delivery via a coronary stent with programmable release pharmacokinetics," Circulation, vol. 107, pp. 777-784, 2003.
14. H.-M. Hsiao, Y.-H. Chiu, K.-H. Lee, and C.-H. Lin, "Computational modeling of effects of intravascular stent design on key mechanical and hemodynamic behavior," Computer-Aided Design, vol. 44, pp. 757-765, 2012.

15. H.-M. Hsiao, C.-T. Yeh, C. Wang, L.-H. Chao, and D.-R. Li, "Effects of stent design on new clinical issue of longitudinal stent compression in interventional cardiology," Biomedical Microdevices, vol. 16, pp. 599-607, 2014.

16. 16.H.-M. Hsiao, Y.-H. Chiu, T.-Y. Wu, J.-K. Shen, and T.-Y. Lee, "Effects of through-hole drug reservoirs on key clinical attributes for drug-eluting depot stent," Medical Engineering & Physics, vol. 35, pp. 884-897, 2013.

17. H.-M. Hsiao and M.-T. Yin, "An intriguing design concept to enhance the pulsatile fatigue life of self-expanding stents," Biomedical Microdevices, vol. 16, pp. 133-141, 2014.

18. H. M. Hsiao, A. Nikanorov, S. Prabhu, and M. K. Razavi, "Respirationinduced kidney motion on cobaltchromium stent fatigue resistance," Journal of Biomedical Materials Research Part B: Applied Biomaterials, vol. 91, pp. 508-516, 2009.

19. M. De Beule, P. Mortier, S. G. Carlier, B. Verhegghe, R. Van Impe, and P. Verdonck, "Realistic finite element-based stent design: the impact of balloon folding," Journal of Biomechanics, vol. 41, pp. 383-389, 2008.

20. F. Gervaso, C. Capelli, L. Petrini, S. Lattanzio, L. Di Virgilio, and F. Migliavacca, "On the effects of different strategies in modelling balloon-expandable stenting by means of finite element method," Journal of Biomechanics, vol. 41, pp. 1206-1212, 2008.

21. L. Shanjin and W. Yang, "An investigation of pulsed laser cutting of titanium alloy sheet," Optics and Lasers in Engineering, vol. 44, pp. 1067-1077, 2006.

22. C. Wandera, "Laser cutting of austenitic stainless steel with a high quality laser beam," LAPPEENRANTA UNIVERSITY OF TECHNOLOGY, 2006.

23. W. Steen, K. G. Watkins, and J. Mazumder, Laser material processing: Springer Science & Business Media, 2010.

13 Chapter

DIABETIC NEUROPATHY AND THERAPEUTIC APPROACHES: EMERGING CHALLENGES AND APPLICATIONS

1. INTRODUCTION: AN OVERVIEW

Diabetes mellitus (DM) is the predominant condition leading to neuropathy globally. In the past century, despite increased information regarding the clinical manifestations of diabetic neuropathy, comprehensive understanding of its mechanism remains elusive.

Diabetic neuropathy is characterized as a peripheral neuropathy that can manifest at both clinical and subclinical levels, arising in the context of diabetes mellitus without the influence of other peripheral neuropathy causes.

Neuropathy is observed in 10% of diabetes individuals at diagnosis, increasing to 50% after 20 years. Research indicates that neuropathy commences within nine years following the diagnosis of Type 2 diabetes. It may encompass signs related to the somatic and/or autonomic components of the peripheral nervous system.

The association between diabetes mellitus and neuropathy has been recognized for over a century. The categorization was initially proposed by Leyden in 1893, encompassing hyperesthetic (painful), paralytic (motor), and ataxic variants. Neuropathy may impact large sensory, tiny sensory, autonomic, and motor fibers. The results may exhibit symmetry or asymmetry. Distal sensorimotor polyneuropathy is the most prevalent type of neuropathy. The predominant mononeuropathy is carpal tunnel syndrome (CTS). The acknowledgment of certain rare conditions, such as diabetic lumbosacral radiculoplexus neuropathy, which can induce discomfort and paralysis, is crucial for mitigating morbidity.

The yearly occurrence of neuropathy is closely linked to the established duration of diabetes. Height, maximum body mass index, smoking status, systolic and diastolic blood pressures, estradiol levels, and cholesterol levels exhibited no significant differences between those with neuropathy and those without neuropathy.

Considering that diabetes is projected to impact approximately 246 million individuals globally, it can be inferred that 20–30 million individuals are afflicted with symptomatic diabetic neuropathy. This figure is projected to quadruple by 2030 [1].

The impact of neuropathy on mortality is minimal. Disability was observed in 44% of patients with Type 1 diabetes mellitus with confirmed neuropathy, while 74% of individuals with Type 2 diabetes mellitus and sensory neuropathy experienced some activity restriction [2,3]. Hypertension, irrespective of diabetes duration, has been identified as the primary factor contributing to neuropathy, according to a study from the Pittsburgh Epidemiology of Diabetes Complications (EDC) examining the impacts of hypertension, height, and smoking on the occurrence of distal symmetric polyneuropathy in patients with prolonged and poorly managed diabetes [4].

Diabetic cardiac autonomic neuropathy is a significant consequence observed in one-fourth of individuals with Type 1 and Type 2 diabetes. It leads to elevated mortality and asymptomatic myocardial ischemia. Autonomic dysfunction has been identified as a contributing factor to the risk of cardiovascular disease and sudden mortality in individuals with Type 2 diabetes. The activation of cytokines indicates inflammation in patients with diabetes. These alterations have been linked to disturbances of the sympathetic-vagal balance. Patients report orthostatic hypotension, exercise intolerance, diminished stability after surgery, silent myocardial infarction, and ischemia. The application of heart rate variability (HRV) and the Valsalva maneuver has been shown in the diagnosis of cardiac autonomic neuropathy [5]. Hyperleptinemia and diminished adiponectin levels in sleep apnea, prevalent in diabetes and metabolic syndrome, were associated with excessive sympathetic system activation and the initiation of the inflammatory cascade. Ultimately, adverse consequences observed in the autonomic nervous system due to impaired cardiovascular function lead to increased morbidity and mortality in diabetic patients [6].

2. THE CAUSES OF DIABETES NEUROPATHY

Diabetic neuropathy arises from the involvement of various nerves to differing extents in distinct individuals. Histopathological examinations in patients with diabetic neuropathy revealed that the lesions were located in the peripheral nerve axons. Neuropathies also impact Schwann cells, perineural cells, and endoneurial vascular systems. Wallerian degeneration, segmental and paranodal demyelination, and endoneurial connective tissue proliferation transpired with the loss and injury of both thick and thin myelinated nerve fibers. Type 1 diabetes leads to significant axonal shrinkage, extensive fiber degeneration, and alterations in nodal and paranodal structures. The structural alterations in Type 2 diabetes are less severe. Mild axonal atrophy, isolated fiber loss, segmental demyelination, and Wallerian degeneration are noted. Primary axonal alterations are more pronounced in Type 1 diabetes, but primary Schwann cell pathology is more apparent in Type 2 diabetes.

The severity and duration of hyperglycemia are closely linked to the onset of diabetic neuropathy. The onset of neuropathy can be postponed or averted with effective metabolic regulation. In a research, the incidence of clinical diabetic neuropathy was reduced by 69% in the primary preventive group and 57% in the secondary intervention group following 5 years of comprehensive diabetes management in individuals with Type 1 diabetes. Six interrelated elements are believed to play a significant influence in the etiology of diabetes mellitus.

Numerous pathways have been proposed in the etiology of diabetic neuropathy. These are metabolic processes that entail direct nerve injury, endoneurial microvascular impairment, autoimmune inflammation, and diminished neurotrophic support.

Epidemiological studies indicate that the duration and severity of hyperglycemia are significant risk factors for the development of neuropathy in people with Type 1 and Type 2 diabetes mellitus. The prevailing view on the onset of diabetic symmetric polyneuropathy (DSP) is that early nerve damage originates from the short, thin, myelinated A-delta fibers and the unmyelinated C fibers. A skin biopsy is the gold standard for evaluating morphological alterations in short nerve fibers. Nonetheless, the absence of information on nerve function, cost, and superficiality, coupled with its ineffectiveness in all individuals with Type 1 diabetes, constrains this approach. A valid clinical approach for the early identification of short fiber disease by imaging techniques has been recently published [8].

2.1. Metabolic Factors

2.1.1. Increased Glycosylation End Products

The glycosylation of the plasma and tissue proteins plays a major role in diabetic microvascular complications by causing the formation of advanced glycation end products (AGEs). Excess glucose combines with amino acids on circulating and tissue proteins in the presence of chronic hyperglycemia. This non-enzymatic process initially leads to the formation of reversible early glycosylation end products and, later, to irreversible advanced glycosylation end products. Advanced glycosylation products change their function by modifying intracellular proteins and extracellular matrix proteins that interact with extracellular integrins. AGE precursors modify plasma proteins by binding IGU receptors RAGE (receptor of advanced glycation end products) in mesangial endothelial cells, microglia, and macrophages. Thus, they initiate the production of reactive oxygen species (ROS). The activation of NF-κB initiates proinflammatory gene expression. Cytokines and growth factors are expressed by macrophages and mesangial cells [9]. Significantly increased serum concentrations of AGEs have been reported to lead to the development of diabetic complications by their proinflammatory effect in diabetic patients. The other effects of AGEs are increasing in vascular permeability, procoagulant activity, adhesion molecule expression, and monocyte invasion [10].

Sorbitol: Glucose, which enters into the cell, is metabolized to sorbitol by the enzyme aldose reductase. Glucose is converted to sorbitol and fructose by the enzyme aldose reductase due to excessive activation of this pathway owing to hyperglycemia. The accumulation of sorbitol in the cell results in the reduction of myoinositol and taurine, and this leads to decrease in Na–K adenosine triphosphatase (ATPase) activity and reduction of nerve conduction velocity. As a result of the accumulation of sorbitol in the cell, nicotinamide adenine dinucleotide phosphate (NADPH) associates with reduced cell metabolism, increased cell osmolarity, and decreased intracellular myoinositol, and the cell has a tendency to oxidative stress. Hyperglycemia may cause an increase in glucose in some intracellular tissues (such as nerves, lenses, kidneys, and blood vessels) that do not require insulin for glucose transport. Sorbitol and fructose that increase in these tissues cause two undesirable effects. First, accumulated sorbitol and fructose lead to an influx of water and eventually to osmotic cell injury by increasing intracellular osmolarity. Second, sorbitol accumulation results in reduction in the myoinositol content and impairment of Na–K ATPase. This mechanism may be responsible for the damage in Schwann cells and retinal capillary pericytes and causes peripheral neuropathy and microaneurysms. Although the relationship between oxidative stress and diabetic retinopathy, nephropathy, and neuropathy is well known, the therapeutic efficacy of many antioxidants (including aldose reductase inhibitors, vitamins C and E) tested in clinical trials has not yet been established.

Hexosamine: Uridine diphosphate-*N*-acetyl glucosamine (UDPGlcNAc), which regulates transcription factors needed for normal cell functions, is produced in hexosamine pathway. Excess glucose is replaced with glycolytic mediators in hexosamine pathway, and thus, glucose flux to hexosamine pathway results in cell injury and increased oxidative stress. The effects of aldose reductase inhibitors in animal models were found to be more effective than clinical trials. One of the reasons is being lower dose used in clinical trials compared with dose used in animal studies.

Protein kinase C: Excess glucose is converted to diacylglycerol that activates protein kinase C. The activation of protein kinase C increases in contractility, permeability, and vascular cell proliferation and enhances the production of extracellular matrix and cytokines. Thus, vasoconstriction and nerve ischemia occur. These neurovascular changes also contribute to diabetic neuropathy. Diacylglycerol-protein kinase C activation was also shown to be associated with many vascular abnormalities in retinal, renal, and cardiovascular tissues in diabetes and insulin resistance period. High glucose enhances ROS formation by causing NF-κB activation in endothelial cells. This condition may be prevented by PKC (protein kinase C) inhibitors [9].

Poly (ADP-ribose) polymerase: Nuclear enzyme poly (ADP-ribose) polymerase (PARP) becomes activated in response to high glucose. This enzyme helps to repair DNA by separating nicotinamide adenine dinucleotide (NAD+) into the remains of nicotinamide and adenine ribose. Over activation of PARP results in increased free radical formation, harmful changes in gene transcription, protein kinase C activation, and increased AGEs.

2.2. Oxidative Stress

As mentioned above, hyperglycemia causes accumulation of ROS and oxidative stress eventually by interacting with many different ways. The free radical is a chemical species usually having very reactive unpaired electron in the molecular or atomic orbit. Although free radical reactions are necessary for defense mechanisms of immune system cells including neutrophils and macrophage, the overproduction of free radicals results in tissue injury and cell death. Free radicals affect all essential components of cells such as lipids, proteins, DNA, and carbohydrates and lead to the deterioration of their structure. The formation and elimination rates of free radicals are in balance in the organism, which are known as oxidative balance. The organism is not affected by free radicals as long as oxidative stability is provided. Studies in which the relationship between diabetes and diabetes complications and the ROS are shown, it is highlighted that tissue injury due to non-enzymatic glycation, metabolic stress caused by changes in energy metabolism, sorbitol path activity, hypoxia, and ischemia–reperfusion, increases the production of free radical and alters the antioxidant defense system. There are studies, which support that the formation of free radical is a direct result of hyperglycemia, as well as experimental trials that show that the formation of free radical starts when the endothelial and smooth muscle cells were incubated in the medium containing high concentrations of glucose. Hyperglycemia-mediated ROS production occurs via three mechanisms. The first mechanism is the auto-oxidation of glucose and superoxide production. Glucose is converted to reactive keto aldehydes and superoxide anion in the presence of a transition element. The chain of reactions results in the transformation of superoxide radical into extremely reactive hydroxyl radical via hydrogen peroxide. The intracellular glucose oxidation leads to the release of NADH. NADH is used for providing needed energy for ATP production by the oxidative phosphorylation way in the respiratory chain. Superoxide radical is released during this reaction in the respiratory chain. The production of superoxide radicals increases in this way in the presence of high glucose concentration. Mitochondrial respiratory chain is the main intracellular source of ROS production. It is considered that superoxide radical occurs continuously during normal respiration chain of events. Recent studies showed that much pathology in diabetes was associated with increased mitochondrial ROS production. The second mechanism in the hyperglycemia-mediated ROS production is the glycation of proteins and the formation of AGE products. When the proteins exposed to high glucose concentrations, glucose leads to uncontrolled glycation reactions by binding to protein without requiring the mediation of an enzyme. The glycated protein causes the formation of ROS by donating an electron to molecular oxygen. AGE products are formed after this non-enzymatic reaction. Advanced glycosylation products lead to endothelial damage by increasing vasoconstriction via endothelin-1 and have the capacity to generate free radicals through complex biochemical mechanisms. Toxic effects of AGEs also include being able to change the structure and function of proteins and to induce oxidative stress with its receptors. The third mechanism of ROS production is polyol pathway. High glucose concentration causes the sorbitol production by polyol pathway. As NADH is used for the activity of enzyme aldose reductase in this pathway, intracellular NADH is consumed. NADH is required for converting oxidized glutathione to reduced form and nitric oxide (NO) synthesis. Therefore, being active of the sorbitol way and the absence of NADPH ultimately mean a limitation of cell's antioxidant capacity. The decrease in reduced glutathione and NO synthesis that has a function in vasodilatation leads to the reduction of endoneurial blood flow, consequently endoneurial hypoxia or ischemia. Due to this event, the damage occurs in neuronal cells, Schwann cells.

2.3. Vascular Hypotheses

Swellings of the capillary vascular endothelial cells, thickening of the blood vessel wall, and undergoing aggregation or fibrin and occlusion with platelets of capillary lumen were shown in various studies. The sudden onset of clinical signs of focal neuropathies in diabetes supports the vascular cause. Decrease in NO production, abnormalities in eicosanoid production, and an increase in oxidative pathway lead to vasoconstriction in endoneurial microvascularization and nerve hypoxia.

2.4. Immunological Mechanisms

Autoantibodies against the sympathetic ganglia develop in patients with insulin-dependent diabetes. Endoneurial or epineural lymphocytic infiltration has been displayed in the sural nerve biopsy of diabetic patients. Coexistence of diabetic neuropathy and chronic inflammatory demyelinating polyneuropathy is also a suggestive finding of immune or cytotoxic factors [11].

2.5. Neurotrophic Factors

Neurotrophins are proteins that ensure the growth, permanence, survival, and differentiation into different specific populations of the neurons. There are studies, which show that impaired neurotrophic support is involved in the pathogenesis of diabetic polyneuropathy. Since nerve growth factor (NGF), a typical growth factor for the nerve, is needed for the survival and the continuity of sympathetic and thin sensory nerve fibers, it was examined particularly well. NGF also regulates the expression of the neuropeptides including calcium gene-related peptide and substance P in sympathetic nerves and sensory neurons of dorsal root ganglion. Retrograde axonal transport from target tissue to neuronal cell body is impaired in diabetes. There is evidence, which shows that NGF expression is decreased in the skin, submandibular glands, and the sympathetic ganglia in experimental diabetic neuropathy. NGF, when administered to rats with streptozotocin-induced diabetes, prevented the protection of the response to thermal painful stimuli (tail flick threshold) and the decrease in levels of neuropeptides including calcitonin gene-related peptide and substance P measured in the cervical dorsal root ganglia. In diabetic autonomic neuropathy model, dystrophic changes in sympathetic ganglia following the administration of NGF indicate that there may be a different dosing effect. Neurotrophin-3 (NT-3) supports the differentiation and survival of sensory neurons. Decreased messenger RNA (mRNA) was shown in the leg muscle of NT-3 diabetic mice. Due to their neurotrophic effect in the treatment of diabetic neuropathy in recent years, glucagon-like peptide-1 (GLP-1) analogues (exendin-4) and peptides such as ghrelin were also found to give successful results in animal models [12].

3. DIAGNOSIS

Symptoms and physical examination results must be assessed collectively for an accurate diagnosis of diabetic peripheral neuropathy (DPN). The standardization and simplicity of diagnostic methods are crucial for their widespread accessibility. There is no definitive standard for detecting the presence of diabetic neuropathy. The San Antonio consensus panel advises doing a minimum of one assessment across five distinct diagnostic areas. The assessments include symptom scoring, physical examination scoring, quantitative sensory testing (QST), cold allodynia frequency test (cAFT), and the Epworth Sleepiness Scale (EDS). Neurological tests of patients frequently disclose a gloves and socks sensory deficiency, hyporeflexia or areflexia, an elevated threshold for vibration sense perception, and mild atrophy and weakening, especially in the intrinsic muscles of the foot.

Neuropathic pain is a prevalent complaint often overlooked by both patients and physicians. Among the patients, 12.5% with painful diabetic peripheral neuropathy said that they had never disclosed their discomfort to physicians, while 40% indicated that they had not gotten any treatment for it. Numerous interrogation techniques exist to assess pain associated with diabetic polyneuropathy; however, none have been recognized as the definitive standard.Visual Analog Scale (VAS) is an easy method applied by grading the pain on a scale of 1–10 by the patient. Another method of pain assessment is "The Leeds Assessment of Neuropathic Symptoms and Signs" (LANSS) pain inquiry. Having a LANSS score of 12 or more is diagnostic for neuropathic pain. The Michigan Neuropathy Screening Instrument is one of the other commonly used interrogation methods, which is used in the diagnosis of neuropathic pain. Neuropathy Disability Score (NDS), which was first developed by Dick for the standardization of examination findings and correct interpretation of the findings and was simplified and modified in the following years, is regarded as a reliable and easy method that does not require experience in neurology. NDS = 0 is considered normal, NDS = 10 indicates maximum deficits, and NDS = 6 or more indicates the risk of developing diabetic foot ulcers. Touch pressure, vibration, hot-cold sensation, thermal pain, cold pain, and mechanical pain detection thresholds are tested in quantitative sensory testing.

The tests related to the vasomotor control, baroreceptor reflex, sudomotor function, pupil, bladder, and bowel innervation are used in autonomic function tests. Electrodiagnostic studies are one of the most common and objective methods used in the diagnosis of DPN. Weakness of electrodiagnostic studies is not showing the early stages of thin fiber damage. Unmyelinated C fiber injury, the most common cause of painful DPN, does not provide any electrophysiological findings, but thick myelinated Aα and Aβ fiber involvements have EDS findings.

Staining of a 3-mm skin sample using protein gene product-9.5 allows the assessment of intraepidermal thin fibers and early diagnosis of neuropathic damage. Although its sensitivity is high, its use is limited because it is an invasive procedure [13].

4. TREATMENT IN DIABETIC NEUROPATHY

Preventing the onset of diabetic polyneuropathy or achieving its final therapy is unfeasible. Nevertheless, several interventions can be implemented to decelerate the progression of neuropathy, alleviate symptom severity, and avert consequences associated with the condition. Patients should be afforded normal or near-normal blood glucose regulation. Maintaining a HbA1c level below 7, controlling cholesterol, ceasing smoking, reducing alcohol consumption, preventing obesity, and practicing foot care can impede the growth of neuropathy. Neuropathy can be identified at an early stage by evaluating the structural connection between membrane ion channel malfunction and axonal loss, utilizing clinical biomarkers that may indicate first alterations in ion channels. Consequently, the opportunity presents itself to initiate treatment without causing irreparable nerve injury [14].

4.1. Metabolic Control

The most important treatment for the prevention of diabetic PNP (peripheral neuropathy) is to control blood glucose. According to Diabetes Control and Complications Center (DCTT) data, the reduction of neuropathy by 57% has been shown in Type 1 DM after 5 years of tight blood glucose control.

4.2. Myoinositol

The addition of myoinositol to the diet was shown to improve nerve Na–K ATPase activity and nerve conduction values in laboratory studies; however, no improvement was found in electrophysiological parameters in humans. Their potential benefits are being able to inhibit nerve damage. Thus, its administration is recommended at an early stage.

4.3. Vitamin Addition

Vitamin treatment is often a non-specific therapy in neuropathy. Controlled studies show that receiving thiamine, vitamin B12, pyridoxine, or pantothenic acid in diabetic neuropathy is of no use [2,15].

4.4. ROS Inhibitors

Alpha lipoic acid: High doses of alpha-lipoic acid were shown to have therapeutic efficacy in the treatment of diabetic polyneuropathy and insulin resistance in experimental and clinical trials [2,9]. The patients (with symptomatic diabetic neuropathy) were given randomized IV ALA 5 days a week (600 mg) or placebo in Sydney trials. After this treatment, a significant improvement was noted in TSS of the patients treated with ALA compared to those given placebo (5.7 vs. 1.8 points $p \leq 0.001$) [16].

Nicotinamide: It inhibits oxidative stress–PARP activation cascade.

Resveratrol: It regulates NCV, diabetic neuropathic pain and inhibits NF-κB.

Routine: It prevents protein glycosylation.

Taurine: It reduces oxidative and nitrosative stress in Schwann cells. It reverses neurovascular insufficiency and reduces increased pain sensitivity [9,17,18].

NO agonist: NO is one of the factors that play a role in the pathogenesis of DPN and l-arginine, a NO agonist, was shown to increase Na–K ATPase activity [9].

Aldose reductase inhibitors: Many aldose reductase inhibitor drugs that are effective through the polyol pathway were reported in the DPN treatment. Sorbinil, an aldose reductase inhibitor, prevents sorbitol accumulation by inhibiting the enzyme aldose reductase in those with diabetes and corrects neuronal dysfunction due to the change in the myoinositol content. It leads to increase in NCV. Tolrestat is the other aldose reductase inhibitors and repairs impaired NCV. Ponalrestat is effective in the delayed treatment of DPN. It normalizes NCV and prevents the impaired neural induction of ornithine decarboxylase. Fidarestat induces the maturation of the nerve fibers, stimulates the repair of nerve fibers, and stops the destruction of nerve fibers. Epalrestat prevents the progression of MNCV, regulates the polyol pathway, and suppresses the production of IGU [9].

PKC inhibitors: Ruboxistaurin, a PKC-β inhibitor, was found to be successful in treating neuropathic sensory symptoms. It improves nerve fiber functions and microvascular blood flow and increases life quality in those with DPN [9,19,20].

Immunosuppressive therapy: Inflammatory vasculopathy is thought to be important in the pathogenesis of cases in which proximal diabetic neuropathy or amyotrophy was detected. The treatment that is appropriate to the natural progress of diabetic amyotrophy and whose validity was accepted is the treatment with immunomodulatory agents including IVIG or corticosteroid. Better response is achieved with corticosteroid therapy and its cost of treatment is less compared to IVIG. However, blood glucose regulation may be difficult with corticosteroid. Starting with the dose of 0.75 mg/kg/day 3–4 times a week and discontinuing gradually are recommended [21].

Pain treatment in diabetic neuropathy: Antidepressants, particularly tricyclic drugs, are the most frequently used. Amitriptyline, imipramine, and nortriptyline may be used. Anticonvulsants such as carbamazepine, gabapentin, pregabalin, and lamotrigine are among the treatment options. Antiarrhythmics, mexiletine, and lidocaine are other pharmacological agents that are used in case of unresponsiveness to other drugs. Capsaicin derived from paprika may be preferred to as a topical agent for treating pain [21].

Tricyclic antidepressants: A great percentage of patients were given at an average dose of 105 mg of amitriptyline or at an average dose of 111 mg desipramine in a double-blind, randomized, placebo-controlled trial of the patients with painful diabetic peripheral neuropathy (PDPN). Decrease in pain by 74%, 61%, and 41% was observed in patients who received amitriptyline, desipramine, and placebo, respectively. Number needed to treat (NNT) is 2.1 (1.9–2.6) and number needed to harm (NNH) value is 2.8 for minor adverse events and 19 for major adverse events. TCAs may promote orthostatic hypotension and may prolong QT (**Q wave** and **T wave**) interval. An increase in the risk of sudden death has been reported with TCAs by taking more than 100 mg amitriptyline or its equivalent [22].

Selective serotonin reuptake inhibitors (SSRIs) : Alternatively, the patients are treated with SSRIs because of many side effects of TCAs. These agents inhibit the presynaptic serotonin reuptake selectively [9]. Unlike the tricyclics, SSRIs lack the postsynaptic receptor-blocking effect. NNT to achieve 50% pain relief is 6.8 (3.4–441), and NNH is not known. While the benefit was observed with paroxetine and citalopram, no benefit was obtained with fluoxetine [22].

Serotonin-norepinephrine reuptake inhibitors (SNRIs): The direction of the treatment of DPN was shifted toward SNRIs because SSRIs are less effective in the treatment than TCAs and SNRIs inhibit both serotonin and norepinephrine reuptake. Duloxetine and venlafaxine are examples of SNRIs. Venlafaxine was argued to decrease the pain, and the effect on norepinephrine is presumed to be more specific in a study in which high dose of venlafaxine was used. Duloxetine is more effective in terms of the affinity in noradrenergic and serotonergic reuptake inhibition. Many people were given duloxetine in the randomized, placebo-controlled studies and 60 mg and 120 mg daily doses were reported to be effective in DPN [9,23,24].

Anticonvulsants: Antiepileptic drugs act by blocking sodium channels (felbamate, lamotrigine, oxcarbazepine, topiramate, and zonisamide), potentiating the activity of GABA (tiagabine and topiramate), blocking calcium channel (felbamate, lamotrigine, topiramate, and zonisamide), antagonizing glutamate at *N*-methyl-d-aspartate (NMDA) α-receptors (felbamate), and behaving as the antagonist of AMPA (a-amino-3-hydroxy-5-methyl-4-isoxazole) receptors (felbamate and topiramate). Rational polytherapy by which we can obtain a synergistic effect comes to the fore through understanding the mechanisms of these drugs. For example, lamotrigine can be given for sodium channel blocking and felbamate may be added to antagonize glutamate receptors or different mechanisms can be targeted with a single medication, for instance, topiramate, and chance of success may be increased. It was reported that a patient who was unresponsive to one of the antiepileptic drugs will respond to another drug or combination treatment consisted of two or more drugs [25,26].

*Topical capsaicin (capsaicin = 8-methyl-*N*-vanillyl-trans-6-nonenamide):* C fibers use neuropeptide P as a neurotransmitter, the reduction of axonal substance P causes pain relief. Storage of substance P, which is released from sensory nerve terminals, finishes with the application of capsaicin. Thus, the transmission of painful stimulus from peripheral nerve terminals is reduced or completely eliminated. A significant improvement was observed in patients with painful neuropathy treated with Capsaicin cream (0.075%) for 8 weeks. The treatment with capsaicin should be limited to 8 weeks, because it is noted that adverse event may be observed in sensory nerves at the end of this period. Eight percent capsaicin patch may be used in postherpetic neuralgia; however, it is contraindicated in diabetic neuropathy, because it desensitizes the nociceptive sensory nerve endings, so it is reported that the risk of development of diabetic foot ulcers may be increased [25,27].

Topical lidocaine: Use of topical lidocaine in painful neuropathy is associated with postherpetic neuralgia [16]. Lidocaine has been shown to be as effective as pregabalin in reducing pain without causing the side effects in a multicenter, randomized, open-label, parallel group study conducted by treating a group ($n = 99$) with 5% lidocaine for 2 weeks and treating another group ($n = 94$) with pregabalin for 4 weeks. This therapy may be continued with oral mexiletine in order to succeed. Relief of superficial pain caused by overstimulation is targeted with oral mexiletine [25].

Acetyl-l-carnitine: It was reported that the pain and the slowed nerve conduction velocity were improved, and nerve regeneration was increased with acetyl-l-carnitine in rats with streptozotocin-induced diabetic neuropathy. It was reported that the pain disappeared with acetyl-l-carnitine, and the pain was resolved by prophylactic treatment in paclitaxel-treated rats [28].

5. CURRENT THERAPEUTIC STRATEGIES IN DIABETIC NEUROPATHY

DPN is a prevalent manifestation of chronic neuropathic pain in clinical settings. Diverse therapeutic approaches are employed in individuals with diabetic neuropathy. Tramadol, an opioid, is a mild opioid analgesic employed for alleviating intense pain. Randomized controlled trials conducted over a duration of 6 weeks shown superior efficacy compared to placebo, with symptomatic alleviation persisting for a minimum of 6 months. The probability of side effects, similar to other opioid-like substances, is prevalent. Nonetheless, the emergence of drug tolerance and the onset of addiction with prolonged tramadol therapy are infrequent. NMDA receptors are crucial in the sensitization of neuropathic pain; nevertheless, the utilization of these medications is limited due to their dose-dependent adverse effects [25]. In recent years, NMDA receptor antagonists have been employed to modulate excitatory transmission at the synapses of primary afferent spinothalamic neurons. The pain terminates with the inhibition of excitatory glutamatergic NMDA receptors in the spinal cord. Dextromethorphan exemplifies a category of analgesic medicines. NMDA receptor antagonists have demonstrated efficacy comparable to that of opioid analgesics in managing chronic pain disorders. A diagnosis of diabetic neuropathy was established using clinical evaluation (including medical history, motor, sensory, and reflex examinations) and electrophysiological assessments for 24 patients with Type 2 diabetes and diabetic neuropathy. The patients' pain complaints were evaluated using a VAS prior to and following the treatment. A notable enhancement in VAS scores was shown in both treatment groups relative to the control group, with a significant difference identified between the treatment groups. In conclusion, Memantine, an NMDA receptor antagonist, enhances the management of neuropathic pain in diabetic polyneuropathy [29].

Flavonoids, which have been shown to provide numerous beneficial benefits on human health, possess antioxidant, anti-inflammatory, cholesterol-lowering, antibacterial, antihyperglycemic, and antiallergic properties. It may be referred to as P factor or

P vitamin due to its effects on regulating capillary circulation and decreasing blood pressure. The primary flavonoid in this context is proanthocyanidin, which is present in grape seeds. Grape seed extract was administered at doses of 25 mg/kg and 50 mg/kg via oral gavage for 6 weeks in a trial where diabetes was established in BALB/C mice. The pain threshold was assessed utilizing the Hot Plate Test, a thermal pain paradigm, in these animals at the conclusion of the second and sixth weeks. Histological examination of the sciatic nerve and abdominal aorta tissue from animals at the conclusion of the trial revealed substantial differences in hot plate measures between the group administered grape seed extract and the other groups. UCE was observed to reduce damage in diabetes-induced microvascular and macrovascular problems during histological assessments [30].

5.1. DPP-4 Inhibitors

Dipeptidyl peptidase-4 incretin hormones are secreted from intestinal endocrine cells. It plays a key role in regulating blood glucose levels by stimulating glucose-dependent insulin secretion, decreasing glucagon secretion, and slowing gastric emptying. DPP-4 inactivates GLP-1 and glucose-dependent insulin tropical polypeptides (GIP) in vivo by destroying them. These peptides are short lived in the circulation because they are destroyed by DPP-4. Alogliptin is a DPP-4 inhibitor. The effects of this medication on vascular and neural complications were evaluated in male Sprague–Dawley rats with STZ-induced diabetes. Alogliptin was observed to regulate MNCV and thermal response latency after a 12-week treatment. No improvement in the decrease in intraepidermal nerve fiber density was detected while SNCVs of the mice were regulating. PKF 275-055, new analog of Vildagliptin, was given to STZ-induced diabetic rats in the study of Bianchi et al., and it was found that it displays an anabolic effect by preventing changes in nociceptive threshold, Na–K ATPase, and NCP. DPP-4 inhibitors were stated to prevent some neural and vascular complications associated with diabetes in the studies conducted [9,31,32,33].

5.2. Cannabinoid CB1 Receptor Antagonists

Nabilone is a CB1 predominant receptor agonist. It was used in neuropathic pain based on the anecdotal evidence and uncontrolled case series [34]. Pain reduction has been reported to occur in 30% of the patients in a single center, randomized, double-blind, placebo-controlled, flexible 5-week study conducted by administering a dose ranges from 1 to 4 mg per day or placebo. DPN symptoms disappeared, and their impaired sleep and standard of living were improved in those received flexible dose. Nabilone is a well tolerated and successful adjuvant in patients with DPN. Rimonabant is a CB1 receptor antagonist; it accelerates skin blood flow and decreases TNF-α level in diabetic rats. It was stated that Rimonabant may be beneficial in the treatment of DPN due to its micro and macro blood vessel protection and inflammatory effects [9,34,35].

5.3. Natural Products

Metanx: It is a product designed for endothelial function disorders, comprising l-methyl folate, pyridoxal 5′ phosphate, and methylcobalamin. It inhibits endothelial nitric oxide synthesis, induces oxidative stress in the endothelium, and affects peripheral neurons. A notable enhancement in numbness, tingling, discomfort, burning, severe pain, and allodynia was observed in diabetic neuropathy patients administered Metanx in a placebo-controlled study over 24 weeks. An enhancement in emotional, social functioning, and energetic aspects of mental health was also seen. Adverse effects occurred in less than 2% of cases during this response. The negative effects primarily included dermatitis and gastrointestinal issues, which were comparable to those observed with placebo [25].

Botulinum toxin has been investigated for trigeminal neuralgia and has been demonstrated to provide a prolonged antinociceptive effect in carpal tunnel syndrome without inducing electrophysiological repair [25].

REFERENCES

1. Satılmış, I. Diyabetes Mellitusda İnsülin Tedavisinin Periferik Sinir Sistemine Etkileri: Klinik ve Elektrofozyolojik Değerlendirme, Sağlık Bakanlığı Şişli Etfal Eğitim ve Araştırma Hastanesi 2. Nöroloji Kliniği, Uzmanlık Tezi, İstanbul, 2007.
2. Terzi M, Cengiz N, Onar MK. Diyabetik Nöropati. OMÜ Tıp Dergisi. 2004;21(1):39–49.
3. Jennifer AT, James BD. The Spectrum of Diabetic Neuropathies. Phys Med Rehabil Clin N Am. 2008;19(1):1–26.
4. Habib AA, Brannapan 3 TH. Therapeutic Strategies for Diabetic Neuropathy, Springer Science + Business media, LLC, 2010.
5. Vinik AI, Erbas T, Casellini CM, Diabetic Cardiac Autonomic Neuropathy, İnflammation and Cardiovascular Disease, J Diabet. 2013;4(1):4-18.
6. Vinik AI, Maser RE, Ziegler D. Autonomic İmbalance; Prophet of Doom or Scope for Hope? Diabet Med. 2011;28:643–651.
7. Şahin C. Diyabetik Sıçanlarda Meydana Gelen Sinir Yaralanmaları Onarımında Perinörotomi Uygulamasının Etkisi, Genelkurmay Başkanlığı Gata Haydarpaşa Eğitim Hastanesi Plastik VE Rekonstrüktif Cerrahi Servis Şefliği, Tıpta Uzmanlık Tezi, 2011.
8. Nouri MN, Ahmed A, Bril V, Orszag A, Ng E, Nwe P, Perkins BA. Diabetic Neuropathy and Axon Reflex Mediated Neurogenic Vasodilatation in Type 1 Diabetes. PLoS ONE 2012;7(4):e34807. doi:10.371/journal.Done.0034807
9. Sing R, Kishore L, Kaur N. Diabetic Peripheral Neuropathy: Current Perspective and Future Directions. Pharmacolog Res. 2014;80:21–35.
10. Singh R, Barden A, Mori T, Beilin L. Advanced Glycation End-Products: A Review. Diabetologia. 2001;44(2):129–146.
11. Kılıç E, Fisetin ve Alfa Lipoik Asidin Ağrılı Diyabetik Nöropati Üzerine Etkilerinin İncelenmesi: Fare Modelinde İn Vivo Davranışsal Çalışma, Ondokuz Mayıs Üniversitesi Tıp Fakültesi İç Hastalıkları Anabilim Dalı Endokrinoloji Bilim Dalı, Uzmanlık Tezi, Samsun, 2013.
12. Erbaş O. Diyabetik Nöropatili Sıçanlarda Oksitosin,Mesna ve Glutamin' in, Nöropati Üzerine Etkilerinin Elektrofizyolojik (EMG) ve Histolojik Yöntemlerle Araştırılması, Ege

Üniversitesi Tıp Fakültesi Fizyoloji Anabilim Dalı Tıpta Uzmanlık Tezi, İzmir, 2012.

13. Cengizhan E. Diyabetik Hastalarda Mıchıgan Nöropati Tarama Enstrümanı Bulgularının Elektrofizyolojik Bulgularla Bağıntısı, Süleyman Demirel Üniversitesi Tıp Fakültesi Nöroloji Anabilim Dalı Tıpta Uzmanlık Tezi, Isparta, 2010.
14. Kiernan MC.Emergence of a Predicitive Clinical Biomarker for Diabetic Neuropathy. Diabetes 2012;61:1346-1347.
15. Ağırman M. Diyabetik Hastalarda Polinöropati ve Karpal Tünel Sendromu Tanısında Ultrasonun Elektrofizyolojiye Göre Tanıdaki Yerinin Araştırılması, Marmara Üniversitesi Tıp Fakültesi Fiziksel Tıp ve Rehabilitasyon Anabilim Dalı, Uzmanlık Tezi, İstanbul, 2012.
16. Dam PSV, Cotter MA, Bravenboer B, Cameron NE. Pathogenesis of Diabetic Neuropathy: Focus on Neurovascular Mechanisms. Eur J Pharmacol. 2013;719:180–186.
17. Sharma SS, Kumar A, Arora M, Kaundal RK. Neuroprotective Potential of Combination of Resveratrol and 4-Amino 1,8 Naphthalimide in Experimental Diabetic Neuropathy: Focus on Functional, Sensorimotor and Biochemical Changes. Free Radic Res. 2009;43:400–408.
18. Li F, Obrosova IG, Abatan O, Tian D, Larkin D, Stuenkel EL, et al. Taurine Replacement Attenuates Hyperalgesia and Abnormal Calcium Signaling in Sensoryneurons of STZ-D Rats. Am J Physiol Endocrinol Metab 2005;288:E29–E36.
19. Hotta N, Toyota T, Matsuoka K, Shigeta Y, Kikkawa R, Kaneko T, et al. Clin-ical efficacy of fidarestat, a novel aldose reductase inhibitor, for diabeticperipheral neuropathy: a 52-week multicenter placebo-controlled double-blind parallel group study. Diabet Care 2001;24:1776–82.
20. Hotta N, Akanuma Y, Kawamori R, Matsuoka K, Oka Y, Shichiri M, et al. Long-Term Clinical Effects of Epalrestat, an Aldose Reductase İnhibitor, on Diabetic Peripheral Neuropathy: The 3-Year, Multicenter, Comparativealdose Reductase İnhibitor-Diabetes Complications Trial. Diabet Care. 2006;29:1538–1544.
21. Said G. Focal and Multifocal Diabetic Neuropathies. Arq Neuropsiquiatr. 2007;65(4):1272–1278.
22. Tahrani AA, Aswith T, Stevens MJ. Emerging Drugs for Diabetic Neuropathy. Expert Opin Emerg Drugs 2010;15(4):661–683.
23. Rowbotham MC, Goli V, Kunz NR, Lei D. Venlafaxine Extended Release in the Treatment of Painful Diabetic Neuropathy: A Double-Blind, Placebo-Controlled Study. Pain 2004;110:697–706.
24. Sultan A, Gaskell H, Derry S, Moore RA. Duloxetine for Painful Diabetic Neuropathy and Fibromyalgia Pain: Systematic Review of Randomised Trials. BMC Neurol. 2008;8:29.
25. Vinik AI, Nevoret ML, Casellini C, Parson H. Diabetic Neuropathy. Endocrinal Metab Clin N Am 2013;42:747–787.
26. Raskin P, Donofrio PD, Rosenthal NR, et al. Topiramate vs Placebo in Painful Diabetic Neuropathy: Analgesic and Metabolic Effects. Neurol. 2004;63:865–873.
27. Mason L, Moore RA, Derry S, et al. Systematic Review of Topical Capsaicin for the Treatment of Chronic Pain. BMJ 2004;328:991.
28. Bennett GJ, Doyle T, Salvemini D. Mitotoxicity in Distal Symmetrical Sensory Peripheral Neuropathies. Nat Rev Neurol. 2014;10:326–336.
29. Gökçe F. Diyabetik Polinöropatik Hastalarda Memantinin Ağrı Üzerine Etkinliği. Orijinal Araştırma 2014;36:474–478.

30. Yurt A. Streptozosinle Diyabet Oluşturulan Farelerde Üzüm Çekġrdeği Ektresinin Nöropatik Ağrı Üzerine Etkiler, İnönü Üniversitesi Sağlık Bilimleri Enstitüsü Yüksek Lisans Tezi, Malatya, 2015.

31. Neumiller JJ, Wood L, Campbell RK. Dipeptidyl Peptidase-4 İnhibitors for the Treatment of Type 2 Diabetes Mellitus. Pharmacother. 2010;30:463–484.

32. Lam S, Saad M. Saxagliptin: A New Dipeptidyl Peptidase-4 İnhibitor for Type 2 diabetes. Cardiol Rev. 2010;18:213–217.

33. Davidson EP, Coppey LJ, Dake B, Yorek MA. Treatment of Streptozotocin-İnduced Diabetic Rats with Alogliptin: Effect on Vascular and Neuralcomplications. Exp Diabet Res. 2011:8104–8169.

34. Toth C, Mawani S, Brady S, Chan C, Liu C, Mehina E, et al. Anenriched-Enrolment, Randomized Withdrawal, Flexible-Dose, Double-Blindplacebo-Controlled, Parallel Assignment Efficacy Study of Nabilone As Adjuvant in the Treatment of Diabetic Peripheral Neuropathic Pain. Pain. 2012;153:2073–2082.

35. Liu WJ, Jin HY, Park JH, Baek HS, Park TS. Effect of Rimonabant, the Cannabinoid CB1 Receptor Antagonist, on Peripheral Nerve in Streptozotocin-İnduced Diabetic Rat. Eur J Pharmacol. 2010;637:70–76.

INDEX

www.ingramcontent.com/pod-product-compliance
Lightning Source LLC
LaVergne TN
LVHW062217200926
848484LV00006B/1421